# Toxicological Effects of Mycotoxins on Target Cells

# Toxicological Effects of Mycotoxins on Target Cells

Editor

**Ana Juan-García**

MDPI • Basel • Beijing • Wuhan • Barcelona • Belgrade • Manchester • Tokyo • Cluj • Tianjin

MDPI

*Editor*
Ana Juan-García
Laboratory of Food Chemistry and Toxicology Faculty of Pharmacy
University of Valencia
Spain

*Editorial Office*
MDPI
St. Alban-Anlage 66
4052 Basel, Switzerland

This is a reprint of articles from the Special Issue published online in the open access journal *Toxins* (ISSN 2072-6651) (available at: https://www.mdpi.com/journal/toxins/special_issues/mycotoxin_target_cells).

For citation purposes, cite each article independently as indicated on the article page online and as indicated below:

| |
|---|
| LastName, A.A.; LastName, B.B.; LastName, C.C. Article Title. *Journal Name* **Year**, *Article Number*, Page Range. |

**ISBN 978-3-03936-926-3 (Hbk)**
**ISBN 978-3-03936-927-0 (PDF)**

Cover image courtesy of Ana Juan-García.

# Contents

# About the Editor

**Ana Juan-García** is Associate Professor of Toxicology at University of Valencia in the Department of Preventive Medicine, Public Health, Food Science, Toxicology, and Forensic Medicine. She holds a degree in Pharmacy and a European PhD in Food Science, both from University of Valencia. She was Postdoc Researcher at Purdue University (IN, USA) for two years with a Fulbright Grant, and more recently a Visiting Scholar at Harvard University (MA, USA). Prof. Juan-García focuses most of her research on the toxic effects of compounds/contaminants present in food and feed, and more specifically on pesticides, antibiotics, and mycotoxins. Her research focusses on evaluating mycotoxins toxicity, mostly through in vitro but also in vivo assays, by using different techniques and biological models.

toxins

MDPI

Editorial

# Introduction to the Toxins Special Issue on Toxicological Effects of Mycotoxins on Target Cells

**Ana Juan-García**

Laboratory of Food Chemistry and Toxicology, Faculty of Pharmacy, University of Valencia, E-46100 Valencia, Spain; ana.juan@uv.es

Received: 19 May 2020; Accepted: 6 July 2020; Published: 10 July 2020

---

Mycotoxins are toxic secondary metabolites produced by filamentous fungi from *Fusarium*, *Alternaria* and *Penicillium spp.* spread naturally worldwide. Mycotoxins are also natural contaminants present in food and feed and several health problems have been evidenced not only for humans, but also for animals. In 2018, the Rapid Alert System for Food and Feed (RASFF) reported 569 notifications for mycotoxins which were situated among the top 10 food and product hazard categories.

Oral exposure of mycotoxins in humans and animals occurs through food although levels found are low and acute effects are scarce. Nonetheless, chronic exposure effects are of great concern which really pose a significant risk to consumers who are eating these products. Several studies have shown mycotoxins are capable of causing various forms of systemic toxicity such as neurotoxicity, hepatotoxicity, nephrotoxicity, mammalian cytotoxicity, etc. However, these toxicological effects of mycotoxins are evaluated through the extrapolation of results from in vivo and in vitro assays. Studies of mycotoxins' effects at the cellular level precede those in organs and systems. All these studies are key steps for risk assessment and following legislation for mycotoxins.

This Special Issue of *Toxins* comprises 10 original contributions and two reviews. The issue reports new findings regarding toxic mechanisms, use of innovative techniques to study the potential toxicity of mycotoxins not only individually but in combination reflecting a real scenario according to nowadays occurrence studies of mycotoxins.

Related with this highlighted scenario, Kifer et al. [1] review the last mathematical models used for evaluating the toxicological effects of mixtures/box/combos/ of mycotoxins. Most of those models are described on the assumption that mycotoxin dose-effect curves are linear; in this review advantages and disadvantages of mathematical models that deal with assessing mycotoxins´ interactions are discussed.

Another review is presented in this Special Issue by Reddy et al. [2], related to less common group of mycotoxins: tremorgenic mycotoxins. Such group of mycotoxins are produced by fungal species often present in association with pasture grasses; indole-diterpenes which may cause toxicity in grazing animals more than in humans directly. Reddy et al., highlight the wide-ranging biological versatility presented by this group of compounds and their role in agricultural and pharmaceutical fields.

Studies of mycotoxins in different cell lines are presented in this issue: intestinal porcine epithelial cells (IPEC-J2), hepatocarcinoma cells (HepG2), mouse macrophage cell line (RAW 264.7), human embryonic kidney cells (HEK 293T), differentiated human intestinal cells (Caco-2 cells), embryonic stem cells (hESCs), human chondrocytes, chicken hepatocytes, wild-type FM3A cells and Bombyx mori (Bm12) cell line.

Transcriptomic analysis based on RNA-seq addressing deoxynivalenol (DON) cytotoxicity in intestinal porcine epithelial cell line (IPEC-J2) showed immune-related pathways to be the main pathway exhibiting more related differentially expressed genes (DEGs). Zhang et al. [3] demonstrated that differentially expressed genes in IPEC-J2 cells treated with DON induced proinflammatory gene expression, including cytokines, chemokines and other inflammation-related genes, by activating p38 and ERK1/2.

Multi-mycotoxin occurrence of 28 mycotoxins in pig feed samples was evaluated by using an LC-MS/MS method. Novak et al. [4] give an overall insight into the amount of fungal secondary metabolites found in pig feed samples compared to their cytotoxic effects in vitro using IPEC-J2 cells. The main mycotoxins, DON and zearalenone (ZEN), were found only at ranks 8 and 10 among all samples analyzed.

Cytotoxicity, genotoxicity and disturbance of cell cycle of two mycotoxins, ochratoxin A (OTA) and beauvericin (BEA), were evaluated in HepG2 cells by Juan-García et al [5]. Effects were evaluated individually and combined through isobologram method and flow cytometry following TG 487 for in vitro micronuclei (MN) assay. BEA showed higher toxicity than OTA in HepG2 cells and combination effects were additive and synergistic. Cell cycle arrest and MN induction were also observed in different scenarios. This study underlines the importance of studying real exposure scenarios of chronic exposure to mycotoxins as mixture of mycotoxins.

Fourteen mycotoxins were individually evaluated in vitro and in different combinations in RAW 264.7 cells, in HepG2 cells and in HEK 293T cells and in silico through ACD/Percepta; the bioavailability potential in differentiated Caco-2 cells is presented (Tran et al. [6]). The mitigation effect with silibinin was also tested. The acute toxicity of these mycotoxins in binary combinations exhibited antagonistic effects in the combinations of T-2 with DON, ENN-A1, or ENN-B, while the rest showed synergistic or additive effects.

OTA is one of the most common and important mycotoxins present in food especially for its potential toxicity. In the work presented by Yang et al. [7], the mechanism underlying the intestinal toxicity of OTA was shown in a dose-dependent manner in differentiated Caco-2 cells. Transcriptome analysis was used to estimate damage to the intestinal barrier; also the protein–protein interaction network by STRING (Search Tool for Retrieval of Interacting Genes) was analyzed, and the validation of eight genes by qRT-PCR analysis was used. Intestinal toxicity of OTA was shown; genome-wide view of biological responses was provided evidencing the theoretical basis for OTA´s enterotoxicity.

A study for evaluating embryotoxicity has been performed by Erceg et al. [8] in embryonic stem cells (hESCs). Results showed mild cytotoxic effects for OTA in these cells by inhibiting cell attachment, survival, and proliferation in a dose-dependent manner.

Two of the most toxic mycotoxins, T-2 and HT-2 toxin, were studied to evaluate apoptosis and autophagy in human chondrocytes through oxidative stress and viability and protein expression (Yu et al. [9]). Decrease of viability was observed for both mycotoxins; while oxidative stress and apoptosis increased but it was higher for T-2 toxin than for HT-2 toxin. The expression levels of apoptosis and autophagy related proteins, Bax, caspase-9, caspase-3, and Beclin1 in chondrocytes induced by T-2 toxin were significantly higher when compared with those levels induced by HT-2 toxin.

Yin et al. [10] in turn studied the toxicological effect of T-2 toxin on apoptosis and autophagy in chicken hepatocytes. At molecular mechanism level, the gene expression level in chicken hepatocytes treated with T-2 toxin induced oxidative stress, apoptosis and cytoprotective autophagy in chicken hepatocytes. This revealed a molecular mechanism of T-2 toxin inducing apoptosis and autophagy in chicken hepatocytes.

Wild-type FM3A cells and G3 cells (transfected cells with Tri101) were exposed to ITDol, isotrichodermin ITD and trichothecenes (DON, 3-ADON) by Tanaka et al [11]. It was observed that wild-type FM3A cells hardly grew, while G3 cells survived and cytotoxicity was lower in G3 cells exposed to ITDol and ITD than in wild-type FM3A cells. More modest results were detected for in deoxynivalenol and 3-acetyldeoxynivalenol. It indicates that he expression of Tri101 conferred trichothecene resistance in cultured mammalian cells.

Destruxin A (DA) was studied in the Bombyx mori Bm12 cell line through three proteins (BmTudor-sn, BmPiwi, and BmAGO2) (Wang et al. [12]). Among all three, it was revealed that only BmTudor-sn had an affinity interaction with DA which means there was a susceptibility to DA. When that protein was knocked down, cell viability increased under DA treatment.

**Acknowledgments:** The guest editor of this Special Issue, Ana Juan-García is grateful to the authors for their contributions and particularly to the referees for their invaluable work. Without their effort this special issue would have not been possible. The valuable contributions, organization, and editorial support of the MDPI management team and staff are greatly appreciated.

**Conflicts of Interest:** The author declares no conflict of interest.

## References

1. Kifer, D.; Jakšić, D.; Šegvić Klarić, M. Assessing the Effect of Mycotoxin Combinations: Which Mathematical Model Is (the Most) Appropriate? *Toxins* **2020**, *12*, 153. [CrossRef] [PubMed]
2. Reddy, P.; Guthridge, K.; Vassiliadis, S.; Hemsworth, J.; Hettiarachchige, I.; Spangenberg, G.; Rochfort, S. Tremorgenic Mycotoxins: Structure Diversity and Biological Activity. *Toxins* **2019**, *11*, 302. [CrossRef] [PubMed]
3. Zhang, H.; Deng, X.; Zhou, C.; Wu, W.; Zhang, H. Deoxynivalenol Induces Inflammation in IPEC-J2 Cells by Activating P38 Mapk And Erk1/2. *Toxins* **2020**, *12*, 180. [CrossRef] [PubMed]
4. Novak, B.; Rainer, V.; Sulyok, M.; Haltrich, D.; Schatzmayr, G.; Mayer, E. Twenty-Eight Fungal Secondary Metabolites Detected in Pig Feed Samples: Their Occurrence, Relevance and Cytotoxic Effects In Vitro. *Toxins* **2019**, *11*, 537. [CrossRef] [PubMed]
5. Juan-García, A.; Tolosa, J.; Juan, C.; Ruiz, M.-J. Cytotoxicity, Genotoxicity and Disturbance of Cell Cycle in HepG2 Cells Exposed to OTA and BEA: Single and Combined Actions. *Toxins* **2019**, *11*, 341. [CrossRef] [PubMed]
6. Tran, V.N.; Viktorova, J.; Augustynkova, K.; Jelenova, N.; Dobiasova, S.; Rehorova, K.; Fenclova, M.; Stranska-Zachariasova, M.; Vitek, L.; Hajslova, J.; et al. In Silico and In Vitro Studies of Mycotoxins and Their Cocktails; Their Toxicity and Its Mitigation by Silibinin Pre-Treatment. *Toxins* **2020**, *12*, 148. [CrossRef] [PubMed]
7. Yang, X.; Gao, Y.; Yan, Q.; Bao, X.; Zhao, S.; Wang, J.; Zheng, N. Transcriptome Analysis of Ochratoxin A-Induced Apoptosis in Differentiated Caco-2 Cells. *Toxins* **2020**, *12*, 23. [CrossRef] [PubMed]
8. Erceg, S.; Mateo, E.M.; Zipancic, I.; Rodríguez Jiménez, F.J.; Pérez Aragó, M.A.; Jiménez, M.; Soria, J.M.; Garcia-Esparza, M.Á. Assessment of Toxic Effects of Ochratoxin A in Human Embryonic Stem Cells. *Toxins* **2019**, *11*, 217. [CrossRef] [PubMed]
9. Yu, F.-F.; Lin, X.-L.; Wang, X.; Ping, Z.-G.; Guo, X. Comparison of Apoptosis and Autophagy in Human Chondrocytes Induced by the T-2 and HT-2 Toxins. *Toxins* **2019**, *11*, 260. [CrossRef] [PubMed]
10. Yin, H.; Han, S.; Chen, Y.; Wang, Y.; Li, D.; Zhu, Q. T-2 Toxin Induces Oxidative Stress, Apoptosis and Cytoprotective Autophagy in Chicken Hepatocytes. *Toxins* **2020**, *12*, 90. [CrossRef] [PubMed]
11. Tanaka, N.; Takushima, R.; Tanaka, A.; Okada, A.; Matsui, K.; Maeda, K.; Aikawa, S.; Kimura, M.; Takahashi-Ando, N. Reduced Toxicity of Trichothecenes, Isotrichodermol, and Deoxynivalenol, by Transgenic Expression of the *Tri101* 3-*O*-Acetyltransferase Gene in Cultured Mammalian FM3A Cells. *Toxins* **2019**, *11*, 654. [CrossRef] [PubMed]
12. Wang, J.; Hu, W.; Hu, Q. BmTudor-sn Is a Binding Protein of Destruxin A in Silkworm Bm12 Cells. *Toxins* **2019**, *11*, 67. [CrossRef] [PubMed]

*toxins*

MDPI

*Review*

# Tremorgenic Mycotoxins: Structure Diversity and Biological Activity

**Priyanka Reddy [1,2], Kathryn Guthridge [1], Simone Vassiliadis [1], Joanne Hemsworth [1], Inoka Hettiarachchige [1], German Spangenberg [1,2] and Simone Rochfort [1,2,*]**

1 Agriculture Victoria, AgriBio, Centre for AgriBioscience, Bundoora, Victoria 3083, Australia; Priyanka.reddy@ecodev.vic.gov.au (P.R.); Kathryn.guthridge@ecodev.vic.gov.au (K.G.); simone.vassiliadis@ecodev.vic.gov.au (S.V.); Joanne.hemsworth@ecodev.vic.gov.au (J.H.); Inoka.Hettiarachchige@ecodev.vic.gov.au (I.H.); german.spangenberg@ecodev.vic.gov.au (G.S.)

2 School of Applied Systems Biology, La Trobe University, Bundoora, Victoria 3083, Australia

* Correspondence: simone.rochfort@ecodev.vic.gov.au

Received: 24 April 2019; Accepted: 22 May 2019; Published: 27 May 2019

**Abstract:** Indole-diterpenes are an important class of chemical compounds which can be unique to different fungal species. The highly complex lolitrem compounds are confined to *Epichloë* species, whilst penitrem production is confined to *Penicillium* spp. and *Aspergillus* spp. These fungal species are often present in association with pasture grasses, and the indole-diterpenes produced may cause toxicity in grazing animals. In this review, we highlight the unique structural variations of indole-diterpenes that are characterised into subgroups, including paspaline, paxilline, shearinines, paspalitrems, terpendoles, penitrems, lolitrems, janthitrems, and sulpinines. A detailed description of the unique biological activities has been documented where even structurally related compounds have displayed unique biological activities. Indole-diterpene production has been reported in two classes of ascomycete fungi, namely Eurotiomycetes (e.g., *Aspergillus* and *Penicillium*) and Sordariomycetes (e.g., *Claviceps* and *Epichloë*). These compounds all have a common structural core comprised of a cyclic diterpene skeleton derived from geranylgeranyl diphosphate (GGPP) and an indole moiety derived from tryptophan. Structure diversity is generated from the enzymatic conversion of different sites on the basic indole-diterpene structure. This review highlights the wide-ranging biological versatility presented by the indole-diterpene group of compounds and their role in an agricultural and pharmaceutical setting.

**Keywords:** mycotoxins; endophyte; fungi; neurotoxin; lolitrems

**Key Contribution:** Understanding the biological activity of individual compounds within the indole-diterpene pathway is important for the development of pasture grasses in the agriculture industry. This review provides a detailed description of the reported activities of indole diterpenes in animal models and cell-based assays. Furthermore, we describe detailed reports of these molecules as potential leads for pharmaceutical drug discovery.

---

## 1. Introduction

Perennial ryegrass (*Lolium perenne* L.) is used for forage in temperate regions throughout the world including Northern Europe, Pacific North West of USA, Japan, South-eastern Australia, and New Zealand [1–5]. It is the most commonly utilized pasture grass on dairy farms in Australia and has a high economic importance [6]. The asexual form of the endophytic fungus *E. festucae* var. *lolii* (previously known as *Neotyphodium lolii* and *Acremonium lolii*) is known to establish a symbiotic relationship with perennial ryegrass [7]. These interactions are beneficial to the pastoral agriculture industry as compounds produced by the endophyte confer resistance to biotic and abiotic stresses.

For example, a select number of indole-diterpene class compounds, such the lolitrems A, B, and E that are present in endophyte-infected ryegrasses, are toxic to the larvae of the Argentine stem weevil (*Listronotus bonariensis*) [8,9]. The grass–endophyte association also produces secondary metabolites that are detrimental to grazing animals. The major toxins of concern are the alkaloids ergovaline and lolitrem B, which are present in old naturalized perennial ryegrass pastures containing the Standard Endophyte (SE) strain. Although both toxins are produced by endophyte-infected perennial ryegrass, ergovaline is normally most abundant in endophyte-infested tall fescue grass and causes the vasoconstrictive conditions fescue foot or summer slump disease [10,11]. The indole-diterpenes are predominant in endophyte-infected perennial ryegrass and lolitrem B is the end-point of the complex indole-diterpene biochemical pathway (Figure 1) [12]. Many of the indole-diterpene class of compounds, particularly the lolitrems, are reported as anti-mammalian alkaloids that significantly affect animal health. In particular, lolitrem B has been identified as a causative agent for perennial ryegrass staggers disease, a nervous disorder, notably of sheep and cattle that causes tremors [12]. However, despite the prevalence of perennial ryegrass in various geographic locations the toxicity reports are generally limited. Neurological signs associated with ryegrass staggers disease has been reported in animals, particularly sheep, grazing on perennial ryegrass in Australia, New Zealand, as well as Pacific northwest of USA and Europe [13,14]. This imposes a negative impact on industry, particularly dairy, meat, and wool production involving grazing animals [15]. Thus, forage improvement programs have been involved in selecting novel endophytes that do not produce the known toxins; however, complex mixtures of the intermediate compounds are still present in marketed forage grasses.

Symptoms of ryegrass staggers include initial head tremors, muscle fasciculation of the neck and legs, and hypersensitivity to external stimuli as a result of the neurotoxic effect. To date, no physical effects or gross lesions have been reported, and animals completely recover when the toxin is eliminated from their systems. Although, affected animals suffer poor weight gain and they may be difficult to handle due to their hypersensitivity [16–18]. Death is rarely a consequence unless an accident, such as drowning, occurs during an episode in which the animal loses voluntary control [18]. One of the methods to control the disease centers on offering alternative feed sources or removal of animals from drought-stressed and overgrazed pastures during summer and early autumn when the toxin levels are elevated [19] and neurological signs appear [18].

Lolitrem B is the most abundant of the indole-diterpene series of compounds produced by perennial ryegrass endophytes belonging to *Epichloë festucae* var. *lolii* (termed *Lp*TG-1). Lolitrem B has many analogues and precursors that are also known to elicit tremors in animals (Table 1) [20–22]. Although the structure–activity relationship is unclear, the literature suggests that lolitrem analogues, and biosynthetic intermediates such as paxilline and terpendole C, cause tremors in grazing animals [22]. Penitrems have also shown to exhibit clinical signs that are similar to ryegrass staggers disease, though intoxication is commonly documented as a result of exposure to moldy foods [23,24]. Additionally, it would be unwise to assign a single compound as the causative agent when a complex mixture of related compounds exists in grass–endophyte associations. Typically, the presence and absence of the major compounds are used in the screening of endophyte-infected grasses and the effect of individual intermediate compounds and their synergistic effects are largely ignored [25]. Furthermore, some of the indole-diterpenes produced could be innocuous to grazing animals and beneficial in deterring insects at the same time [15]. This is an important factor to consider when novel grass–endophyte associations are in development.

There is a growing need to understand the toxicity of all compounds within the indole-diterpene group, including intermediates and analogues, as shown in the biosynthetic map in Figure 1. However, obtaining these compounds to test on animal models is challenging due to the difficulty involved in compound isolation and purification such that large kilogram (kg) quantities of starting material is required to obtain milligrams of some of the intermediates [26,27]. For example, Munday-Finch et al. enriched fractions obtained from extraction of 360 kg of seed and were then able to identify lolicine A, lolicine B, lolitriol, and lolitrem N, as well as the naturally occurring 31-epilolitrem N and 31-epilolitrem F [27,28]. No biological activities were determined for these compounds other than 31-epi-lolitrem F [27]. Thus, it would be more effective to understand structure–activity associations as tools for predicting the toxicity of novel or previously uncharacterized compounds.

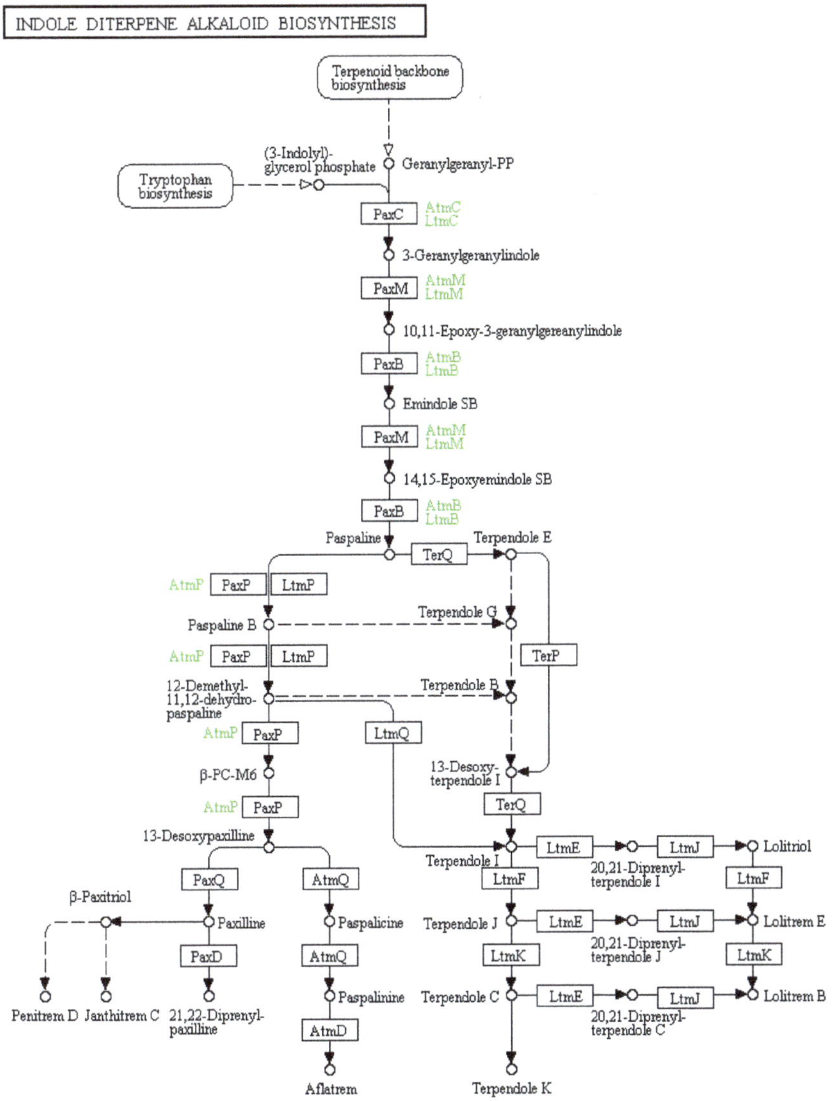


**Figure 1.** Indole-diterpene biosynthetic map sourced from KEGG pathways showing the enzymes responsible for producing indole-diterpene compounds at each step. Reproduced from [29–31].

The purpose of this review is to provide an exhaustive compilation of biological activities reported for indole-diterpene compounds produced by *Epichloë* endophytes. Where known, biological activities of some indole-diterpenes produced by other fungal genera such as *Aspergillus* and *Penicillium* are also presented.

## 2. Reported Animal Toxicity for Indole-Diterpenes

In 1986, Gallagher and Hawkes established mouse model assays to assess the tremorgenicity of lolitrems using a visual rating scale and a positive control (lolitrem B or paxilline) [16]. The mouse model assay showed good correlation to large animal models as seeds, deemed toxic through mouse studies, were also neurotoxic to sheep that were orally fed with pellets containing the toxin [32]. Mouse model assays established by Gallagher and Hawkes were used to assess tremor intensity of most of the indole-diterpenes described in Table 1 [16].

Another technique to test toxicity in larger animal models is electromyography (EMG), a method for measuring and evaluating the electrical activity of muscles. McLeay et al. carried out toxicity studies on sheep in which EMG activity of skeletal muscles and the smooth muscles of the reticulum and rumen were measured, in response to single doses of penitrems (mixture of 88.3% penitrem A, 6.4% penitrem B, 5.3% penitrem E), paxilline, lolitrem B, and 31-epilolitrem B [33] (Table 1). It was found that the reticulum and rumen muscles showed inhibition of normal electrical activity, which coincided with the induction of tremoring associated with skeletal muscle activity in penitrems, paxilline, and lolitrem B [33]. These findings indicate that disruption of digestion may occur in animals grazing endophyte-infected pasture, especially in the case of lolitrem B, in which perturbations in muscle electrical activity lasted 12 h [33].

Studies to further understand the mode of action of indole-diterpenes were conducted based on evidence relating to potassium channel inhibition as a potential mechanism of tremorgens and observed symptoms of hyperexcitation of the central nervous system [34–38]. In particular, Big Potassium (BK) channel receptor inhibition was tested in response to a series of compounds, as shown in Table 1, since BK channels have major roles in smooth muscle function and neuronal excitability [39].

It has been reported that mice deficient in BK ion channels are unaffected by these neurotoxins at concentrations that are lethal to wild-type mice [37]. This suggests that motor function deficits induced by lolitrems are mediated by BK channels [37]. These BK channels are independently activated by depolarizing membrane voltages and elevated intracellular calcium and magnesium [39]. The BK channel is suggested as the major molecular target for these compounds as they are reported to cause inhibition of the BK channel currents. The indole-diterpenes show differences in their interaction with BK channels in vitro and these differences are also apparent when comparing in vivo response of these compound such as duration of tremor and effects on motor function. Paxilline shows BK current inhibition to be calcium-dependent and there is reduced inhibition with increased calcium concentration [40] which is reported to rightward shift the conductance–voltage (G–V) [40,41]. It is also later reported that the G–V shift induced by paxilline is dependent on calcium concentration and an open state preference for BK (*hSlo*) channels [39]. In contrast, inhibition by lolitrem B does not affect G–V relationship [41], Although, both compounds are reported to possess a calcium concentration-dependence to their inhibitory effects and show higher apparent affinity for the open state of the BK channel in comparison to the closed state [41].

The concentration at which half-maximal inhibition ($IC_{50}$) is achieved is reported in Table 1. However, lolitrem E and paspalicine although showing potent BK channel activity, elicit a nontremorgenic effect on animals. This could be related to structural changes occurring in vivo, rendering it less active [41]. Knaus et al., suggested that although some pharmacological properties could be explained by BK channel inhibition, tremorgenicity may not be directly related to channel block [36].

Postulations regarding structure–activity relationship have been reported for motor and coordination deficits previously shown in mouse models and BK channel activity [37,39,41–43]. For example, the key attributes that have been postulated for the tremorgen lolitrem B as a potent neurotoxin include the presence of the acetal-linked isoprene unit on the right-hand side of the molecule, presence of the A/B rings and the position of the hydrogens in the junction of the rings (Figure 2). The presence of the A/B rings in particular are thought to be responsible for the slow-onset and long-acting tremorgenic activity of the lolitrem toxins [28,41]. Loss of the isoprene unit and opening of the ring attached to this isoprene unit removes the tremorgenic potency, as seen in lolitrem M and when lolitrem B loses its tremorgenicity when it degrades to lolitriol [28]. Table 1 describes in detail the results obtained from the assays described above for compounds belonging to indole-diterpene biosynthetic pathways.

**Table 1.** A summary of the biological activities reported for intermediaries isolated from the indole-diterpene biosynthetic pathway and some synthetic derivatives.

| Compound Name | Toxicity as Per Biological Activity on Mice (mg of Compound/kg of Body Weight) | Observation on Mice | Biological Activity on BK/Maxi or *hSlo* Channel | Biological Activity on Animal Model (EMG Activity/Observation in Sheep) | Reference |
|---|---|---|---|---|---|
| Lolitrem A | 2 mg/kg | Severe and prolonged tremor | - | - | [44] |
| Lolitrem B | 0.5 to 8.0 mg/kg | Severe and prolonged tremor | $IC_{50}$ = 4 nM (No recovery after wash out) | At 70 µg/kg dose, tremors were observed after 15 min and slowly increased in severity lasting for duration of 12 h. The reticulum and rumen showed inhibition after 20–30 min, coinciding with tremors. | [16,35,41] |
| 31-*epi*-lolitrem B | 4 mg/kg | Nontremorgenic | $IC_{50}$ = 50 nM (>50% recovery after 10 min) | The lolitrem B isomer was administered at a dose of 70 µg/kg and there was no effect either on the skeletal muscle EMG activity or EMG activity of the reticulum and rumen. | [33,41,45] |
| Lolitrem E | 2 mg/kg | Nontremorgenic | $IC_{50}$ = 6 nM (No recovery after wash out) | - | [20,41] |
| Lolitrem E acetate | 16 mg/kg | Weakly tremorgenic | $IC_{50}$ = 2 nM (No recovery after wash out) | - | [28,41] |
| 31-*epi*-lolitrem F[a] | 4 mg/kg | Slightly less tremorgenic than lolitrem B | - | - | [46] |
| Lolitrem F[a] | 4 mg/kg | Slightly less tremorgenic than lolitrem B | $IC_{50}$ = 8 nM (No recovery after wash out) | - | [41,46] |
| Lolitrem M | | Nontremorgenic | $IC_{50}$ = 78 nM (>50% recovery after 10 min) | - | [41] |
| Paxilline | 4 to 8 mg/kg and an 80 mg/kg dose | Severe but short term tremorgenicity compared to lolitrem B | Complete inhibition = 1 µM (recovery after wash out)<br>Fraction current blocked by 10 nM = 70% (recovery after wash out) | At 1.0 mg/kg dose, moderate to strong tremors; the onset was immediate after 2 min administration; tremors gradually disappeared over the next hour. EMG activity showed both excitatory and inhibitory on the reticulum and rumen. Also, within a minute of infusion, elevations of the EMG activity coincided with induction of marked tremoring. | [33,36,38,47] |
| 13-Desoxypaxilline | 8 mg/kg | Nontremorgenic | < 50% inhibition = 30 µM | - | [38] |

**Table 1.** *Cont.*

| Compound Name | Toxicity as Per Biological Activity on Mice (mg of Compound/kg of Body Weight) | Observation on Mice | Biological Activity on BK/Maxi or *hSlo* Channel | Biological Activity on Animal Model (EMG Activity/Observation in Sheep) | Reference |
| --- | --- | --- | --- | --- | --- |
| α-Paxitriol | 100 mg/kg | Lethargy and rough coats, also normal activities such as walking, rearing and preening were greatly reduced for several hours. Animals recovered to normal by 24 h post-injection. | - | - | [47] |
| β-Paxitriol | 100 mg/kg | Lethargy and rough coats, also normal activities such as walking, rearing and preening were greatly reduced for several hours. Animals recovered to normal by 24 h post-injection. | - | - | [47] |
| Lolitriol | 20 mg/kg | Nontremorgenic | $IC_{50}$ = 196 nM (>50% recovery after 10 min) | - | [47] |
| Lolitriol acetate | - | Nontremorgenic | $IC_{50}$ = 43 nM (>50% recovery after 10 min) | - | [41] |
| Lolitriol and β-Paxitrol | As a mixture: 16 mg/kg and 100 mg/kg respectively (200 µL dosage) | The single administration of both β-paxitriol and the nontremorgenic lolitriol proved lethal after an initial period of lethargy | - | - | [47] |
| Lolilline | 8 mg/kg | Nontremorgenic | - | - | [43] |
| 6,7-dehydroterpendole A | 8 mg/kg | Produced more intense tremors than terpendole C and K at the same dose level | - | - | [48,49] |
| Terpendole C | 4 mg/kg and 8 mg/kg | A fast-acting tremorgen that produced more intense tremors than paxilline, 11-hydroxy12,13-epoxyterpendole K and 6,7-dehydro-11-hydroxy-12, 13 epoxyterpendole A at the same dose level, but the activity ceased after 2 h, as compared to paxilline which ceased after 6 h. | | - | [43,48] |

**Table 1.** *Cont.*

| Compound Name | Toxicity as Per Biological Activity on Mice (mg of Compound/kg of Body Weight) | Observation on Mice | Biological Activity on BK/Maxi or *hSlo* Channel | Biological Activity on Animal Model (EMG Activity/Observation in Sheep) | Reference |
|---|---|---|---|---|---|
| Terpendole D, E, F, G, H and I | 8 mg/kg | Nontremorgenic | - | - | [28] |
| Terpendole K | 8 mg/kg | Produced more intense tremors than paxilline, 11-hydroxy12,13-epoxyterpendole K and 6,7-dehydro-11-hydroxy-12,13 epoxyterpendole A at the same dose level | - | - | [48] |
| Terpendole M | 8 mg/kg | Weakly tremorgenic | - | - | [50] |
| 6,7-dehydro-11-hydroxy-12,13 epoxyterpendole A and 11-hydroxy12,13-epoxyterpendole K | 8 mg/kg | Mild tremors | - | - | [48,49] |
| Mixture of 88.3% Penitrem A, 6.4% Penitrem B, 5.3% Penitrem E | | - | - | A dose of 5.5 mg/kg showed no significant skeletal EMG activity, although exhibited strong inhibition on the reticulum and rumen. This was apparent at 15 to 30 min and lasted 2 h. The maximum period of inhibition coincided with the period of greatest tremoring. | [33,51] |
| Penitrem A | 0.75 mg/kg (dose range 0.5 mg/kg to 1.5 mg/kg) | Elicited moderate tremors. Tremor duration reported as several hours. | Fraction current blocked by 10 nM = 100% (no recovery after wash out) | Tremorgenic observation in sheep when given at a dose of 20 µg/kg intravenously. | [36,52–54] |
| Penitrem E | 2.25 mg/kg (dose range 1.0 mg/kg to 3.6 mg/kg) | Elicited moderate tremors. Tremor duration reported as several hours. No difference to penitrem A in the rates of onset of tremors observed, and the symptomatology were like-wise similar. | - | - | [54] |
| Paspaline | - | - | Slight inhibition at concentrations up to 1 µM | - | [38] |
| Paspalinine | 8 mg/kg | Short duration tremors | Fraction current blocked by 10 nM = 100% (no recovery after wash out) | - | [28,36,55,56] |
| Paspalicine | 250 mg/kg | Nontremorgenic | Fraction current blocked by 10 nM = 83% (recovery after wash out) | - | [36,55,57] |
| Paspalitrems | 14 mg/kg | Short duration tremors | Fraction current blocked by 10 nM of paspalitrem A and paspalitrem C = 98% and 100% respectively (no recovery after wash out) | - | [36,55] |

**Table 1.** *Cont.*

| Compound Name | Toxicity as Per Biological Activity on Mice (mg of Compound/kg of Body Weight) | Observation on Mice | Biological Activity on BK/Maxi or *hSlo* Channel | Biological Activity on Animal Model (EMG Activity/Observation in Sheep) | Reference |
|---|---|---|---|---|---|
| Aflatrem | 1 mg/kg (dose range 0.5 mg/kg to 4.0 mg/kg) | Short duration tremors | Fraction current blocked by 10 nM = 100% (no recovery after wash out) | - | [16,36] |
| Janthitrem A | 4 mg/kg | Tremor duration was reported as 8 h and peaked at 15 min. Tremors produced were more intense than janthitrem B, from 2 h post exposure. | - | - | [58] |
| Janthitrem B | 6 mg/kg | Tremor duration reported as 6 h and peaked at 30 min. Un-coordination and hypersensitivity to sound and touch is also reported. | - | - | [58–60] |

a) Lolitrem F and 31-*epi*-lolitrem F have been reported to have a similar but slightly reduced tremorgenic activity compared to that reported for lolitrem B; however, Munday-Finch et al. assume that impurities present in lolitrem F and 31-*epi*-lolitrem F could have caused the slightly reduced activity [46].

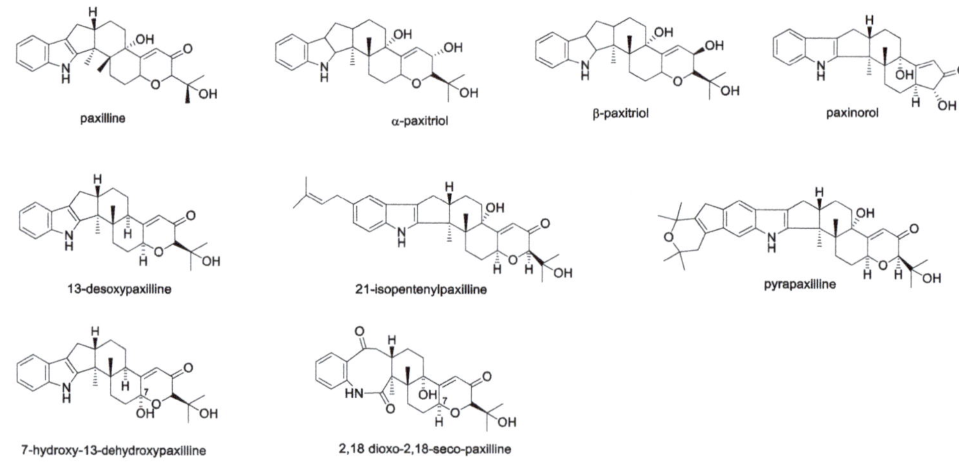


**Figure 2.** Structures of paxilline and selected derivatives.

## 2.1. *Classes of Indole-Diterpenes and Their Reported Activities*

### 2.1.1. Paxilline

Paxilline is produced by many types of fungi and was originally identified in *Penicillium paxilli* [61]. In 1975, the structure of paxilline was elucidated and the biological activity tested in mice [62]. It was found to induce tremors that sustained for several hours, yet it was evidently less toxic than other tremorgens exhibiting a $LD_{50}$ of 150 mg/kg body weight [62]. In comparison to lolitrem B, it is reported to produce shorter and less intense tremors in mice [43] and other vertebrate animals [63]. It is also a potent and selective BK channel inhibitor [36,40,64,65].

There are many other paxilline derivatives, such as α-paxitriol and β-paxitriol (Figure 2), which are proposed precursors of terpendoles and lolitrems as well as janthitrems and penitrems, respectively [66]. Structurally related compounds of paxilline are also reported to possess unique biological activities. For example, pyrapaxilline and 21-isopentenylpaxilline have been reported to inhibit the production of the neurotransmitter nitrogen monoxide (NO), though with less potency than paxilline [67]. The suppression of NO production is important for treating inflammatory diseases such as rheumatoid arthritis and atherosclerosis, a disease in which plaque builds up inside arteries [67]. Paxilline and paxilline derivatives were shown to be readily produced by various fungi in culture. For example, paxilline acetate, 13-desoxypaxilline (13-dehydroxypaxilline), from *Emericella striata* [68], 7-hydroxy-13-dehydroxypaxilline, 13-desoxypaxilline, 2,18-dioxo-2,18-seco-paxilline from *Eupenicillium shearii* [69] and paxinorol from *Penicillium paxilli* [70]. The structure of paxilline and several of its derivatives are indicated in Figure 2 and associated biological activities for mammalian toxicity (where known) are indicated in Table 1.

### 2.1.2. Lolitrems

In 1981, Gallagher et al. reported that lolitrems were the causative agents of ryegrass staggers in animals grazing perennial ryegrass pastures [71]. This study, and later reports, show that seeds containing lolitrems had the same toxic effect in symptomatology and the same reversible nature of neurotoxicity as observed for ryegrass staggers [32,71]. Later, in 1984, Gallagher reported the properties of lolitrem A–D and described full characterization studies of the major compound, lolitrem B [72]. Lolitrems A–N (Figure 3) and the derivatives epilolitrems, lolicines, and lolitriols (Figure 4) have been isolated and their structures elucidated [20,27,28,43,44,46,47]. The epi-lolitrems, are lolitrem B and lolitriol analogues which differ only in their stereochemistry at C-31 and C-35 position [27,46].

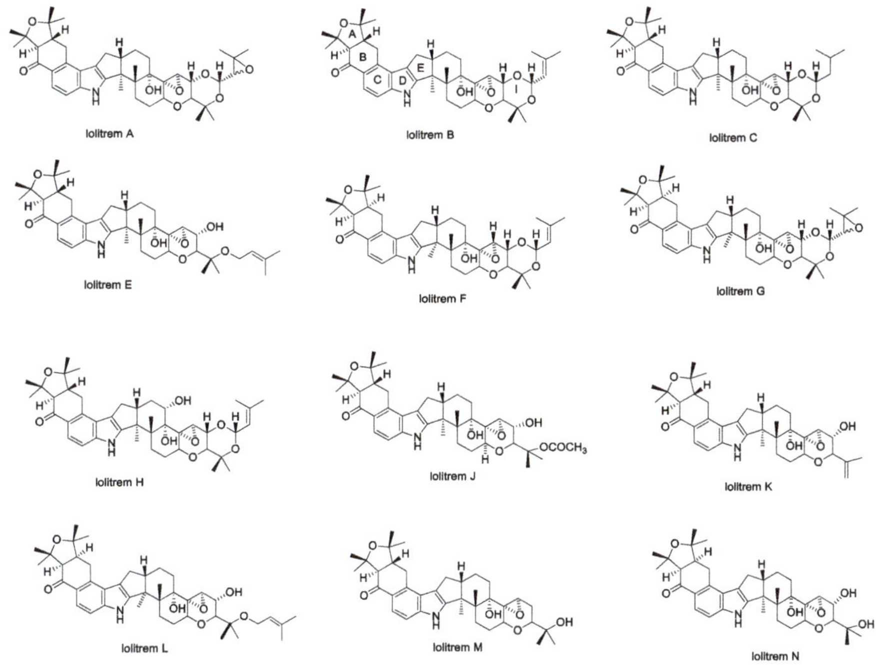


**Figure 3.** Structures of lolitrems A–N.

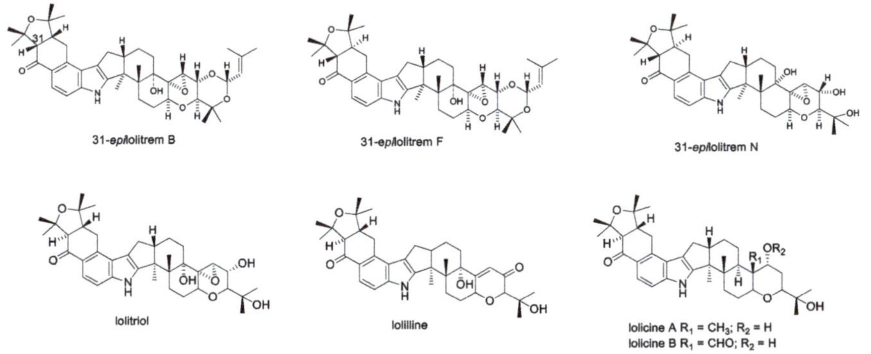


**Figure 4.** Structures of lolitrem derivatives.

The prolonged duration of tremors elicited by lolitrem B and its complete reversible response is considered to be of pharmacological importance [16]. The mode of action of the indole diterpenes, mainly as BK channel inhibitors, have allowed them to be used as lead compounds for pharmaceutical drug discovery.

Indole diterpenes, including nontremorgenic alkaloids have been reported to significantly inhibit the production of cytokines particularly those with a proinflammatory response. Cytokine proteins are produced by cells in response to an infection or trigger. The over-response of the immune system in humans to foreign substances, i.e., anaphylactic reaction, can cause fatalities. In the case of lolitrem B and 31-epi-lolitrem B, the production of cytokines IL-6 and TNFa was significantly inhibited in murine macrophage cells. It is also found that these compounds showed no toxicity against the host cells by means of cell proliferation assay at concentrations 100 and 250 times higher. Thus, it is suggested that these compounds would make good candidates for drug design [34].

### 2.1.3. Penitrems

Penitrems are found in several species of fungi and have been described particularly well in the case of *Penicillium crustosum* [73,74]. Penitrem A is the most tremorgenic and abundant of the penitrems (Figure 5) [54,75]. It causes severe sustained tremors in mice when given intraperitoneally at a dose of 1 mg/kg [52]; and in sheep when given intravenously at dose of only 20 μg/kg (Table 1). Furthermore, sheep dosed intravenously with 5.5 mg/kg of a penitrem mixture showed strong inhibition on the reticulum and rumen despite no significant skeletal EMG activity (Table 1). Penitrem A is also known to cause neuronal death, in particular of Purkinje neurons, located in the cerebellum, that are critical for coordination and movement [75].

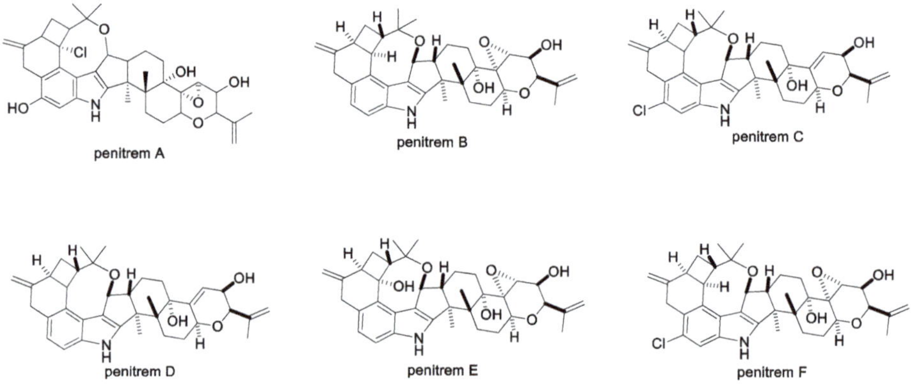


**Figure 5.** Structures of penitrems A–F.

Early work investigating the mode of action of the mycotoxins penitrem A and verruculogen shows that these toxins interfere with amino acid neurotransmitter release mechanisms in the central nervous system [76–78]. Penitrem A as well as another mycotoxin verruculogen are known to interfere with amino acid neurotransmitters release mechanisms in the central nervous system [76–79]. Norris et al. conducted a study in which toxins were administered in vivo and synaptosomes were subsequently prepared from cerebrocortical and spinal cord medullary regions of rat, and corpus striatum of sheep [77]. In this study, penitrem A increased and spontaneous release of glutamate [77], GABA, and aspartate from the cerebral cortex and midbrain region was observed [77]. However, no change was observed in the synthesis or release of dopamine and other amino acids and neurotransmitters in the central nervous system [77,78]. The tremorgen verruculogen increased the spontaneous release of glutamate and aspartate and decreased and inhibited uptake of GABA in mice in the central nervous system [77,78,80–82].

BK channels are important for cancer development and progression. Thus, BK channel blockers such as the indole diterpenes would be regarded as potential candidates for cancer therapeutic drugs [83–85]. Penitrems A, B, D, E, and F (Figure 5) as well as 6-bromopenitrem B and 6-bromopenitrem E are reported to show in vitro inhibition of proliferation, migration, and invasion properties against human breast cancer cells [86]. This effect was also observed for less complex biosynthetic intermediates emindole SB and paspaline [86]. These compounds were identified as potential candidates for future studies as they do not inhibit BK channels, thus eliminating any associated toxicity in relation to tremorgenicity [86]. A blockade of the α-subunit of the BK channels would also interfere with downstream biological functions such as neurotransmitter release and activation in the central and peripheral nervous system. A more targeted approach on β-catenin in human breast cancer cells was reported to have success with specific structural analogues of penitrems [87]. Additionally, combination therapy with other agents has been shown to reduce the associated toxicity [88]. Penitrem B also showed in vitro growth inhibition of the human tumor cell line screen representing leukemia [86]. This test was carried out using 60 cell lines representing various cancers (e.g., leukemia, melanoma, and cancers of the lung, colon, brain, ovary, breast, prostate, and kidney) [86]. Selective activity was exhibited by penitrem B against all cancer cells representing leukemia [86].

### 2.1.4. Paspaline

Paspaline and paspaline B have been isolated from *Pencillium paxilli* [89,90]. Paspaline, paspalinine, and paspalicine (Figure 6) were also isolated from *Claviceps paspali* and all three compounds were shown to possess no toxic or tremorgenic activity [90]. Although, paspalicine [36,89] and paspalitrem C (Figure 6) [65] potently block BK channels (refer to Table 1). This may be related to degradation or structural rearrangement occurring in vivo, thus reducing its potency [41].

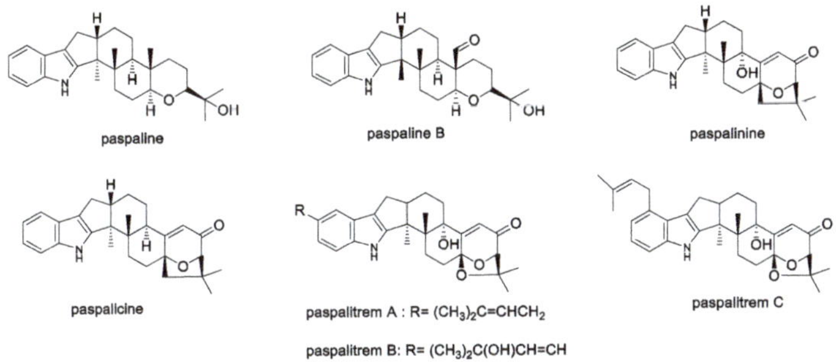


**Figure 6.** Structures of paspaline and paspaline derivatives.

### 2.1.5. Terpendoles

In 1994, the first reported terpendoles (A–D) (Figure 7) were isolated from culture of the then newly discovered species *Albophoma yamanshiensis* [91]. The compounds paspaline and emindole SB were also reported from this fungus [91]. Terpendoles inhibit acyl-CoA:cholesterol acyl transferase (ACAT) activity in rat liver microsomes [91,92]. The ACAT enzymes are membrane-bound proteins that utilize long-chain fatty acyl-CoA and cholesterol as substrates to form cholesteryl esters. The terpendoles are likely to inhibit ACAT activity by competing with the cholesterol substrate as the two groups exhibit structural similarity. Thus, inhibition of ACAT would be expected to improve or limit the development of atherosclerosis [93]. Terpendole C showed the most potent ACAT inhibition followed by terpendoles D, A, and B [91]. Terpendoles J, K, L and emindole SB exhibited moderate ACAT inhibitory activity, and paspaline and terpendoles E–I showed weak activity [92]. The subsequent identification of two ACAT isoenzymes present in mammals showed that the selectivity of potential inhibitors toward the two ACAT isoenzymes is important for the development of new anti-atherosclerotic agents. Although, terpendole C was found to inhibit both ACAT isoenzymes to a similar extent [94,95].

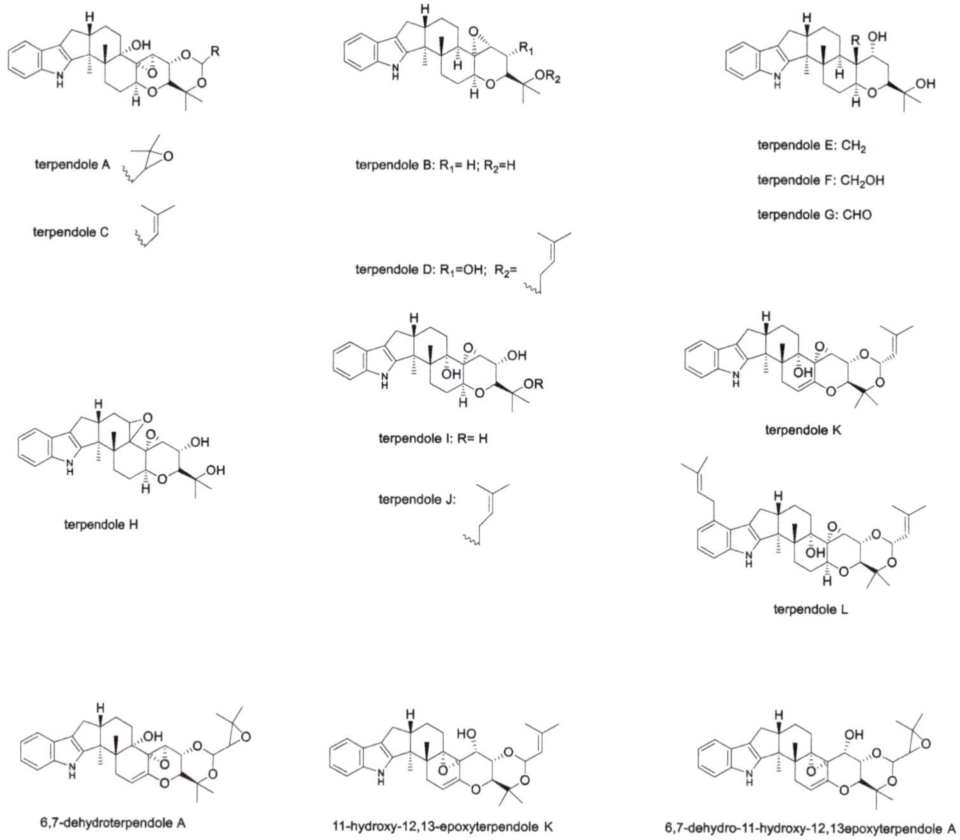


**Figure 7.** Structures of terpendoles A–L and derivatives.

A wide range of microorganisms were selected to test bioactivity of terpendoles A, B, C, and D, and in a separate study, terpendoles E–L [91,92]. The terpendoles did not exhibit any antimicrobial activity [91,92]. However, terpendole E exhibits unique properties; it has been found to be a novel and specific/selective inhibitor of human kinesin, Eg5. In contrast, terpendoles C, H, and I showed no inhibitory activity. Mitotic kinesin activity has been used as a specific target for antitumor compounds [96,97], since cancer therapeutic drugs such as Taxol® (NSC 125973) lack specificity and interfere with other cell functions, causing significant side effects [96].

Small animal toxicity studies showed that the terpendole A derivative, 6,7-dehydroterpendole A, elicited the most intense tremors compared to other terpendoles that were tested for tremorgenicity in mice (Table 1) [48]. Terpendole C was found to be a potent and fast-acting tremorgen; terpendole M displayed only weak tremorgenic activity in mice [50]. Since the majority of terpendoles exhibited no toxicological effects on mice, there is an opportunity to further investigate this class of compounds for pharmaceutical and agricultural purposes.

### 2.1.6. Sulpinines

Sulpinines A-C, secopenitrem (Figure 8) and penitrem B (Figure 5) isolated from the sclerotia of *Aspergillus sulphureus* [98] exhibit insecticidal properties and are active against the first instar larvae corn earworm (*Helicoverpa zea*). Feeding trials showed that sulpinine A possesses the strongest bioactivity, observed as reduced weight gain in the insects [98,99]. Sulpinine A also possesses cytotoxicity towards human lung carcinoma, breast adenocarcinoma, and colon adenocarcinoma [98].

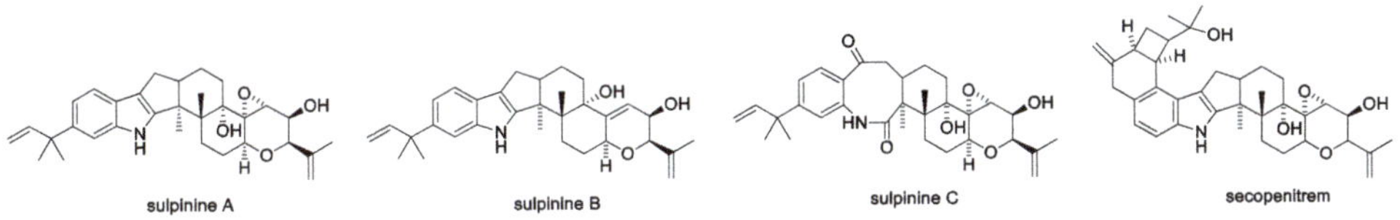


**Figure 8.** Structures of sulpinines A–C and secopenitrem.

### 2.1.7. Emindoles and Asporyzins

Emindoles were first reported in 1987 by Nozawa et al. from the *Emericella* spp. They were named emindole DA, emindole DB, emindole SA, and emindole SB (Figure 9) [68]. Emindoles reported from the mycelium of *Emericella purpurea* include emindoles PA, PB and PC (Figure 9) [100]. Emindole SC (Figure 9) was isolated from *Aspergillus sclerotiicarbonarius* (IBT 28362) and is reported to possess insecticidal properties towards *Drosophila melanogaster* larvae; however, it was found to be inactive against the fungus *Candida albicans* [101]. Emindoles including emindole SB [68] and related compounds emeniveol [102] and JBIR-03 [103] have also been isolated from many other fungal species including *Aspergillus oryzae*, *Dichotomomyces cejpii*, *Emericella nivea*, and *Emericella striata* [104]. Emeniveol was reported to inhibit pine pollen germination and tea pollen growth [102]. JBIR-03 is reported to have antibacterial activity against methicillin-resistant *Staphylococcus aureus* (MRSA); and also exhibits antifungal activity against the apple Valsa canker-causing fungus, *Valsa ceratosperma* [103]. In a study comparing JBIR-03, emindole SB, emeniveol, and related compounds asporyzin A, asporyzin B, asporyzin C (Figure 10), JBIR-03 was found to possess more potent insecticidal activity against brine shrimp (*Artemia salina*); while asporyzin C showed the most potent antibacterial activity against *Escherichia coli* [104].

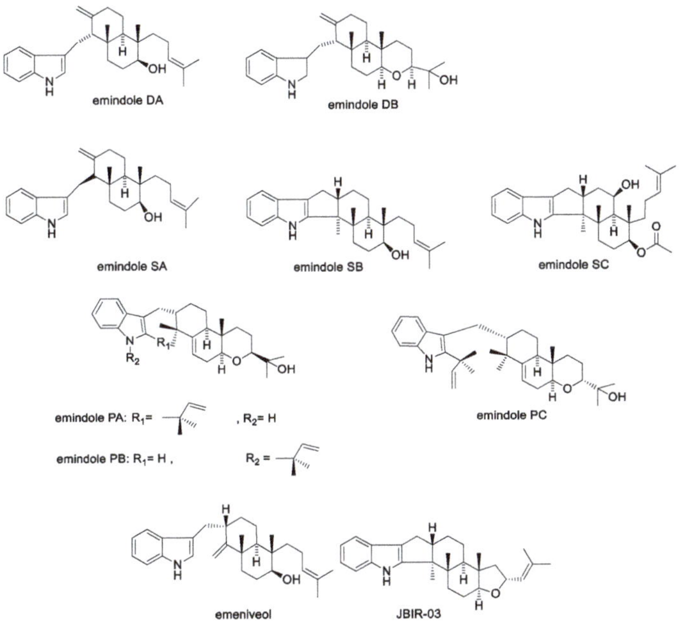


**Figure 9.** Structures of emindoles.

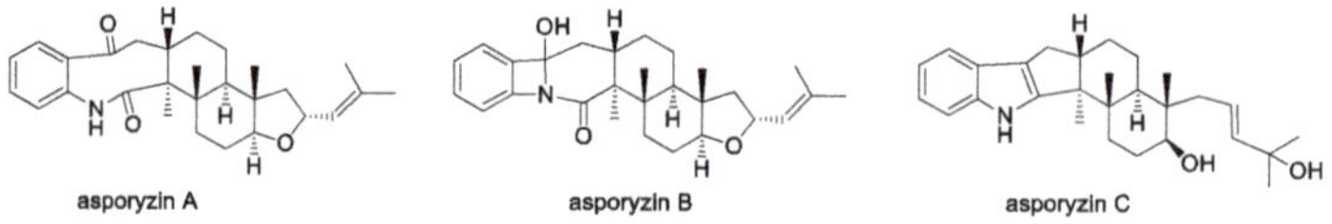


**Figure 10.** Structures of asporyzins.

### 2.1.8. Aflatrems

Aflatrem and β-aflatrem (Figure 11) are produced by the soil fungus *Aspergillus flavus*. Although, aflatrem is reported as a potent tremorgenic mycotoxin that causes a fast and sharp onset of tremors, it does not exhibit the same level of sustained tremors as lolitrem B (Table 1) [16]. β-aflatrem is reported to cause a significant reduction in the growth rate of the corn earworm *H. zea* [105]. Studies on precursors of aflatrem, such as paspalinine and paspalicine, indicated weaker activity on BK channels compared to aflatrem. Paspalicine an analogue of paspalinine does not exhibit tremorgenic activity but potently blocks BK channels (Table 1) [36].

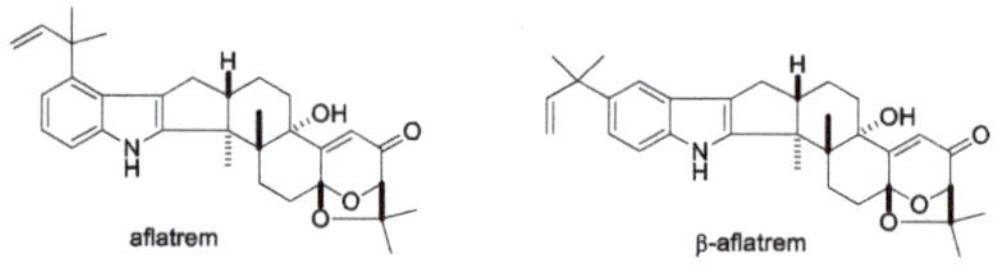


**Figure 11.** Structures of aflatrems.

### 2.1.9. Janthitrems

In 1980, Gallagher first identified, by high resolution mass spectrometry, the fluorescent tremorgenic mycotoxins janthitrems A, B, and C (Figure 12) in *Penicillium janthinellum* isolates obtained from ryegrass pastures in which ryegrass staggers had been observed [60].

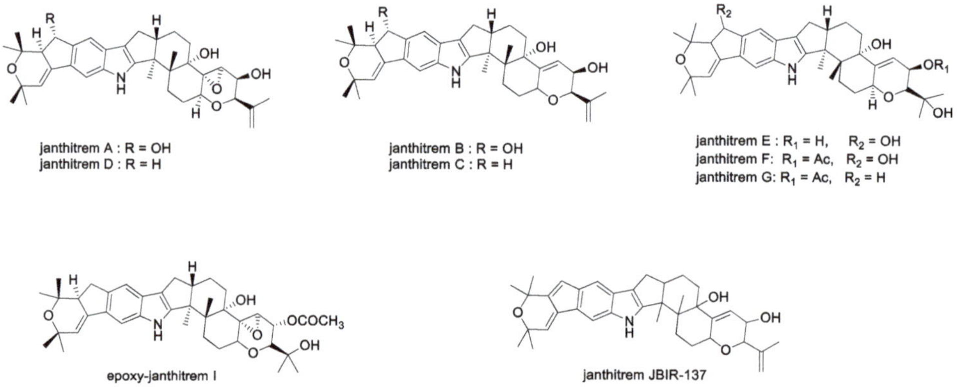


**Figure 12.** Structures of janthitrems.

Janthitrems B and C were isolated from isolates of *P. janthinellum* as the two most abundant tremorgenic mycotoxins [106]. Full structure elucidation of janthitrem B [106,107] and C [106] were carried out by NMR spectroscopy and later the NMR assignments for janthitrem C were revised [58]. The janthitrems are challenging to isolate as they are reported to be unstable and decompose at 4 °C [59,60].

Janthitrem A is reported to be the more potent tremorgen compared to the structurally similar compound janthitrem B (Table 1) [58]. Tremorgenic potency could be attributed to the 11,12-epoxy group as this is the only structural difference [58]. This could explain the tremors observed in animals grazing ryegrass pastures with AR37 endophyte, an *Epichloë* spp. (*Lp*TG-3) strain that is known to produce epoxy-janthitrems [58,108]. Janthitrems A and B also show antifeedant activity against porina (*Wiseana cervinata*) larvae, although janthitrem A is more potent than janthitrem B [58].

Using characteristic properties of the janthitrems, high throughput methods of quantitation were developed in 1982 by Lauren and Gallagher, and a fourth compound was identified as janthitrem D [59,60]. Although in 1984, [109] and later in 1993 [106] janthitrems E–G (Figure 12) was isolated and structures determined, the tremorgenicity of janthitrems E–G remain unknown.

In 2012, Kawahara et al. described the development of an in-house library by analyzing purified natural compounds from cultures of microorganisms using an ultra-performance liquid chromatography coupled with UV detection (UPLC-UV)-evaporative light-scattering (ELS)-MS system [110]. Compounds which are present in microbial cultures that are registered in the library are automatically identified within the system. The high-throughput screening assay allows the detection of unregistered secondary metabolites in microbial cultures. The *Aspergillus* species was targeted in this scheme due to the large number of bioactive compounds it produced [110]. As a result, a new janthitrem derivative, JBIR-137 was isolated (Figure 12) [110]. The cytotoxic activity reported against human ovarian adenocarcinoma SKOV-3 cell showed that JBIR-137 and janthitrem B exhibit weak cytotoxic activities [110].

#### 2.1.10. Shearinines

Shearinines are very similar to the janthitrem class of compounds and were first isolated from the aseostromata of *Eupenicillium shearii*. Shearinines A–C (Figure 13) exhibit insecticidal activity as shown in dietary bioassays testing the effect of purified compounds on corn earworm *H. zea* and the dried-fruit beetle *Carpophilus hemipterus* [69]. Shearinine A also exhibited antifeeding activity in a topical assay against *H. zea*, and shearinine B caused significant mortality in the fall armyworm *Spodoptera frugiperda*, when exposed to treated leaf disks [69].

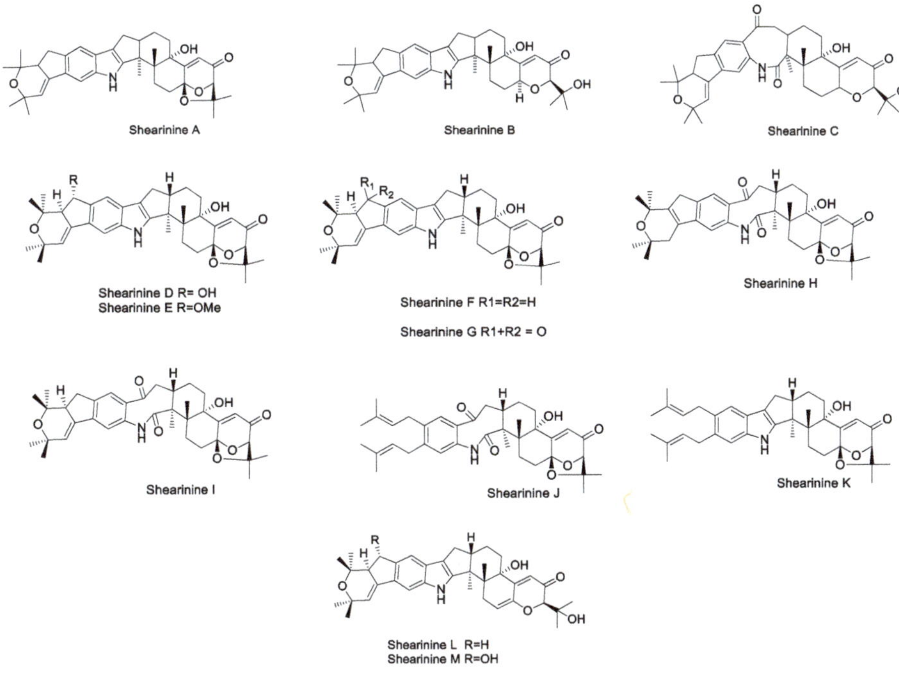


**Figure 13.** Structures of shearinines A–M.

Shearinines D–K have been isolated from *Pencillium* spp., resident endophytic fungus from the mangrove plant *Aegiceras corniculatum* L. Shearinine A, paspalitrem A, and paspaline were also identified. Shearinines D, E, and G (which have reduced potency) showed significant in vitro blocking activity on BK channels [111]. Shearinines also exhibit biological activity against fungal diseases in humans, specifically the *Candida* spp. *Candida albicans* are a common cause of mycoses (fungal diseases) and their ability to form biofilms in human tissues and indwelling medical devices shields the fungus from attack from the immune system and antibiotics [112]. Shearinines D and E have shown to inhibit biofilm formation at a relatively late stage of biofilm development, although they show weaker activity on existing biofilms [112]. Shearinines, in combination with the antifungal drug amphotericin B, augment the potency eight-fold on existing and developing biofilms [112].

Shearinines L and M (Figure 13) were isolated from the fungal pathogen *Escovopsis weberi* [113]. Certain ant and fungal species can form mutualistic symbiosis, such as in the case of leaf-cutting ants and their garden fungus (*Leucoagaricus gongylophorus*). The fungal pathogen *E. weberi* was found to degrade the hyphae of *L. gongylophorus* without direct physical interaction by secreting toxins. To investigate the source of the pathogenicity, Dhodary et al. identified and isolated the secondary metabolites produced by the pathogen. The study found that secondary metabolites cycloarthropsone and emodin strongly inhibited the growth of the garden fungus. Shearinine L did not affect the growth of the garden fungus; however, the ants (*Acromyrmex octospinosus*) learned to avoid shearinine L-treated substrate in dual choice behavioural assays [113].

#### 2.1.11. Other Pharmaceutical Applications of Indole-Diterpenes

The indole-diterpenes as active BK channel blockers have opened pharmaceutical applications, including the treatment of glaucoma, a degenerative eye disease that begins with intraocular pressure [114–116]. Goetz et al. patented the application of indole-diterpenes for the treatment of glaucoma, as the compounds were shown to reduce intraocular pressure and hence any further degenerative conditions [114–116].

A number of indole-diterpenes also show significant activity against the H1N1 virus, particularly emindole SB, 21-isopentenylpaxilline, paspaline, paxilline, and dehydroxypaxilline [117]. The H1N1 virus is an aggressive influenza virus strain that can cause fatalities in humans [117]. To date, there are very few drugs which treat H1N1 viral infections [117].

In summary, there is a common trend to utilize non-tremorgenic indole-diterpenes for pesticides in an agricultural setting. Although, the indole-diterpene group of compounds have proven valuable in applications even beyond the agricultural scope. This could be attributed to their selectivity to receptor binding sites, particularly as BK channel blockers. Minor stereochemical changes have proven to drastically change their effect on the behavioral phenotype in animal models, such as in the case of lolitrem B when it loses its tremorgenicity in its epimeric form (31-epilolitrem B). The unique selectivity exhibited by these compounds have allowed them to be exploited as potential candidates for pharmaceutical drug discovery. However, discrepancies regarding structure–activity relationships remain questionable, particularly in relation to BK channel inhibition and tremorgenicity, which need to be addressed. Lolitrem E and paspalicine, for example, exhibit strong BK channel activity; however, they do not exhibit tremorgenicity. Thus, further investigation would be required into the mode of action of these compounds.

## 3. Toxicity of Ergovaline and Lolitrem B in the Field

The ergot alkaloid largely responsible for mammalian toxicity in tall fescue (*Festuca arundinacea*) pastures is ergovaline—where it accounts for approximately 90% of total plant ergopeptide alkaloid content [10]. Toxicity of ergot alkaloids, although present in endophyte-infected perennial ryegrass, is not as commonly reported as ryegrass staggers disease [118]. The threshold levels for fescue toxicosis is 300–500 parts per billion (ppb), depending on the season [119].

There are difficulties in characterizing all compounds in a grass–endophyte association, thus thresholds are set for major toxins. Ergovaline is well studied in tall fescue and has a toxic threshold of 300–400 ppb for cattle and sheep [120]. The Oregon State University College of Veterinary Medicine found the threshold levels of ergovaline in tall fescue, subject to weather, are 300–500 ppb (for horses), 400–750 ppb (for cattle), and 500–800 ppb (for sheep). Threshold levels for lolitrem B in perennial ryegrass staggers for cattle and sheep is 1800–2000 ppb and 500 ppb for camels [119].

In Australia and New Zealand, the concentrations of lolitrem B and ergovaline in naturalized populations of perennial ryegrass are usually lowest in winter/spring from June to November and highest in summer from December to February [19]. A seasonal variation study was carried out by Repussard et al. on lolitrem B and ergovaline concentrations in *Lp*TG-1 infected perennial ryegrass in southern France. Here, concentrations within the leaves, base and inflorescence were analyzed to assess the effect of temperature, rainfall and maturity [120]. Ergovaline was found to accumulate in the inflorescence of the plant whilst lolitrem B varied with the maturity of the plant, whereby concentrations were highest in the oldest leaves. In general, ergovaline and lolitrem B concentrations exhibited similar trends in peaks and troughs (i.e., low or high concentrations), but these similarities vary in different perennial ryegrass varieties/ecotypes [120].

In an effort to identify new host plant–endophyte associations that exhibit nontoxic effects on sheep, Oliveira et al. used two perennial ryegrass genotypes (EI19 and EI24) which were infected with the same lolitrem B-free fungal endophyte [121]. These were sowed on two sites, with different soil types and seasons, in north-west Spain. Low levels of ergovaline were produced and no animal toxicity was reported. A mean value of less than 0.4 ppm ergovaline (mg/kg of dry mass) was reported across the matrix, the highest level being 0.57 ppm [121]. Despite significant seasonal variation in concentrations of ergovaline, grass–endophyte associations safe for agricultural use can be developed.

## 4. Indole-Diterpenes Reported in the Environment

The presence of these indole-diterpene-type compounds is ubiquitous in the natural environment. Moldy food products produced by the *Penicillium* spp. are a common source for these compounds. For example, fungal metabolites such as janthitrems, paspalinine, paxilline, and 3-*O*-acetoxypaxilline were found to be produced by *Pencillium tularense* found in fresh tomatoes homegrown and from supermarkets, with developing fungal lesions [122]. Also, *Pencillium crustosum* a commonly occurring foodborne fungus that is responsible for spoilage of a wide variety of foods, is known for producing the tremorgenic mycotoxin penitrem A. Humans have developed tremors followed by headache, vomiting, diplopia, weakness, and bloody diarrhea by ingesting *P. crustosum* in moldy food [23] or inhaling moldy hay dust [123]. Also, domestic animals such as dogs exposed to moldy food items have been reported to be poisoned by penitrem A [124,125]. Penitrem A intoxication are characteristic of indole-diterpene intoxication; these include tremors and ataxia that may progress to seizures and death in high levels of exposure. Poisoning has also been documented in cattle, sheep, and horses in the field [24].

## 5. High Throughput Methods for Determining Endophyte Toxicity

This review highlights the requirement to screen grass–endophyte associations to determine endophyte toxicity, particularly for novel endophytes that are in the evaluation phase prior to commercialization. Concentrations of metabolites produced by the endophyte, specifically the major toxins lolitrem B and ergovaline, need to be monitored and thoroughly investigated for toxicity to animals. This information is critical for the generation of safer endophyte-infected pastures, and utilizing compounds known to cause limited or no neurotoxic effects whilst still maintaining the competitive advantage for the plant (such as insect control).

Understanding the toxicity of the indole-diterpene and ergot alkaloid families and their derivatives would provide an avenue in the development of high-throughput screening assays which are required for the selection of novel grass–endophyte associations. Animal models are expensive, time consuming and considered unviable for testing a large number of grass–endophyte associations selected in the breeding program.

In the past, high throughput methods were developed solely based on information on the toxicity of the major mycotoxin lolitrem B. For example, a high-performance liquid chromatography (HPLC) method was developed in 1985 by Gallagher for the quantitation of lolitrem B using the unique profile of 268 nm absorbance of lolitrem B. Although, compounds in the plant matrix with similar UV absorbance's interfered with the reliable detection of the lolitrems at low levels [126]. Later, Gallagher discovered that the lolitrems had strong fluorescence properties and developed a new sensitive quantitation method using a HPLC fluorescence detector, which remains one of the most sensitive methods used for the detection of lolitrems [127,128].

With the advent of metabolomics and mass spectrometry (MS), sample preparation has become much simpler and many compounds can be simultaneously quantitated based on MS and MSMS studies [129]. Currently, liquid chromatography–mass spectrometry (LCMS) is the most widely used tool for identification and quantitation of endophyte-produced alkaloids [10,22,130,131]. However, with the development of facile and rapid methods provided by advanced MS techniques, the limitation now remains on the availability of analytical standards.

In conclusion, current pasture improvement programs involve maintenance of beneficial endophyte infection in perennial ryegrass, whilst reducing the negative effects of particular compounds on mammalian health. It has been long established that lolitrem B and ergovaline, derived from the indole-diterpene and ergot alkaloid pathways, respectively, are the major compounds that cause toxicity syndromes in grazing animals. The contribution of some analogues and intermediates within the indole-diterpene pathway have also more recently been studied for biological activity and mode of action. Currently, information regarding the toxicity status of many of the compounds within the indole-diterpene pathway is lacking, and this information is imperative for the agriculture industry. This is due to naturally varied concentrations of the compounds found in marketed forage grasses. Further, there are limited studies exploring the effect of individual compounds on animal models. The primary challenge is obtaining these compounds through complex isolation and purification methods before any studies can be carried out. Research focused on characterizing the toxicity and biochemical effects of fungal metabolites in animal models will provide greater confidence in dairy and meat products containing these compounds.

**Funding:** The research described here was funded by the Dairy Futures Cooperative Research Centre and DairyBio.

**Acknowledgments:** We thank the Molecular Phenomics and Molecular Genetics group at Agriculture Victoria.

**Conflicts of Interest:** The authors declare no conflict of interest.

## References

1. Forster, J.W.; Cogan, N.O.I.; Dobrowolski, M.P.; Francki, M.G.; Spangenberg, G.C.; Smith, K.F. Functionally associated molecular genetic markers for temperate pasture plant improvement. In *Plant Genotyping II: SNP Technology*; Henry, R.J., Ed.; CABI: Wallingford, UK, 2008; pp. 154–186.
2. Young, C.A.; Hume, D.E.; McCulley, R.L. Forages and pastures symposium: Fungal endophytes of tall fescue and perennial ryegrass: Pasture friend or foe? *J. Anim. Sci.* **2013**, *91*, 2379–2394. [CrossRef]
3. Cunningham, P.J.; Foot, J.Z.; Reed, K.F.M. Perennial ryegrass (*Lolium perenne*) endophyte (*Acremonium lolii*) relationships: the Australian experience. *Agric. Ecosyst. Environ.* **1993**, *44*, 157–168. [CrossRef]
4. Tian, P.; Le, T.N.; Ludlow, E.J.; Smith, K.F.; Forster, J.W.; Guthridge, K.M.; Spangenberg, G.C. Characterisation of novel perennial ryegrass host-*Neotyphodium* endophyte associations. *Crop Pasture Sci.* **2013**, *64*, 716–725. [CrossRef]
5. Van Zijll De Jong, E.; Dobrowolski, M.P.; Bannan, N.R.; Stewart, A.V.; Smith, K.F.; Spangenberg, G.C.; Forster, J.W. Global genetic diversity of the perennial ryegrass fungal endophyte *Neotyphodium lolii*. *Crop Sci.* **2008**, *48*, 1487–1501. [CrossRef]

6. Moate, P.J.; Williams, S.R.O.; Grainger, C.; Hannah, M.C.; Mapleson, D.; Auldist, M.J.; Greenwood, J.S.; Popay, A.J.; Hume, D.E.; Mace, W.J.; et al. Effects of wild-type, AR1 and AR37 endophyte-infected perennial ryegrass on dairy production in Victoria, Australia. *Anim. Prod. Sci.* **2012**, *52*, 1117–1130. [CrossRef]
7. Leuchtmann, A.; Bacon, C.W.; Schardl, C.L.; White Jr, J.F.; Tadych, M. Nomenclatural realignment of *Neotyphodium* species with genus *Epichloë*. *Mycologia* **2014**, *106*, 202–215. [CrossRef] [PubMed]
8. Popay, A.J.; Hume, D.E.; Mainland, R.A.; Saunders, C.J. Field resistance to Argentine stem weevil (*Listronotus bonariensis*) in different ryegrass cultivars infected with an endophyte deficient in lolitrem B. *New Zeal. J. Agr. Res.* **1995**, *38*, 519–528. [CrossRef]
9. Prestidge, R.A.; Ball, O.J.P. The role of endophytes in alleviating plant biotic stress in New Zealand. In *Proceedings of the Second International Symposium on Acremonium/Grass Interactions*; Hume, D.E., Latch, G.C.M., Easton, H.S., Eds.; AgResearch: Palmerston North, New Zealand, 1993; pp. 141–151.
10. Porter, J.K. Analysis of endophyte toxins: Fescue and other grasses toxic to livestock. *J. Animal. Sci.* **1995**, *73*, 871–880. [CrossRef] [PubMed]
11. Hovermale, J.T.; Craig, A.M. Correlation of ergovaline and lolitrem B levels in endophyte-infected perennial ryegrass (*Lolium perenne*). *J. Vet. Diagn. Invest.* **2001**, *13*, 323–327. [CrossRef]
12. Weedon, C.M.; Mantle, P.G. Paxilline biosynthesis by *Acremonium loliae*; a step towards defining the origin of lolitrem neurotoxins. *Phytochemistry* **1987**, *26*, 969–971. [CrossRef]
13. CHAPTER 14—Neurological Diseases. In *Diagnostic Techniques in Equine Medicine*, 2nd ed.; Taylor, F.G.R.; Brazil, T.J.; Hillyer, M.H. (Eds.) W.B. Saunders: Edinburgh, UK, 2009; pp. 287–304.
14. CHAPTER 14—Diseases of the Nervous System. In *Veterinary Medicine*, 11th ed.; Constable, P.D.; Hinchcliff, K.W.; Done, S.H.; Grünberg, W. (Eds.) W.B. Saunders: Edinburgh, UK, 2017; pp. 1155–1370.
15. Kozák, L.; Szilágyi, Z.; Tóth, L.; Pócsi, I.; Molnár, I. Tremorgenic and neurotoxic paspaline-derived indole-diterpenes: Biosynthetic diversity, threats and applications. *Appl. Microbiol. Biotechnol.* **2019**, *103*, 1599–1616. [CrossRef]
16. Gallagher, R.T.; Hawkes, A.D. The potent tremorgenic neurotoxins lolitrem B and aflatrem: A comparison of the tremor response in mice. *Experientia* **1986**, *42*, 823–825. [CrossRef] [PubMed]
17. Latch, G.C.M. Trichothecenes and other mycotoxins. In Proceedings of the International Mycotoxin Symposium, Sydney, Australia, August 1984.
18. Plumlee, K.H.; Galey, F.D. Neurotoxic mycotoxins: A review of fungal toxins that cause neurological disease in large animals. *J. Vet. Intern. Med.* **1994**, *8*, 49–54. [CrossRef]
19. Thom, E.R.; Clark, D.A.; Waugh, C.D. Growth, persistence, and alkaloid levels of endophyte-infected and endophyte-free ryegrass pastures grazed by dairy cows in northern New Zealand. *New Zeal. J. Agr. Res.* **1999**, *42*, 241–253. [CrossRef]
20. Miles, C.O.; Munday, S.C.; Wilkins, A.L.; Ede, R.M.; Towers, N.R. Large-scale isolation of lolitrem B and structure determination of lolitrem E. *J. Agric. Food Chem.* **1994**, *42*, 1488–1492. [CrossRef]
21. Russell, C.A. Letter: "Rye grass staggers". *Vet. Rec.* **1975**, *97*, 295. [CrossRef]
22. Young, C.A.; Tapper, B.A.; May, K.; Moon, C.D.; Schardl, C.L.; Scott, B. Indole-diterpene biosynthetic capability of *Epichloë* endophytes as predicted by ltm gene analysis. *Appl. Environ. Microbiol.* **2009**, *75*, 2200–2211. [CrossRef]
23. Lewis, P.R.; Donoghue, M.B.; Cook, L.; Granger, L.V.; Hocking, A.D. Tremor syndrome associated with a fungal toxin: sequelae of food contamination. *Med. J. Aust.* **2005**, *182*, 582–584. [CrossRef] [PubMed]
24. Evans, T.J.; Gupta, R.C. Chapter 74—Tremorgenic Mycotoxins. In *Veterinary Toxicology*, 3rd ed.; Gupta, R.C., Ed.; Academic Press: Amsterdam, Netherlands, 2018; pp. 1033–1041.
25. Bluett, S.J.; Thom, E.R.; Clark, D.A.; Macdonald, K.A.; Minneé, E.M.K. Effects of perennial ryegrass infected with either AR1 or wild endophyte on dairy production in the Waikato. *New Zeal. J. Agr. Res.* **2005**, *48*, 197–212. [CrossRef]
26. Reddy, P.; Deseo, M.A.; Ezernieks, V.; Guthridge, K.; Spangenberg, G.; Rochfort, S. Toxic indole diterpenes from endophyte-infected perennial ryegrass *Lolium perenne* L.: Isolation and stability. *Toxins* **2019**, *11*, 16. [CrossRef]
27. Munday-Finch, S.C.; Wilkins, A.L.; Miles, C.O. Isolation of lolicine A, lolicine B, lolitriol, and lolitrem N from *Lolium perenne* infected with *Neotyphodium lolii* and evidence for the natural occurrence of 31-epilolitrem N and 31-epilolitrem F. *J. Agric. Food Chem.* **1998**, *46*, 590–598. [CrossRef]
28. Munday-Finch, S. Aspects of the chemistry and toxicology of indole-diterpenoid mycotoxins involved in tremorganic disorder of livestock. *Mycotoxin Res.* **1997**, *13*, 88. [CrossRef]
29. Kanehisa, M.; Furumichi, M.; Tanabe, M.; Sato, Y.; Morishima, K. KEGG: New perspectives on genomes, pathways, diseases and drugs. *Nucleic. Acids. Res.* **2017**, *45*, D353–D361. [CrossRef] [PubMed]

30. Kanehisa, M.; Goto, S. KEGG: Kyoto encyclopedia of genes and genomes. *Nucleic. Acids. Res.* **2000**, *28*, 27–30. [CrossRef] [PubMed]
31. Kanehisa, M.; Sato, Y.; Furumichi, M.; Morishima, K.; Tanabe, M. New approach for understanding genome variations in KEGG. *Nucleic. Acids. Res.* **2019**, *47*, D590–D595. [CrossRef]
32. Gallagher, R.T.; Campbell, A.G.; Hawkes, A.D.; Holland, P.T.; McGaveston, D.A.; Pansier, E.A. Ryegrass staggers: The presence of lolitrem neurotoxins in perennial ryegrass seed. *N. Z. Vet. J.* **1982**, *30*, 183–184. [CrossRef] [PubMed]
33. McLeay, L.M.; Smith, B.L.; Munday-Finch, S.C. Tremorgenic mycotoxins paxilline, penitrem and lolitrem B, the nontremorgenic 31-epilolitrem B and electromyographic activity of the reticulum and rumen of sheep. *Res. Vet. Sci.* **1999**, *66*, 119–127. [CrossRef]
34. Dalziel, J.E.; Dunlop, J.; Finch, S.C.; Wong, S.S. Immune Response Inhibition Using Indole Diterpene Compound. WO2006115423A1, 2006. Available online: https://patents.google.com/patent/WO2006115423A1/ko (accessed on 2 November 2018).
35. Dalziel, J.E.; Finch, S.C.; Dunlop, J. The fungal neurotoxin lolitrem B inhibits the function of human large conductance calcium-activated potassium channels. *Toxicol. Lett.* **2005**, *155*, 421–426. [CrossRef]
36. Knaus, H.-G.; McManus, O.B.; Lee, S.H.; Schmalhofer, W.A.; Garcia-Calvo, M.; Helms, L.M.H.; Sanchez, M.; Giangiacomo, K.; Reuben, J.P.; Smith, A.B.; et al. Tremorgenic indole alkaloids potently inhibit smooth muscle high-conductance calcium-activated potassium channels. *Biochemistry* **1994**, *33*, 5819–5828. [CrossRef]
37. Imlach, W.L.; Finch, S.C.; Dunlop, J.; Meredith, A.L.; Aldrich, R.W.; Dalziel, J.E. The molecular mechanism of "ryegrass staggers," a neurological disorder of K+ channels. *J. Pharmacol. Exp. Ther.* **2008**, *327*, 657–664. [CrossRef]
38. McMillan, L.K.; Carr, R.L.; Young, C.A.; Astin, J.W.; Lowe, R.G.; Parker, E.J.; Jameson, G.B.; Finch, S.C.; Miles, C.O.; McManus, O.B.; et al. Molecular analysis of two cytochrome P450 monooxygenase genes required for paxilline biosynthesis in *Penicillium paxilli*, and effects of paxilline intermediates on mammalian maxi-K ion channels. *Mol. Genet. Genomics.* **2003**, *270*, 9–23. [CrossRef] [PubMed]
39. Imlach, W.L.; Finch, S.C.; Zhang, Y.; Dunlop, J.; Dalziel, J.E. Mechanism of action of lolitrem B, a fungal endophyte derived toxin that inhibits BK large conductance Ca2+-activated K+ channels. *Toxicon* **2011**, *57*, 686–694. [CrossRef] [PubMed]
40. Sanchez, M.; McManus, O.B. Paxilline inhibition of the alpha-subunit of the high-conductance calcium-activated potassium channel. *Neuropharmacology* **1996**, *35*, 963–968. [CrossRef]
41. Imlach, W.L.; Finch, S.C.; Dunlop, J.; Dalziel, J.E. Structural determinants of lolitrems for inhibition of BK large conductance $Ca^{2+}$-activated $K^+$ channels. *Eur. J. Pharmacol.* **2009**, *605*, 36–45. [CrossRef]
42. Imlach, W.L.; Finch, S.C.; Miller, J.H.; Meredith, A.L.; Dalziel, J.E. A role for BK channels in heart rate regulation in rodents. *PLoS One* **2010**, *5*, e8698. [CrossRef] [PubMed]
43. Munday-Finch, S.C.; Wilkins, A.L.; Miles, C.O.; Tomoda, H.; Omura, S. Isolation and structure elucidation of lolilline, a possible biosynthetic precursor of the lolitrem family of tremorgenic mycotoxins. *J. Agric. Food Chem.* **1997**, *45*, 199–204. [CrossRef]
44. Munday-Finch, S.C.; Miles, C.O.; Wilkins, A.L.; Hawkes, A.D. Isolation and structure elucidation of lolitrem A, a tremorgenic mycotoxin from perennial ryegrass infected with *Acremonium lolii*. *J. Agric. Food Chem.* **1995**, *43*, 1283–1288. [CrossRef]
45. Munday-Finch, S.C.; Wilkins, A.L.; Miles, C.O. Isolation of paspaline B, an indole-diterpenoid from *Penicilium paxilli*. *Phytochemistry* **1996**, *41*, 327–332. [CrossRef]
46. Munday-Finch, S.C.; Wilkins, A.L.; Miles, C.O.; Ede, R.M.; Thomson, R.A. Structure elucidation of lolitrem F, a naturally occurring stereoisomer of the tremorgenic mycotoxin lolitrem B, isolated from *Lolium perenne* infected with *Acremonium lolii*. *J. Agric. Food Chem.* **1996**, *44*, 2782–2788. [CrossRef]
47. Miles, C.O.; Wilkins, A.L.; Gallagher, R.T.; Hawkes, A.D.; Munday, S.C.; Towers, N.R. Synthesis and tremorgenicity of paxitriols and lolitriol: Possible biosynthetic precursors of lolitrem B. *J. Agric. Food Chem.* **1992**, *40*, 234–238. [CrossRef]
48. Gardner, D.R.; Welch, K.D.; Lee, S.T.; Cook, D.; Riet-Correa, F. Tremorgenic indole diterpenes from *Ipomoea asarifolia* and *Ipomoea muelleri* and the identification of 6,7-dehydro-11-hydroxy-12,13-epoxyterpendole A. *J. Nat. Prod.* **2018**, *81*, 1682–1686. [CrossRef]
49. Lee, S.T.; Gardner, D.R.; Cook, D. Identification of indole diterpenes in *Ipomoea asarifolia* and *Ipomoea muelleri*, plants tremorgenic to livestock. *J. Agric. Food Chem.* **2017**, *65*, 5266–5277. [CrossRef]

50. Gatenby, W.A.; Munday-Finch, S.C.; Wilkins, A.L.; Miles, C.O. Terpendole M, a novel indole-diterpenoid isolated from *Lolium perenne* infected with the endophytic fungus *Neotyphodium lolii*. *J. Agric. Food Chem.* **1999**, *47*, 1092–1097. [CrossRef]
51. De Jesus, A.E.; Gorst-Allman, C.P.; Steyn, P.S.; Van Heerden, F.R.; Vleggaar, R.; Wessels, P.L.; Hull, W.E. Tremorgenic mycotoxins from *Penicillium crustosum*. Biosynthesis of penitrem A. *J. Chem. Soc. Perkin. Trans.* **1983**, *1*, 1863–1868. [CrossRef]
52. Ciegler, A. Mycotoxins: Occurrence, chemistry, biological activity. *Lloydia* **1975**, *38*, 21–35. [PubMed]
53. Penny, R.H.; O'Sullivan, B.M.; Mantle, P.G.; Shaw, B.I. Clinical studies on tremorgenic mycotoxicoses in sheep. *Vet. Rec.* **1979**, *105*, 392–393. [CrossRef]
54. Kyriakidis, N.; Waight, E.S.; Day, J.B.; Mantle, P.G. Novel metabolites from *Penicillium crustosum*, including penitrem E, a tremorgenic mycotoxin. *Appl. Environ. Microbiol.* **1981**, *42*, 61–62. [PubMed]
55. Cole, R.J.; Dorner, J.W.; Lansden, J.A.; Cox, R.H.; Pape, C.; Cunfer, B.; Nicholson, S.S.; Bedell, D.M. Paspalum staggers: Isolation and identification of tremorgenic metabolites from sclerotia of *Claviceps paspali*. *J. Agric. Food Chem.* **1977**, *25*, 1197–1201. [CrossRef] [PubMed]
56. Cole, R.J.; Dorner, J.W.; Springer, J.P.; Cox, R.H. Indole metabolites from a strain of *Aspergillus flavus*. *J. Agric. Food Chem.* **1981**, *29*, 293–295. [CrossRef]
57. Gallagher, R.T.; Finer, J.; Clardy, J.; Leutwiler, A.; Weibel, F.; Acklin, W.; Arigoni, D. Paspalinine, a tremorgenic metabolite from *Claviceps paspali* Stevens et Hall. *Tetrahedron. Lett.* **1980**, *21*, 235–238. [CrossRef]
58. Babu, J.V.; Popay, A.J.; Miles, C.O.; Wilkins, A.L.; Di Menna, M.E.; Finch, S.C. Identification and structure elucidation of janthitrems A and D from *Penicillium janthinellum* and determination of the tremorgenic and anti-insect activity of janthitrems A and B. *J. Agric. Food Chem.* **2018**, *66*, 13116–13125. [CrossRef] [PubMed]
59. Lauren, D.R.; Gallagher, R.T. High-performance liquid chromatography of the janthitrems: Fluorescent tremorgenic mycotoxins produced by *Penicillium janthinellum*. *J. Chromatogr. A* **1982**, *248*, 150–154. [CrossRef]
60. Gallagher, F.T.; Latch, G.C.M.; Keogh, R.G. The janthitrems: Fluorescent tremorgenic toxins produced by *Penicillium janthinellum* isolates from ryegrass pastures. *Appl. Environ. Microbiol.* **1980**, *39*, 272–273.
61. Cole, R.J.; Kirksey, J.W.; Wells, J.M. A new tremorgenic metabolite from *Penicillium paxilli*. *Can. J. Microbiol.* **1974**, *20*, 1159–1162. [CrossRef] [PubMed]
62. Springer, J.P.; Clardy, J.; Wells, J.M.; Cole, R.J.; Kirksey, J.W. The structure of paxilline, a tremorgenic metabolite of *Penicillium paxilli* Bainier. *Tetrahedron. Lett.* **1975**, *16*, 2531–2534. [CrossRef]
63. CHAPTER 8—Tremorgen Group. *Handbook of Toxic Fungal Metabolites*; Cole, R.J., Cox, R.H., Eds.; Academic Press: New York, NY, USA, 1981; pp. 355–509.
64. Zhou, Y.; Lingle, C.J. Paxilline inhibits BK channels by an almost exclusively closed-channel block mechanism. *J. Gen. Physiol.* **2014**, *144*, 415–440. [CrossRef]
65. DeFarias, F.P.; Carvalho, M.F.; Lee, S.H.; Kaczorowski, G.J.; Suarez-Kurtz, G. Effects of the K+ channel blockers paspalitrem-C and paxilline on mammalian smooth muscle. *Eur. J. Pharmacol.* **1996**, *314*, 123–128. [CrossRef]
66. Saikia, S.; Parker, E.J.; Koulman, A.; Scott, B. Defining paxilline biosynthesis in *Penicillium paxilli*: Functional characterization of two cytochrome P450 monooxygenases. *J. Biol. Chem.* **2007**, *282*, 16829–16837. [CrossRef]
67. Matsui, C.; Ikeda, Y.; Iinuma, H.; Kushida, N.; Kunisada, T.; Simizu, S.; Umezawa, K. Isolation of a novel paxilline analog pyrapaxilline from fungus that inhibits LPS-induced NO production. *J. Antibiot.* **2014**, *67*, 787–790. [CrossRef]
68. Nozawa, K.; Nakajima, S.; Kawai, K.; Udagawa, S.; Horie, Y.; Yamazaki, M. Novel indoloditerpenes, emindoles, and their related compounds from *Emericella* spp. Proceedings of Tennen Yuki Kagobutsu Toronkai Koen Yoshishu (Symposium on the Chemistry of Natural Products), Sapporo, Japan, 23–26 May 1987; pp. 637–643. Available online: https://www.worldcat.org/title/29-tennen-yuki-kagobutsu-toronkai-koen-yoshishu-sapporo-august-26-28-1987-2/oclc/833622249 (accessed on 5 February 2018).
69. Belofsky, G.N.; Gloer, J.B.; Wicklow, D.T.; Dowd, P.F. Antiinsectan alkaloids: Shearinines A-C and a new paxilline derivative from the ascostromata of *Eupenicillium shearii*. *Tetrahedron* **1995**, *51*, 3959–3968. [CrossRef]
70. Miles, C.O.; Wilkins, A.L.; Garthwaite, I.; Ede, R.M.; Munday-Finch, S.C. Immunochemical techniques in natural products chemistry: Isolation and structure determination of a novel indole-diterpenoid aided by TLC-ELISAgram. *J. Org. Chem.* **1995**, *60*, 6067–6069. [CrossRef]
71. Gallagher, R.T.; White, E.P.; Mortimer, P.H. Ryegrass Staggers: Isolation of Potent Neurotoxins Lolitrem A and Lolitrem B From Staggers-Producing Pastures. *N. Z. Vet. J.* **1981**, *29*, 189–190. [CrossRef] [PubMed]

72. Gallagher, R.T.; Hawkes, A.D.; Steyn, P.S.; Vleggaar, R. Tremorgenic neurotoxins from perennial ryegrass causing ryegrass staggers disorder of livestock: structure elucidation of lolitrem B. *J. Chem. Soc. Chem. Commun.* **1984**, *9*, 614–616. [CrossRef]
73. De Jesus, A.E.; Steyn, P.S.; Van Heerden, F.R.; Vleggaar, R.; Wessels, P.L.; Hull, W.E. Structure and biosynthesis of the penitrems A-F, six novel tremorgenic mycotoxins from *Penicillium crustosum*. *J. Chem. Soc. Chem. Commun.* **1981**, *6*, 289–291. [CrossRef]
74. De Jesus, A.E.; Steyn, P.S.; Van Heerden, F.R.; Vleggaar, R.; Wessels, P.L.; Hull, W.E. Tremorgenic mycotoxins from *Penicillium crustosum*. Structure elucidation and absolute configuration of penitrems B—F. *J. Chem. Soc. Perkin.* **1983**, *1*, 1857–1861. [CrossRef]
75. Cavanagh, J.B.; Holton, J.L.; Nolan, C.C.; Ray, D.E.; Naik, J.T.; Mantle, P.G. The effects of the tremorgenic mycotoxin penitrem A on the rat cerebellum. *Vet. Pathol.* **1998**, *35*, 53–63. [CrossRef]
76. Wilson, B.J.; Hoekman, T.; Dettbarn, W.D. Effects of a fungus tremorgenic toxin (penitrem A) on transmission in rat phrenic nerve-diaphragm preparations. *Brain Res.* **1972**, *40*, 540–544. [CrossRef]
77. Norris, P.J.; Smith, C.C.T.; de Belleroche, J.; Bradford, H.F.; Mantle, P.G.; Thomas, A.J.; Penny, R.H. Actions of tremorgenic fungal toxins on neurotransmitter release. *J. Neurochem.* **1980**, *34*, 33–42. [CrossRef]
78. Bradford, H.F.; Norris, P.J.; Smith, C.C.T. Changes in transmitter release patterns in vitro induced by tremorgenic mycotoxins. *J. Environ. Pathol. Toxicol. Oncol.* **1990**, *10*, 17–30.
79. Sobotka, T.J.; Brodie, R.E.; Spaid, S.L. Neurobehavioral studies of tremorgenic mycotoxins verruculogen and penitrem A. *Pharmacology* **1978**, *16*, 287–294. [CrossRef]
80. Cho, Y.; Cha, S.H.; Sok, D.E. Presynaptic effects of verruculogen on gamma-aminobutyric acid(GABA) uptake and release in rat brain. *Korean Biochemical. Journal* **1994**, *27*, 353–356.
81. Hotujac, L.; Stern, P. Pharmacological examination of verruculogen induced tremor. *Acta. Medica. Iugoslavica.* **1974**, *28*, 223–229.
82. Hotujac, L.J.; Muftić, R.H.; Filipović, N. Verruculogen: A new substance for decreasing of gaba levels in CNS. *Pharmacology* **1976**, *14*, 297–300. [CrossRef]
83. Ouadid-Ahidouch, H.; Roudbaraki, M.; Delcourt, P.; Ahidouch, A.; Joury, N.; Prevarskaya, N. Functional and molecular identification of intermediate-conductance Ca 2+-activated K+ channels in breast cancer cells: Association with cell cycle progression. *Am. J. Physiol. Cell. Physiol.* **2004**, *287*, C125–C134. [CrossRef]
84. Goda, A.A.; Siddique, A.B.; Mohyeldin, M.; Ayoub, N.M.; El Sayed, K.A. The Maxi-K (BK) channel antagonist penitrem a as a novel breast cancer-targeted therapeutic. *Marine Drugs* **2018**, *16*, 157. [CrossRef] [PubMed]
85. Lu, W.; Lin, C.; Roberts, M.J.; Waud, W.R.; Piazza, G.A.; Li, Y. Niclosamide suppresses cancer cell growth by inducing Wnt co-receptor LRP6 degradation and inhibiting the Wnt/β-catenin pathway. *PLoS ONE* **2011**, *6*, e29290. [CrossRef] [PubMed]
86. Sallam, A.A.; Houssen, W.E.; Gissendanner, C.R.; Orabi, K.Y.; Foudah, A.I.; El Sayed, K.A. Bioguided discovery and pharmacophore modeling of the mycotoxic indole diterpene alkaloids penitrems as breast cancer proliferation, migration, and invasion inhibitors. *MedChemComm* **2013**, *4*, 1360–1369. [CrossRef]
87. Sallam, A.A.; Ayoub, N.M.; Foudah, A.I.; Gissendanner, C.R.; Meyer, S.A.; El Sayed, K.A. Indole diterpene alkaloids as novel inhibitors of the Wnt/β-catenin pathway in breast cancer cells. *Eur. J. Med. Chem.* **2013**, *70*, 594–606. [CrossRef]
88. Goda, A.A.; Naguib, K.M.; Mohamed, M.M.; Amra, H.A.; Nada, S.A.; Abdel-Ghaffar, A.R.B.; Gissendanner, C.R.; El Sayed, K.A. Astaxanthin and docosahexaenoic acid reverse the toxicity of the maxi-K (BK) channel antagonist mycotoxin penitrem A. *Marine Drugs* **2016**, *14*, 208. [CrossRef]
89. Selala, M.I.; Musuku, A.; Schepens, P.J.C. Isolation and determination of paspalitrem-type tremorgenic mycotoxins using liquid chromatography with diode-array detection. *Anal. Chim. Acta.* **1991**, *244*, 1–8. [CrossRef]
90. Springer, J.P.; Clardy, J. Paspaline and paspalicine, two indole-mevalonate metabolites from *Claviceps paspali*. *Tetrahedron Lett.* **1980**, *21*, 231–234. [CrossRef]
91. Huang, X.H.; Nishida, H.; Tomoda, H.; Tabata, N.; Shiomi, K.; Yang, D.J.; Takayanagi, H.; Omura, S. Correction: Terpendoles, novel AC AT inhibitors produced by *Albophoma yamanashiensis*. II. Structure elucidation of terpendoles A, B, C and D. *J. Antibiot. (Tokyo)* **1995**, *48*, 5–11. [CrossRef] [PubMed]
92. Tomoda, H.; Tabata, N.; Yang, D.-J.; Takayanagi, H.; Omura, S. Terpendoles, novel AC AT inhibitors produced by *Albophoma yamanashiensis*. III. Production, isolation and structure elucidation of new components. *J. Antibiot.* **1995**, *48*, 793–804. [CrossRef] [PubMed]

93. Chiwata, T.; Aragane, K.; Fujinami, K.; Kojima, K.; Ishibashi, S.; Yamada, N.; Kusunoki, J. Direct effect of an acyl-CoA:cholesterol acyltransferase inhibitor, F-1394, on atherosclerosis in apolipoprotein E and low density lipoprotein receptor double knockout mice. *Br. J. Pharmacol.* **2001**, *133*, 1005–1012. [CrossRef]
94. Ohshiro, T.; Rudel, L.L.; Omura, S.; Tomoda, H. Selectivity of microbial acyl-CoA: Cholesterol acyltransferase inhibitors toward isozymes. *J. Antibiot. (Tokyo)* **2007**, *60*, 43–51. [CrossRef] [PubMed]
95. Anderson, R.A.; Joyce, C.; Davis, M.; Reagan, J.W.; Clark, M.; Shelness, G.S.; Rudel, L.L. Identification of a form of acyl-CoA: Cholesterol acyltransferase specific to liver and intestine in nonhuman primates. *J. Biol. Chem.* **1998**, *273*, 26747–26754. [CrossRef] [PubMed]
96. Nakazawa, J.; Yajima, J.; Usui, T.; Ueki, M.; Takatsuki, A.; Imoto, M.; Toyoshima, Y.Y.; Osada, H. A novel action of terpendole E on the motor activity of mitotic Kinesin Eg5. *Chem. Biol.* **2003**, *10*, 131–137. [CrossRef]
97. Rosenfeld, S.S.; Rich, J.; Venere, M. Mitotic Kinesin Eg5 Inhibiting Anticancer Agents. WO2015153967A1, 2015. Available online: https://patents.google.com/patent/US20150352114A1/en (accessed on 3 January 2019).
98. Laakso, J.A.; Gloer, J.B.; Wicklow, D.T.; Dowd, P.F. Sulpinines A-C and secopenitrem B: New antiinsectan metabolites from the sclerotia of *Aspergillus sulphureus*. *J. Org. Chem.* **1992**, *57*, 2066–2071. [CrossRef]
99. Laakso, J.A.; Tepaske, M.R.; Dowd, P.F.; Gloer, J.B.; Wicklow, D.T.; Staub, G.M. Indole Antiinsectan *Aspergillus* Metabolites. US5227396A, 1993. Available online: https://patents.google.com/patent/US5227396A/en (accessed on 5 February 2019).
100. Hosoe, T.; Itabashi, T.; Kobayashi, N.; Udagawa, S.-i.; Kawai, K.-i. Three new types of indoloditerpenes, emindole PA-PC, from *Emericella purpurea*. Revision of the structure of emindole PA. *Chem. Pharm. Bull.* **2006**, *54*, 185–187. [CrossRef] [PubMed]
101. Petersen, L.M.; Frisvad, J.C.; Knudsen, P.B.; Rohlfs, M.; Gotfredsen, C.H.; Larsen, T.O. Induced sclerotium formation exposes new bioactive metabolites from *Aspergillus sclerotiicarbonarius*. *J. Antibiot.* **2015**, *68*, 603–608. [CrossRef] [PubMed]
102. Kimura, Y.; Nishibe, M.; Nakajima, H.; Hamasaki, T.; Shigemitsu, N.; Sugawara, F.; Stout, T.J.; Clardy, J. Emeniveol; A new pollen growth inhibitor from the fungus, *Emericella nivea*. *Tetrahedron Lett.* **1992**, *33*, 6987–6990. [CrossRef]
103. Ogata, M.; Ueda, J.Y.; Hoshi, M.; Hashimoto, J.; Nakashima, T.; Anzai, K.; Takagi, M.; Shin-Ya, K. A novel indole-diterpenoid, JBIR-03 with anti-MRSA activity from *Dichotomomyces cejpii* var. *cejpii* NBRC 103559. *J. Antibiot. (Tokyo)* **2007**, *60*, 645–648. [CrossRef]
104. Qiao, M.F.; Ji, N.Y.; Liu, X.H.; Li, K.; Zhu, Q.M.; Xue, Q.Z. Indoloditerpenes from an algicolous isolate of *Aspergillus oryzae*. *Bioorg. Med. Chem. Lett.* **2010**, *20*, 5677–5680. [CrossRef]
105. TePaske, M.R.; Gloer, J.B.; Wicklow, D.T.; Dowd, P.F. Aflavarin and β-aflatrem: New anti-insectan metabolites from the sclerotia of *Aspergillus flavus*. *J. Nat. Prod.* **1992**, *55*, 1080–1086. [CrossRef]
106. Penn, J.; Swift, R.; Wigley, L.J.; Mantle, P.G.; Bilton, J.N.; Sheppard, R.N. Janthitrems B and C, two principal indole-diterpenoids produced by *Penicillium janthinellum*. *Phytochemistry* **1993**, *32*, 1431–1434. [CrossRef]
107. Wilkins, A.L.; Miles, C.O.; Ede, R.M.; Gallagher, R.T.; Munday, S.C. Structure elucidation of janthitrem B, a tremorgenic metabolite of *Penicillium janthinellum*, and relative configuration of the A and B rings of janthitrems B, E, and F. *J. Agric. Food Chem.* **1992**, *40*, 1307–1309. [CrossRef]
108. Tapper, B.; Lane, G.A. Janthitrems found in a *Neotyphodium* endophyte of perennial ryegrass. In Proceedings of the 5th International Symposium on *Neotyphodium*/Grass Interactions, Fayetteville, AR, USA, 23–26 May 2004; p. 301.
109. De Jesus, A.E.; Steyn, P.S.; Van Heerden, F.R.; Vleggaar, R. Structure elucidation of the janthitrems, novel tremorgenic mycotoxins from *Penicillium janthinellum*. *J. Chem. Soc. Perkin. 1* **1984**, 697–701. [CrossRef]
110. Kawahara, T.; Nagai, A.; Takagi, M.; Shin-Ya, K. JBIR-137 and JBIR-138, new secondary metabolites from *Aspergillus* sp. fA75. *J. Antibiot.* **2012**, *65*, 535–538. [CrossRef]
111. Xu, M.; Gessner, G.; Groth, I.; Lange, C.; Christner, A.; Bruhn, T.; Deng, Z.; Li, X.; Heinemann, S.H.; Grabley, S.; et al. Shearinines D-K, new indole triterpenoids from an endophytic *Penicillium* sp. (strain HKI0459) with blocking activity on large-conductance calcium-activated potassium channels. *Tetrahedron* **2007**, *63*, 435–444. [CrossRef]
112. You, J.; Du, L.; King, J.B.; Hall, B.E.; Cichewicz, R.H. Small-molecule suppressors of *Candida albicans* biofilm formation synergistically enhance the antifungal activity of amphotericin B against clinical *Candida* isolates. *ACS. Chem. Biol.* **2013**, *8*, 840–848. [CrossRef] [PubMed]
113. Dhodary, B.; Schilg, M.; Wirth, R.; Spiteller, D. Secondary metabolites from *Escovopsis weberi* and their role in attacking the garden fungus of Leaf-cutting ants. *Chem. Eur. J.* **2018**, *24*, 4445–4452. [CrossRef]

114. Goetz, M.A.; Kaczorowski, G.J.; Monaghan, R.L.; Strohl, W.R.; Tkacz, J.S. Maxi-K Potassium Channel Blockers for Treatment of Glaucoma and as Ocular Neuroprotective Agents. WO2003105868A1, 2003. Available online: https://patents.google.com/patent/WO2003105868A1/ru (accessed on 22 March 2018).
115. Garcia, M.L.; Goetz, M.A.; Kaczorowski, G.J.; McManus, O.B.; Monaghan, R.L.; Strohl, W.R.; Tkacz, J.S. Indole Diterpene Compound Maxi-K Potassium Channel Blockers, Methods Using Them for the Treatment of Glaucoma and Other Conditions, and Fermentation Process for Production. WO2003105724A2, 2003. Available online: https://patents.google.com/patent/WO2003105724A2 (accessed on 22 March 2018).
116. Brnardic, E.; Doherty, J.B.; Dorsey, J.; Ellwood, C.; Fillmore, M.; Malaska, M.; Nelson, K.; Soukri, M. Preparation of Indole Diterpene Alkaloids as Maxi-K Channel Blockers for the Treatment of Glaucoma. WO2009048559A1, 2009. Available online: https://patents.google.com/patent/WO2009048559A1/en (accessed on 22 March 2018).
117. Fan, Y.; Wang, Y.; Liu, P.; Fu, P.; Zhu, T.; Wang, W.; Zhu, W. Indole-diterpenoids with anti-H1N1 activity from the aciduric fungus *Penicillium camemberti* OUCMDZ-1492. *J. Nat. Prod.* **2013**, *76*, 1328–1336. [CrossRef] [PubMed]
118. Easton, H.S.; Lane, G.A.; Tapper, B.A.; Keogh, R.G.; Cooper, B.M.; Blackwell, M.; Anderson, M.; Fletchers, L.R. Ryegrass endophyte-related heat stress in cattle. *Proc. N. Z. Grassl. Assoc.* **1996**, *57*, 37–41.
119. Craig, A.M.; Blythe, L.L.; Duringer, J.M. The role of the oregon state university endophyte service laboratory in diagnosing clinical cases of endophyte toxicoses. *J. Agric. Food Chem.* **2014**, *62*, 7376–7381. [CrossRef] [PubMed]
120. Repussard, C.; Zbib, N.; Tardieu, D.; Guerre, P. Ergovaline and lolitrem B concentrations in perennial ryegrass in field culture in Southern France: Distribution in the plant and impact of climatic factors. *J. Agric. Food Chem.* **2014**, *62*, 12707–12712. [CrossRef] [PubMed]
121. Oliveira, J.A.; Rottinghaus, G.E.; González, E. Ergovaline concentration in perennial ryegrass infected with a lolitrem B-free fungal endophyte in north-west Spain. *New Zeal. J. Agr. Res.* **2003**, *46*, 117–122. [CrossRef]
122. Andersen, B.; Frisvad, J.C. Natural Occurrence of Fungi and Fungal Metabolites in Moldy Tomatoes. *J. Agric. Food Chem.* **2004**, *52*, 7507–7513. [CrossRef] [PubMed]
123. Gordon, K.E.; Masotti, R.E.; Waddell, W.R. Tremorgenic encephalopathy: A role of mycotoxins in the production of CNS disease in humans? *Can. J. Neurol. Sci.* **1993**, *20*, 237–239. [CrossRef] [PubMed]
124. Talcott, P.A. Chapter 63—Mycotoxins. In *Small Animal Toxicology*, 3rd ed.; Peterson, M.E., Talcott, P.A., Eds.; W.B. Saunders: Saint Louis, MO, USA, 2013; pp. 677–682.
125. Walter, S.L. Acute penitrem A and roquefortine poisoning in a dog. *Can. Vet. J.* **2002**, *43*, 372–374.
126. Gallagher, R.T.; Hawkes, A.D. High-performance liquid chromatography with stop-flow ultraviolet spectral chracterization of lolitrem neu-rotoxins from perennial ryegrass. *J. Chromatogr. A* **1985**, *322*, 159–167. [CrossRef]
127. Gallagher, R.T.; Hawkes, A.D.; Stewart, J.M. Rapid determination of the neurotoxin lolitrem B in perennial ryegrass by high-performance liquid chromatography with fluorescence detection. *J. Chromatogr. A* **1985**, *321*, 217–226. [CrossRef]
128. Repussard, C.; Tardieu, D.; Alberich, M.; Guerre, P. A new method for the determination of lolitrem B in plant materials. *Anim. Feed. Sci. Tech.* **2014**, *193*, 141–147. [CrossRef]
129. Laganà, A. Introduction to the toxins special issue on LC-MS/MS methods for mycotoxin analysis. *Toxins* **2017**, *9*, 325. [CrossRef] [PubMed]
130. Nicholson, M.J.; Koulman, A.; Monahan, B.J.; Pritchard, B.L.; Payne, G.A.; Scott, B. Identification of two aflatrem biosynthesis gene loci in *Aspergillus flavus* and metabolic engineering of *Penicillium paxilli* to elucidate their function. *Appl. Environ. Microbiol.* **2009**, *75*, 7469–7481. [CrossRef] [PubMed]
131. Rasmussen, S.; Lane, G.A.; Mace, W.; Parsons, A.J.; Fraser, K.; Xue, H. The use of genomics and metabolomics methods to quantify fungal endosymbionts and alkaloids in grasses. In *Plant Metabolomics Methods in Molecular Biology (Methods and Protocols)*; Hardy, N., Hall, R., Eds.; Humana Press: New York City, NY, USA, 2012; Volume 860, pp. 213–226.

*toxins*

MDPI

*Review*

# Assessing the Effect of Mycotoxin Combinations: Which Mathematical Model Is (the Most) Appropriate?

**Domagoj Kifer [1], Daniela Jakšić [2] and Maja Šegvić Klarić [2,*]**

[1] Department of Biophysics, Faculty of Pharmacy and Biochemistry, University of Zagreb, A. Kovačića 1, Zagreb 10000, Croatia; dkifer@pharma.hr

[2] Department of Microbiology, Faculty of Pharmacy and Biochemistry, University of Zagreb, Schrottova 39, Zagreb 10000, Croatia; djaksic@pharma.hr

* Correspondence: msegvic@pharma.hr; Tel.: +385-1-6394-493

Received: 8 January 2020; Accepted: 26 February 2020; Published: 29 February 2020

**Abstract:** In the past decades, many studies have examined the nature of the interaction between mycotoxins in biological models classifying interaction effects as antagonisms, additive effects, or synergisms based on a comparison of the observed effect with the expected effect of combination. Among several described mathematical models, the arithmetic definition of additivity and factorial analysis of variance were the most commonly used in mycotoxicology. These models are incorrectly based on the assumption that mycotoxin dose-effect curves are linear. More appropriate mathematical models for assessing mycotoxin interactions include Bliss independence, Loewe's additivity law, combination index, and isobologram analysis, Chou-Talalays median-effect approach, response surface, code for the identification of synergism numerically efficient (CISNE) and MixLow method. However, it seems that neither model is ideal. This review discusses the advantages and disadvantages of these mathematical models.

**Keywords:** mycotoxin interaction; Loewe additivity; combination index; isobologram; Chou-Talalay method; MixLow

**Key Contribution:** Comments on methods for assessing mycotoxin combination effect.

## 1. Introduction

Mycotoxins are secondary metabolites mainly produced by fungi belonging to the genera of *Aspergillus*, *Penicillium*, or *Fusarium* [1]. Although the role of mycotoxins is not yet fully understood, it has been shown that mycotoxins form an integral part of microbial interactions in ecological niches where they protect fungi from competing or invading microbes (e.g., by antimicrobial activity and/or quorum sensing disruption) [2,3]. Throughout history, these fungal toxic metabolites have been recognized as harmful contaminants in crops, causing acute toxic, carcinogenic, mutagenic, teratogenic, immunotoxic, and oestrogenic effects in humans and animals [1,4]. From the public health point of view, the most important foodborne mycotoxins are aflatoxins (AFs), fumonisins (FBs), trichothecenes (including deoxynivalenol (DON) and T-2 and HT-2 toxins), ochratoxin A (OTA), patulin (PAT) and zearalenone (ZEN) and maximum levels have been set in European Union legislation to control these mycotoxin levels in food and feed [4,5]. Analytical methods based on the liquid chromatography tandem mass spectrometry (LC-MS/MS) have been developed for the simultaneous detection of multiple mycotoxins in foods which facilitated and enabled survey of their co-occurrence in various food matrices [6,7]. This methodology enabled the simultaneous detection of more than one hundred fungal metabolites including major mycotoxins as well as masked (e.g., DON-3-glucoside and ZEN-14 sulfate), modified mycotoxins (e.g., 15-acetyl-DON) and so called emerging mycotoxins (enniatins-ENN, beauvericin-BEA, and fusaproliferin-FUS and moniliformin-MON) [8–13]. The latter is defined as "mycotoxins, which are neither routinely determined, nor legislatively regulated; however, the evidence of their incidence is rapidly increasing" [13]. Recently, for the first time ever, reports were published on the multi-occurrence on major mycotoxins and their derivates as well as modified mycotoxins (such as DON-3-glucoside) and emerging mycotoxins in animal feeds and maize from Egypt. This study emphasized significant levels of $AFB_1$ in this African region, but also suggested that low concentrations of the other detected mycotoxins should also be considered due to their unknown interactions [6]. As mycotoxins often co-occur in food and feed there is a possibility that, due to interactions between one or more mycotoxins, they can act harmfully, even if they are present at or below permitted concentrations (regulated mycotoxins) or are continuously present in low or high levels depending on the region (unregulated/emerging mycotoxins) [10–12]. Assunção et al. [5] underlined the priority of testing the most relevant mycotoxins mixtures taking into account human exposure assessments and the use of adequate mathematical approaches to evaluate interactions in experimental models. Kademi et al. [14] developed a mathematical model using a system of ordinary differential equations to describe the dynamics of AFs from plants (feeds) to animals, plants (plant foods) to humans, and animals to humans (carry-over effects) which showed that the entire dynamics depends on the numerical values of the threshold quantity defined as $R_{01}$ and $R_{02}$ (e.g., if $R_{01} < 1$ and $R_{02} < 1$ then AF concentrations in animals and plants will not reach toxic limit and vice versa). This kind of mathematical modeling can be useful in controlling AFs and other mycotoxin toxicity limits by employing various control measures like biological control and/or decontamination technologies. In addition, mathematical modeling has been applied to predict fungal germination, growth, mycotoxin production, inactivation and also to study the response to environmental factors which can be useful in the prediction of mycotoxin food contamination [15,16]. Taken together, mathematical modeling could be very helpful in the prediction and estimation of mycotoxin impact on human and animal health as well as in controlling contamination below acceptable limits.

In vitro studies of mycotoxin interactions reflect mycotoxin occurrence and co-occurrence in food/feed. Among *Aspergillus*- and/or *Penicillium*-derived mycotoxins, $AFB_1$, OTA, citrinin (CIT), PAT and penicillic acid (PA) have been the most studied, while the most studied mycotoxins produced by *Fusarium* species were ZEN, FBs, nivalenol (NIV), T-2, DON and its derivates. Since in the last decade attention toward unregulated/emerging mycotoxins increased, interactions of these mycotoxins as well as their interactions with major mycotoxins have also been extensively studied [17,18]. The effects of binary, tertiary and multiple mixtures of these mycotoxins in vitro have been studied on cell models originating from the digestive system, i.e., intestinal Caco-2 cells and hepatic HepG2 cells, or kidney cells like i.e., monkey kidney Vero cells, porcine PK15, human kidney HK2, and occasionally immune system-derived cells like THP-1 macrophages [18–21]. A number of studies examined the nature of interaction between mycotoxins both in vivo and in vitro classifying interaction effects into three types: antagonistic effect, additive effect, and synergistic effect [18,19]. The definition of each interaction effect is based on a comparison of observed effects with the expected effects of combination. If the observed effect is greater than expected, it is defined as a synergism, and if the opposite is true, i.e., if the observed effect is lesser than expected, it is defined as an antagonism. The third case, when the expected value is equal to the observed one is called an additive effect [22,23]. These simple definitions leave one problem though: estimations of expected effects for combinations of two non-interacting mycotoxins. Among the several available mathematical models that may be used to describe mycotoxin interactions, the arithmetic definition of additivity was the most commonly used one [24]. Other models included a factorial analysis of variance [25], Bliss independence criterion [26], Loewe's additivity law [27], response surface [28], combination index and isobologram analysis [29], Chou-Talalay's median effect approach [30], and the MixLow method [31]. These models will be discussed later on in this review. Additionally, the highest single agent model [32] and CISNE (code for the identification of synergism numerically efficient) [33], that have not been used so far in mycotoxicology, will also be discussed.

The most comprehensive review on mycotoxin interactions in cell cultures of human and animal origin was given by Alassane-Kpembi et al. [18]; the majority of conducted studies used the arithmetic definition of additivity. In the studies conducted in the last four years (Tables 1 and 2) the interactions between mycotoxins in vitro were evaluated using more appropriate mathematical models than the arithmetic definition of additivity.

## 2. Mathematical Models for Assessing Mycotoxin Interactions

In this paper, *E* will serve as an abbreviation for "effect" in equations. It is also assumed that effect is relative to maximal effect, i.e., percentage of cell viability suppression, where suppression is equal to difference between negative control (100% viability) and treated cells (100%-effect viability).

### 2.1. *Simple Addition of Effects*

The simplest method for estimating interactions between mycotoxins is the assumption of effect additivity known as arithmetic definition of additivity or response additivity (Equation (1)):

$$E_{exp} = E_{M1} + E_{M2} \tag{1}$$

where $E_{exp}$ is the expected effect of combination of mycotoxin $M_1$ in dose $D_1$ and mycotoxin $M_2$ in dose $D_2$, while $E_{M1}$ and $E_{M2}$ are the effects of single tested mycotoxins $M_1$ and $M_2$ in doses $D_1$ and $D_2$, respectively. That simple addition of effect was applied by Šegvić Klarić et al. [34] for assessing the combination effect of beauvericin (BEA) and OTA using Equation (1) and observed synergistic effect for two combinations. Mathematically, this approach would be incorrect most of the time because the dose-effect curve is not linear. Using the data on cytotoxicity of OTA alone of the mentioned paper, it is easy to see that using this method we can prove that OTA applied in combination with itself at concentrations of 5 µM and 5 µM revealed an antagonistic effect; the expected cell viability would be around 20%, while the observed value for cell viability after treatment with 10 µM ochratoxin A was around 50% (Figure 1). Interestingly, despite an inaccurate estimation of expected effects, this model was widely applied; Alassane-Kpembi et al. [18] in their review cited 52 studies out of 83 that used this method.

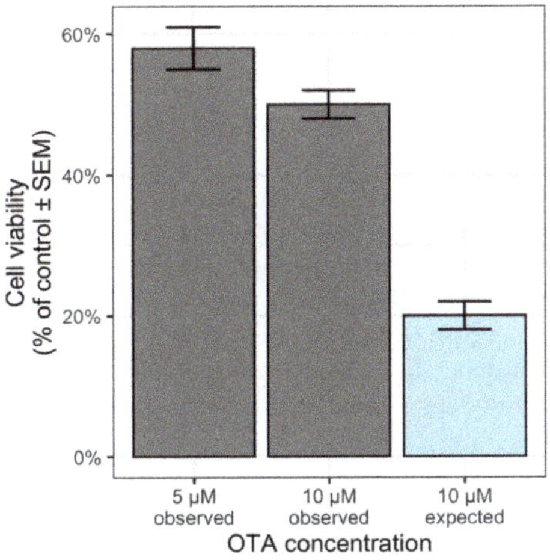


**Figure 1.** Cytotoxicity of OTA (5 µM and 10 µM observed) on PK15 cells after 24 h of exposure [34]; arithmetic additivity calculation shows that upon treatment with 5 + 5 µM of OTA expected viability is much lower than observed viability indicating antagonism (no copyright permission needed as we created this figure).

Some studies presented in Table 1 [35,36] used simple addition of effects according to Weber et al. [24] who modified Equation (1) by subtracting the 100% (or 1) from the sum of the mean effects. Needless to say, the unexplained subtraction of 100% did not account for the non-linearity of the dose response curves.

### 2.2. Factorial Analysis of Variance

This model uses simple 2-way ANOVA for modelling the detection of interactions between two mycotoxins (Equation (2)):

$$E = \beta_0 + \beta_1 \times D_1 + \beta_2 \times D_2 + \beta_3 \times D_1 \times D_2 \quad (2)$$

where $E$ is the estimated effect, $\beta_0$ is the part of the effect achieved by negative control, $\beta_1/\beta_2$ is the coefficient that increases effect for each increase in one unit of dose $D_1/D_2$ of mycotoxin $M_1/M_2$ and $\beta_3$ is the interaction term.

Eight studies that have used this approach to define mycotoxin interactions were reviewed in detail by Alassane-Kpembi et al. [18]. If the interaction term was significantly (in a statistical manner) different than zero, it was concluded that an interaction between mycotoxins occurred. The main problem with this method is that ANOVA can be very misleading, similarly to the simple addition of effects method because ANOVA is based on linear modelling which is not useful for modelling nonlinear dose-effect curves [25]. This method was recently applied in only one study for testing the dual combination effects of ZEN and OTA or α-ZEL in HepG2 cells [37], as summarized in Table 1.

### 2.3. Bliss Independence Criterion

Bliss introduced this model in 1939 for predicting the proportion of animals that will die after combining two toxins under the assumption that there is no interaction between the toxins (i.e., they have completely different mechanisms of action or act in different compartments):

$$E_{exp} = 1 - (1 - E_{M1}) \times (1 - E_{M2}) = E_{M1} + E_{M2} - E_{M1} \times E_{M2} \quad (3)$$

where $E_{exp}$ is the expected effect of a combination of mycotoxin $M_1$ in dose $D_1$ and mycotoxin $M_2$ in dose $D_2$, while $E_{M1}$ and $E_{M2}$ are the effects of single tested mycotoxins $M_1$ and $M_2$ in doses $D_1$ and $D_2$, respectively [26], all effects need to be expressed as proportions ranging from 0 to 1 (Equation (3)).

Similarly to the simple addition of effects, Bliss can result in a detection of an interaction of some mycotoxin with itself but that is not possible in model validation since this would a priori violate the assumption of two toxins acting independently.

Several of the recent studies listed in Table 1 simultaneously used different mathematical models, e.g., response additivity and Bliss independence criterion [38,39] or Bliss independence and Loewe additivity [40] or Chou-Talalay method [39,41]. As expected, these studies obtained different conclusions on mycotoxin interactions depending on the mathematical models that have been applied. For example, Smit et al. [39] obtained a synergism of DON + ZEN at low and medium concentrations by both response additivity and Bliss independence model; while at high concentrations in combinations, an additive effect was obtained with Bliss independence model and antagonism by response additivity.

### 2.4. Loewe's Additivity Law

Loewe's additivity law (also called isobolografic method, concentration additivity or dose additivity) assumes that mycotoxins act within the same compartment on the same biological size by the same mechanism. The only difference is in their potency. This model is based on the dose equivalence principle and the sham combination principle; in short, every dose $D_1$ of mycotoxin $M_1$ gives an equal effect as $D_{2(1)}$ of mycotoxin $M_2$, and vice versa, and any $D_{2(1)}$ can be added to any other dose of $D_2$ to show the additive effect [27] as presented by Equation (4):

$$E\ (D_1 + D_2) = E\ (D_1 + D_{1(2)}) = E\ (D_{2(1)} + D_2) \quad (4)$$

where E is the effect, $D_1$ is the dose of mycotoxin $M_1$, $D_2$ is the dose of mycotoxin $M_2$, $D_{1(2)}$ dose of mycotoxin $M_1$ that provokes same effect as $D_2$ dose of mycotoxin $M_2$, $D_{2(1)}$ dose of mycotoxin $M_2$ that provokes same effect as $D_1$ of mycotoxin $M_1$. For additive effects, the following Equation (5) is valid:

$$D_1/D_{E1} + D_2/D_{E2} = 1, \quad (5)$$

where $D_1$ and $D_2$ are the doses of mycotoxins $M_1$ and $M_2$ applied in combination, and $D_{E1}$ and $D_{E2}$ are the dose of mycotoxin $M_1$ and $M_2$ applied alone. All doses ($D_1$+$D_2$, $D_{E1}$ or $D_{E2}$) result with the same effect E.

Additionally, Loewe's additivity law makes a larger number of assumptions; each mycotoxin in a mixture must have an equal maximum effect and all log(dose)-effect curves must be parallel and have constant relative potency [42,43], according to Equation (6):

$$(R = D_{E1}/D_{E2}) \quad (6)$$

Finding two mycotoxins in a combination that fulfils all of these assumptions seems somewhat impossible. For example, apart from the Bliss independence criterion, Li et al. [44] also used this method (as a concentration addition model) to assess the nature of interaction between OTA and ZEN. Since their dose-effect curves did not meet all of the assumptions, it is easy to see that Equation (4), on which Loewe's additivity law is based, does not hold true when we assign the values $EC_{10}$ (OTA) = 0.8 μM and $EC_{10}$ (ZEN) = 11.84 μM [44], and try to apply the main principles of dose equivalence and sham combination of this model (Equations (7) and (8)):

$$E\ (EC_{10\ OTA} + EC_{10\ ZEN}) = E\ (EC_{10\ OTA} + EC_{10\ OTA}) = E\ (EC_{10\ ZEN} + EC_{10\ ZEN}) \quad (7)$$

$$E\ (2 \times 0.8\ \mu M \text{ of OTA}) = E\ (2 \times 11.84\ \mu M \text{ of ZEN}) \quad (8)$$

This does not seem to be correct according to the dose-response curves for OTA (E (1.60 μM of OTA) ≈ 30%) and ZEN (E (23.68 μM of ZEN) ≈ 50%) presented in aforementioned article [44], which raises the question: can the observed synergies be trusted at all?

Even though this model is mathematically valid, due to the excessive number of assumptions that need to be fulfilled, this model probably remains inapplicable for assessing combinations of mycotoxins [43].

### 2.5. *Response Surface*

Some authors expanded the Loewe's additivity law and Bliss independence criterion to the whole surface defined by all predicted additive concentration combinations (in all ratios, for all effects) [45,46] as presented in Table 1. In mycotoxicology, Assunção et al. [46] implemented model generalization built by Jonker et al. [28]. They estimated the deviation from Loewe's additivity law by Equation (9):

$$D_1/D_{E1} + D_2/D_{E2} = e^G \quad (9)$$

where G is the deviation function defined separately for 4 models. If G = 0, then Equation (9) collapses to Equation (5), suggesting an additive effect. To test for synergism or antagonism G is substituted with (Equation (10)):

$$G\ (z_1, z_2) = a \times z_1 \times z_2 \quad (10)$$

where parameter a is less than zero for synergisms and greater than zero for antagonisms, $z_1$ and $z_2$ are relative contribution to toxicity, i.e., for $z_1$ as presented by Equation (11):

$$z_1 = D_1/D_{E1}\ /\ (D_1/D_{E1} + D_2/D_{E2}) \quad (11)$$

Jonker et al. [28] also define more complicated interaction patterns between two toxins and with the inclusion of parameters $b_1$ for detection of dose ratio-dependent deviation (Equation (12)), and parameters $b_{DL}$ for the detection of dose level-dependent deviations (Equation (13)) from a non-interacting additive model:

$$G(z_1, z_2) = (a + b_1 \times z_1) \times z_1 \times z_2 \tag{12}$$

$$G(z_1, z_2) = a \times (1 - b_{DL} \times (D_1/D_{M1} + D_2/D_{M2})) \times z_1 \times z_2 \tag{13}$$

The procedure by Jonker et al. [28] suggests fitting all four models (defined by four deviation functions) and then choosing the best one to make conclusions about the nature of the interaction at different dose ratios or dose levels based on parameters a, $b_1$, and $b_{DL}$ according to Table 1 of Jonker et al. [28].

This method provides more information than the other methods mentioned in this article, but it comes with a greater cost of the experiment since a checkerboard experimental design is needed, with dense concentration ranges in all combinations.

### 2.6. *Highest Single Agent (HSA) Model*

This model is also referred to as the Gaddums non-interaction [32], it defines the expected effect as the maximum of single mycotoxin effects (Equation (14)):

$$E_{exp} = max\ (E_{M1}, E_{M2}) \tag{14}$$

where $E_{exp}$ is the expected effect of a combination of mycotoxin $M_1$ in dose $D_1$ and mycotoxin $M_2$ in dose $D_2$, while $E_{M1}$ and $E_{M2}$ are the effects of single tested mycotoxins $M_1$ and $M_2$ in doses $D_1$ and $D_2$, respectively.

Because of underestimations of the expected combination effect, this model is not appropriate for detection of synergistic effects, except in cases: (i) where one compound is completely inactive at any concentration for the measured effect (which is rare in the field of mycotoxins); (ii) where a mycotoxin with maximal effect does not reach full effect (i.e., never suppresses viability to 0%). On the other hand, this method is useful for detecting antagonistic effects since observing a combination effect less than the maximal effect of a mycotoxin alone clearly demonstrates an interaction of antagonistic nature. However, underestimations of the expected combination effect can hide milder antagonistic effects. The great advantage of this model is the financial cost of the experiment: to prove an antagonistic effect, it is sufficient to test three concentrations, each mycotoxin alone and a combination of the mycotoxins. Another advantage is that this method is also independent of the mechanism of action, and it does not make any assumptions on the dose-effect curve. However, this simple approach has never been applied in mycotoxicology.

**Table 1.** Interactions between mycotoxin combinations in vitro assessed by simple addition of effects, full factorial analysis, Bliss independence criterion, Loewe additivity law and response surface.

| Mycotoxin Combination | *In Vitro* Model | Mathematical Model Applied for the Endpoint | Endpoint Combined Effect | Reference |
|---|---|---|---|---|
| $AFM_1$ + OTA | Caco-2/ human colon HT29-MTX co-cultures (100/0, 90/10, 75/25 and 0/100) | Simple addition of effects | Cell viability (Enhanced Cell Counting Kit-8, CCK-8):<br>synergism in all cultures<br>TEER:<br>antagonism in all cultures, except additive effect in 90/10 co-culture<br>Intestinal mucin *MUC2* and *MUC5B* mRNA expression:<br>synergistic effect in 75/25 and 0/100 cultures at 4 µg/mL<br>additive effects at the low concentration (0.05 µg/mL) culture,<br>antagonistic effects in 100/0 and 90/10 cultures at 4 µg/mL<br>Intestinal mucin *MUC5AC* mRNA expression:<br>antagonistic effect in 100/0 cultures, an additive effect in 0/100 cultures at two concentrations of the mixtures<br>Intestinal mucin MUC5AC, MUC2 AND MUC5B on protein level:<br>synergism at 0.05 and 4 µg/mL<br>additive effect at 0.05 µg/mL in 75/25 and 90/10 cultures | [35] |
| $AFB_1$ + $FB_1$ | HepG2 cells | Simple addition of effects and factorial analysis (two-way ANOVA) | Cell cycle analysis (flow citometry assay):<br>synergism on apoptosis at 10% and 30% of $IC_{50}$ | [36] |
| ZEN (30 or 60 µM) + OTA (6 or 12 µM)<br>ZEN (30 or 60 µM) + α-ZEL (15 or 30 µM) | HepG2 cells | Full factorial analysis: 3 × 3 two-way ANOVA matrix | Cytotoxicity (MTT test):<br>synergism of ZEN (60 µM) + α-ZEL (15 or 30 µM)<br>antagonism in all other combinations<br>Oxidative stress parameters (MDA, GSH, Gpx, SOD):<br>synergism of ZEN (60 µM) + α-ZEL (15 or 30 µM)<br>antagonism in all other combinations | [37] |
| DON + ZEN | Bi- and tri-culture systems:<br>A) Caco-2 and HepaRG;<br>B) Caco-2 and THP-1;<br>C) HepaRG and THP-1<br>D) Caco-2, HepaRG and THP-1 | Response additivity, $CI_{RA}$) and Bliss independence criterion (independent joint action, $CI_{IjA}$); $IC_{10}$ (1:1) and $IC_{30}$ (1:1) | Cytotoxicity (MTS test):<br>additive effect for combination of $IC_{10}$ in A–D ($CI_{RA}$ and $CI_{IjA}$)<br>synergism for combination of $IC_{30}$ in A–C ($CI_{RA}$ and $CI_{IjA}$)<br>additive effect for combination of $IC_{30}$ in D ($CI_{RA}$ and $CI_{IjA}$) | [38] |

**Table 1.** *Cont.*

| Mycotoxin Combination | *In Vitro* Model | Mathematical Model Applied for the Endpoint | Endpoint Combined Effect | Reference |
|---|---|---|---|---|
| DON + MON<br>DON + $FB_1$<br>DON + ZEN<br>NIV + T-2 | HepaRG cells | Response additivity ($CI_{RA}$) and Bliss independence criterion (independent joint action, $CI_{IjA}$) | Cytotoxicity (MTS):<br>synergism of DON + MON in all combinations except additive effect at highest concentration (1:1) ($CI_{RA}$ and $CI_{IjA}$)<br>synergism of DON + $FB_1$ in all combinations ($CI_{RA}$ and $CI_{IjA}$) except additive effect at highest concentration (1:1) ($CI_{RA}$)<br>synergism of DON + ZEN at low and medium concentrations ($CI_{RA}$ and $CI_{IjA}$); additive effect ($CI_{IJA}$) and antagonism at high concentrations ($C_{RA}$)<br>NIV + T-2 synergism at low concentrations ($CI_{RA}$ and $CI_{IjA}$); additive effect or antagonism ($CI_{IJA}$) and antagonism at medium and high concentrations ($CI_{RA}$) | [39] |
| $AFB_1$ + ZEN<br>AFB1 + DON<br>ZEN + DON<br>AFB1 + ZEN + DON | HepG2 cells | Bliss independence criterion (IA) and Loewe additivity models (CA); CI-Isobologram method | Cell number (high content analysis by fluorescent labelling:<br>IA and CA model: deviation from the obtained results; better consistency was achieved by CA model;<br>CI model: antagonism at low fraction affected (0.05–0.15) changing to additive and synergistic effect as fraction affected increases for all combinations | [40] |
| TeA + ENN B; TeA + ZEN; TeA + DON; TeA + NIV; TeA + AURO; ENN B + ZEN; ENN B + DON; ENN B + NIV<br>ENN B + AURO; ZEN + DON; ZEN + NIV; ZEN + AURO; DON + NIV; DON + AURO | Caco-2 cells | Bliss independence criterion combined with CI calculated by Chou (C) and Chou-Talalay (CT) method | Cytotxicity (WST-1 test):<br>additive effects of binary mixtures at low concentrations calculated by Bliss independence criterion<br>antagonism of binary mixtures ENN B, ZEN and DON as well as binary combinations of *Fusarium* toxins with TeA applied at cytotoxic concentrations as calculated by CI | [41] |
| ATX II + AOH | HepG2, HT29 cells and human corneal epithelial HCEC cells | Bliss independence criterion, constant ratio of 1:10 or 1:1 | Cytotoxicity (WST-1 test):<br>dominant additive effect in all cell lines<br>antagonism in specific doses of ratios 1:10 or 1:1 | [47] |

**Table 1.** *Cont.*

| Mycotoxin Combination | *In Vitro* Model | Mathematical Model Applied for the Endpoint | Endpoint Combined Effect | Reference |
|---|---|---|---|---|
| AOH + DON<br>AOH + ZEN<br>ZEN + DON<br>AOH + DON + ZEN | THP-1 monocytes differentiated into macrophages | Concentration addition (CA) and independent action (IA) model at equal effect concentration | CD14 expression:<br>synergism of AOH + DON applied at low concentrations<br>additive effects of binary and tertiary mixtures of AOH, ZEN and DON, as calculated by both CA and IA | [48] |
| CIT + OTA<br>OTA + PAT<br>OTA + MPA<br>OTA + PA<br>CIT + PAT<br>CIT + MPA<br>CIT + PA<br>PAT + MPA<br>PAT + PA<br>MPA + PA | Bovine peritoneal macrophage BoMacs cells | CA and IA model; *Penicillium* toxins in $IC_{25}$, $\frac{1}{2}$ $IC_{25}$ and $\frac{1}{4}$ $IC_{25}$ | Cell proliferation (CyQUANT® GR dye):<br>CIT + OTA synergism at $\frac{1}{2}$ $IC_{25}$ (CA, IA)<br>OTA + PAT additive effects (CA, IA)<br>OTA + MPA synergism at $IC_{25}$, $\frac{1}{2}$ $IC_{25}$ and $\frac{1}{4}$ $IC_{25}$ (CA)<br>OTA + PA synergism at $IC_{25}$ and $\frac{1}{4}$ $IC_{25}$ (CA)<br>- CIT + PAT antagonism at $\frac{1}{2}$ $IC_{25}$ (CA)<br>CIT + MPA inconclusive (synergism CA, antagonism IA)<br>CIT + PA antagonism at $IC_{25}$, $\frac{1}{2}$ $IC_{25}$ (IA)<br>PAT + MPA antagonism at $IC_{25}$, $\frac{1}{2}$ $IC_{25}$ and $\frac{1}{4}$ $IC_{25}$ (IA)<br>PAT + PA synergism at $\frac{1}{2}$ $IC_{25}$; antagonism at $IC_{25}$<br>MPA + PA inconclusive | [45] |
| OTA + PAT | Caco-2 cells | Concentration addition model (CA) and independent action (IA) model with Jonker's generalization [28] | Cytotoxicity (MTT test):<br>- additive effects (CA)<br>synergism at high concentration of OTA and low of PAT (IA)<br>antagonism at high concentration of PAT and low of OTA (IA)<br>Gastrointestinal barrier integrity (TEER assay):<br>synergism at low concentration and antagonism at high concentration; the change from synergism to antagonism at higher $IC_{50}$ level (CA, IA)<br>Genotoxicity (alkaline comet test):<br>no dose-effect relationship of the single toxins; mathematical modelling was not applicable for the mixture | [46] |

$AFB_1$ and $AFM_1$: aflatoxin $B_1$ and $M_1$, DON: deoxynivalenol, ZEN: zearalenone, α and β-ZEL: α and β-zearalenol, OTA: ochratoxin A, $FB_1$: fumonisn $B_1$, PAT: patulin, CIT: citrinin, MPA: mycophenolic acid, PA: penicillic acid, NIV: nivalenol, ENN A and B: enniatins A and B, AURO: aurofusarin, AOH: alternariol, ATX II: altertoxin II, TeA: tenuasoic acid, $IC_{10-90}$: inhibitory concentration 10–90%, MDA: malondyaldehide, GSH: glutathione, Gpx: glutathione peroxidase, SOD: superoxide dismutase, MTT: (3-(4,5 dimethylthiazol-2-yl)-2,5-diphenyltetrazolium bromide) tetrazolium, TEER: transepithelial/transendothelial electrical resistance, MTS: (3-(4,5-dimethylthiazol-2-yl)-5-(3-carboxymethoxyphenyl)-2-(4-sulfophenyl)-2H tetrazolium.

### 2.7. Combination Index and Isobologram Analysis

Applying Loewe's additivity law or similar methods can allow researchers to use the Interaction/combination index which is based on Equation (5) for describing the nature of the combination effect (Equation (15)):

$$CI = D_1/D_{E1} + D_2/D_{E2}, \quad (15)$$

where CI is the interaction/combination index: CI < 1 indicates synergism, CI = 1 indicates an additive effect and CI > 1 indicates an antagonism [29]. Isobologram analysis is just a "fancy" name for the graphical representation of the combination index for the same effect in different ratios of two mycotoxins. It is a simple plot with the dose/concentration of mycotoxin 1 on the x axis and the dose/concentration of mycotoxin 2 on the y axis. The characteristic line, isobole, connects the y intercept and x intercept which represents the doses needed for achieving a defined effect (i.e., 50%) for single acting mycotoxins. Plotting the dot with coordinates of doses in combination that achieve the same defined effect gives us a clue about the nature of the combination effect. All of the dots below the isobole indicate synergy, the dots above the isobole indicate antagonism, while the dots on the isobole indicate a possible additive effect [49]. The combination index and isobologram method were applied in 15 studies reviewed in Alassane-Kpembi et al. [18] and was the second most used method for assessing mycotoxin interactions and much more appropriate than the arithmetic definition of additivity or factorial design.

The problems of not meeting the assumptions of Loewe's additivity law affect the combination index and isobologram. For example, if the two dose-response curves are not parallel, instead of one linear isobole, there will be two curvilinear isoboles around the former, linear one. The area between the two new curvilinear isoboles is not an area of synergy, nor is it an area of antagonism [43]. A recent study by Anastasiadi et al. [50] generalized the Loewe's model accounting for nonparallel dose-response curves. As a result, Equation (15) was expanded to Equation (16):

$$CI = (D_1/D_{E1})^{m1/m2} + D_2/D_{E2}, \quad m_1 < m_2 \quad (16)$$

where $m_1$ and $m_2$ are the slopes of the dose-response curves for mycotoxin 1 and mycotoxin 2.

Recently we tested the cytotoxicity (MTT test, 24 h) of single CIT, STC and 5-M-STC and dual combinations of CIT with STC and 5-M-STC in A549 cells (Table 2). The cytotoxicity of the mycotoxins was as follows: 5-M-STC ($IC_{50}$ = 5.5 μM) > STC ($IC_{50}$ = 60 μM) > CIT ($IC_{50}$ =128 μM). Mycotoxin interactions of 1:1, 1:2 and 2:1 of $IC_{50}$ concentration ratios were tested by applying a concentration addition model with correction for unparalleled dose-response curves as developed by Anastasiadi et al. [50], as presented in Figure 2.

### 2.8. Chou and Talalay's Median Effect Approach

Chou and Talalay developed a unified general theory for the Michaelis-Menten, Hill, Henderson-Hasselbalch, and Scatchard equations, mathematically presented by Equation (17):

$$E = 1/1 + (D_M/D)^m \quad (17)$$

where E is the effect (between 0 and 1), D is the dose, $D_M$ is the median effective dose (i.e., $EC_{50}$) and m is a parameter for shape definition (if m < 1 dose-effect curve is hyperbolic, and if m ≥ 1 dose-effect curve is sigmoidal) [30]. Using Equation (17), it is possible to estimate the doses needed to achieve a particular effect which can be used in Equation (15) for the estimation of CI, which is then used for assessing the nature of the combination effect. Similarly to Loewe's additivity model, the isobologram can be constructed. The Chou-Talalay model combined with an isobologram has been applied in the majority of the recently published studies [39,51–65] listed in Table 2. Its great advantage is the recent development of a method for the estimation of confidence intervals for the combination index which enables the application of statistics [66]. This method can easily be implemented using the web-based CalcuSyn software which automatically calculates dose-effect curves and combination indices.

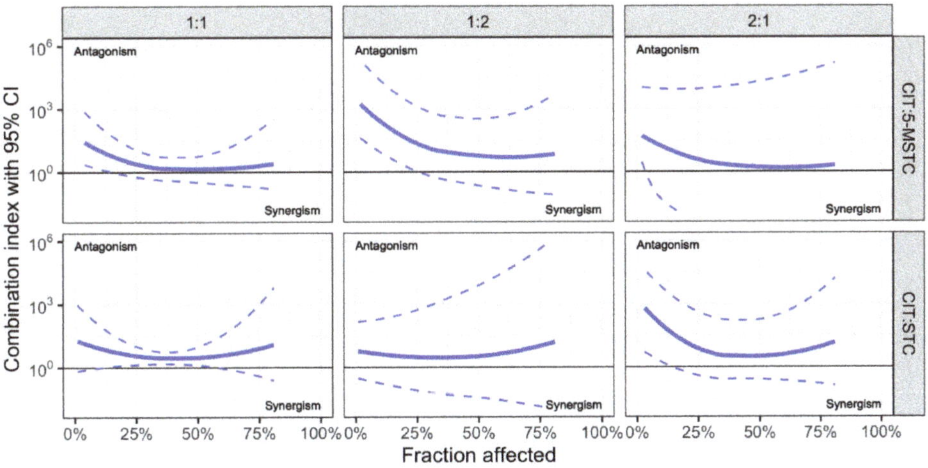


**Figure 2.** Combination indices calculated according to Anastasiadi et al. [50] accounting for different slopes of dose-response curves, 95% confidence interval (CI) was estimated using Monte Carlo simulations (N = 10000). All dose-response curves were fitted using non-linear regression. Results show mostly additive effect, with an exception of CIT + 5-M-STC combination which shows antagonistic effect in the area of up to 20% of cells affected, and CIT + STC combination (only 1 $IC_{50}$: 1 $IC_{50}$ ratio) in the area of 25–50% of cells affected.

**Table 2.** Interactions between mycotoxin combinations in vitro assessed by isobologram and Choul-Talalay method as well as MixLow model.

| Mycotoxin Combination | *In Vitro* Model | Mathematical Model Applied for the Endpoint | Endpoint Combined Effect | Reference |
|---|---|---|---|---|
| AOH (50 nM-10 μM) + ZEN (10 pM-1nM)<br>AOH (50 nM-10 μM) + α-ZEL (1 pM-1nM) | Human endometrial adenocarcinoma cell line, Ishikawa | Chou and Chou-Talalay method | Estrogenic effect (AIP test) according to C:<br>61% synergism, 10% additive effect, 32% antagonism for AOH + ZEN<br>86% synergism, 14% antagonism for AOH + α-ZEL<br>Estrogenic effect (AIP assay) according to CT:<br>ZEN or α-ZEL:AOH (1:250) dominant synergism<br>Cytotoxicity (SRB assay):<br>not possible to calculate CI | [51] |
| DON + T2 | Human chondrocytic C28/I2,<br>human hepatic epithelial L-02 and human tubular epithelial HK-2 cells | CI-Isobologram according to Chou-Talalay method; CI at $IC_{10–90}$ (1:1) | Cytotoxicity (MTT test):<br>synergism at $IC_{10}$ in HK2<br>antagonism in C28/12, L-02 ($IC_{10–90}$) and in HK2 ($IC_{25–90}$) | [58] |
| DON + 15-ADON (1:1)<br>DON + FX (3:1)<br>DON + NIV (3:1)<br>15-ADON + FX (3:1)<br>15-ADON + NIV (3:1)<br>FX + NIV (1:1) | Human gastric epithelial GES-1 cells | CI-Isobologram according to Chou-Talalay method; CI at $IC_{10}$–$IC_{90}$ | Cytotoxicity (OD test):<br>synergism of DON + 15-ADON, DON + NIV, FX + NIV at $IC_{10}$–$IC_{70}$; DON +FX at $IC_{10}$ and $IC_{30}$; 15-ADON + FX at $IC_{10}$<br>additive effect of FX + NIV at $IC_{90}$<br>antagonism of 15A-DON + NIV at $IC_{10}$–$IC_{90}$; 15-ADON + FX at $IC_{30}$-$IC_{90}$; DON + FX at $IC_{50}$-$IC_{90}$; DON +15-ADON, DON + NIV, FX + NIV at $IC_{90}$ | [59] |
| $AFB_1$ + DON<br>$AFB_1$ + ZEN<br>DON + ZEN<br>$AFB_1$ + DON + ZEN | HepG2 and (murine leukemia virus-induced tumor RAW 264.7 cells | CI-Isobologram according to Chou-Talalay method; CI at $IC_{25,50,70}$ (1:1 and 1:1:1) | Cytotoxicity (Resazurin test) in HepG2:<br>synergism of DON + ZEN<br>$AFB_1$ + DON + ZEN at $IC_{25–70}$<br>additive effects of $AFB_1$ + DON at $IC_{25–70}$<br>antagonism of $AFB_1$ + ZEN at $IC_{25–70}$<br>Cytotoxicity in RAW 264.7:<br>synergism of $AFB_1$ + DON at $IC_{25}$; DON + ZEN, $AFB_1$ + DON + ZEN at $IC_{50,70}$<br>additive effects of $AFB_1$ + DON at $IC_{50,70}$, DON + ZEN, $AFB_1$ + DON + ZEN at $IC_{25}$<br>antagonism of AFB1 + ZEN at $IC_{25–70}$ | [60] |

**Table 2.** *Cont.*

| Mycotoxin Combination | *In Vitro* Model | Mathematical Model Applied for the Endpoint | Endpoint Combined Effect | Reference |
|---|---|---|---|---|
| $AFM_1$ + OTA<br>$AFM_1$ + α-ZEL<br>$AFM_1$ + ZEN<br>OTA + ZEN<br>OTA + α-ZEL<br>ZEN + α-ZEL<br>$AFM_1$ + OTA + α-ZEL<br>$AFM_1$ + ZEN + α-ZEL<br>$AFM_1$ + OTA + ZEN<br>OTA + ZEN + α-ZEL<br>$AFM_1$ + OTA + α-ZEL + ZEN | Caco-2 cells | CI-Isobologram according to Chou-Talalay method; CI at $IC_{25,50,75,90}$ (1:1, 1:1:1 and 1:1:1.1) | Cytotoxicity (MTT test):<br>synergism of $AFM_1$ + OTA at $IC_{50}$; OTA + ZEN at $IC_{25,50}$; OTA + α-ZEL at $IC_{25}$; ZEN + α-ZEL at $IC_{75,90}$; $AFM_1$ + ZEN + α-ZEL, $AFM_1$ + OTA + ZEN and OTA + ZEN + α-ZEL at $IC_{25}$; four toxins combination at $IC_{25,50}$<br>additive effects of $AFM_1$ + OTA at $IC_{25,75}$; $AFM_1$ + ZEN at $IC_{25}$; OTA + ZEN and ZEN + α-ZEL at $IC_{50}$; $AFM_1$ + OTA + α-ZEL at $IC_{25,50}$; $AFM_1$ + OTA + ZEN and OTA + ZEN + α-ZEL at $IC_{50}$<br>antagonism at $AFM_1$ + OTA at $IC_{90}$; $AFM_1$ + α-ZEL at $IC_{25–90}$; $AFM_1$ + ZEN at $IC_{50\text{-}90}$; OTA + ZEN at $IC_{75,90}$; OTA + α-ZEL at $IC_{25}$; ZEN + α-ZEL at $IC_{25}$; $AFM_1$ + OTA + α-ZEL, $AFM_1$ + OTA + ZEN, OTA + ZEN + α-ZEL and $AFM_1$ + OTA + α-ZEL + ZEN at $IC_{75,90}$; $AFM_1$ + ZEN + α-ZEL at $IC_{50\text{-}90}$ | [61] |
| ZEN + α-ZEL<br>ZEN + ß-ZEL<br>α-ZEL + ß-ZEL | HepG2 cells | CI-Isobologram according to Chou-Talalay method; CI at $IL_{25}$-$IL_{75}$ (1:1) | Cytotoxicity (NR test):<br>synergistic effect in all combinations, except additive effect for ZEA + β ZEL at $IL_{25}$<br>Expression of pro-inflammatory cytokines (IL-1ß, TNF-α, IL-8):<br>synergism of all mixtures for IL-8 at $IL_{50.75}$; ZEN + α-ZEL ($IL_{50,75}$) and, ZEN + β-ZEL ($IL_{75}$) for IL-1β and TNF-α<br>antagonism of all mixtures for all cytokines at $IL_{25}$ except for ZEN + α-ZEL (synergism); ZEN + β-ZEL ($IL_{50}$) for ILβ; α-ZEL + β-ZEL for IL-1β and TNF-α at $IL_{50,75}$ | [62] |
| 3-ADON + AOH<br>15-ADON + AOH<br>3-ADON + 15-ADON<br>AOH + 3-ADON + 15-ADON | HepG2 cells | CI-Isobologram according to Chou-Talalay method; CI at $IC_{25,50,75,90}$ (1:1) | Cytotoxicity (MTT test) upon 24, 48 and 72 h:<br>dominant synergism, 3-ADON + AOH (24 and 48 h and $IC_{25}$ 72 h), 15-ADON + AOH (24 h), 3-ADON + 15-ADON and AOH + 3-ADON + 15-ADON (all treatments)<br>additive effect of 3-ADON + AOH $IC_{50\text{-}90}$ (72 h); 15-ADON + AOH at $IC_{25,50}$ (48 h) and $IC_{50\text{-}90}$ (72 h)<br>antagonism of 15-ADON + AOH at $IC_{75,90}$ (48 h) and $IC_{25}$ (72 h) | [63] |

**Table 2.** *Cont.*

| Mycotoxin Combination | *In Vitro* Model | Mathematical Model Applied for the Endpoint | Endpoint Combined Effect | Reference |
|---|---|---|---|---|
| $AFB_1$ + DON<br>$AFB_1$ + OTA<br>DON+OTA | Caco-2 and HepG2 cells | CI-Isobologram according to Chou-Talalay method; CI at $IC_{10}$–$IC_{90}$ (1:1) | Cytotoxicity (MTT test) in Caco-2 cells:<br>synergism of DON+OTA at $IC_{10}$–$IC_{90}$; $AFB_1$ + DON at $IC_{60\text{-}90}$; $AFB_1$ + OTA at $IC_{75\text{-}90}$<br>antagonism of AFB1 + OTA at $IC_{10\text{-}50}$; $AFB_1$ + DON at $IC_{10,30}$<br>Cytotoxicity in HepG2 cells:<br>synergism of $AFB_1$ + DON at $IC_{10\text{-}90}$;<br>additive effects of $AFB_1$ + OTA at $IC_{10,90}$; DON + OTA at $IC_{60,90}$<br>antagonism of DON + OTA at $IC_{10\text{-}50}$ | [64] |
| DON + PAT<br>DON + T2<br>PAT + T2<br>DON + T2 + PAT | HepG2 cells | CI-Isobologram according to Chou-Talalay method; CI at $IC_{10}$–$IC_{90}$ (1:1) | Cytotoxicity (MTT test) upon 24, 48 and 72 h:<br>no synergism<br>dominant additive effect of DON + PAT; DON + T2 upon 72 h and at $IC_{75,90}$ (24 h); PAT + T2 upon 72 h and at $IC_{10,\ 50\text{-}90}$ (24 h); DON + T2 + PAT upon 72 h and at $IC_{50\text{-}90}$ (24 h) and $IC_{25\text{–}90}$ (48 h)<br>antagonism of DON + T2 upon 48 h and at $IC_{10\text{-}50}$ (48 h); PAT + T-2 upon 48 h and at $IC_{25}$ (24 h); DON + T2 + PAT at $IC_{10,25}$ (24 h) and $IC_{10}$ (48 h) | [65] |
| DON + NIV (1:0.6)<br>NIV + FX (3:1)<br>DON + FX (1:0.2)<br>DON + NIV + FX (1:0.6:0.2) | Jurkat human T cells | CI-Isobologram according to Chou-Talalay method; CI at $IC_{10}$, $IC_{20}$ and $IC_{30}$ | Cytotoxicity (MTT test):<br>DON + NIV additive effect ($IC_{10}$) and antagonism ($IC_{20,30}$)<br>NIV + FX synergism<br>DON + FX antagonism<br>DON + NIV + FX antagonism | [52] |
| DON + NIV | Differentiated three-dimensional porcine jejunal explants | CI-Isobologram according to Chou-Talalay method; CI at equimolar concentrations (1:1) | mRNA expression of cytokines:<br>synergism in activation of all the tested pro-inflammatory genes (IL-1$\alpha$,$\beta$, IL-8, IL-17A, IL-22) | [53] |

**Table 2.** *Cont.*

| Mycotoxin Combination | *In Vitro* Model | Mathematical Model Applied for the Endpoint | Endpoint Combined Effect | Reference |
|---|---|---|---|---|
| DON + NIV<br>DON + FX<br>NIV + FX<br>DON + NIV + FX | Human alveolar adenocarcinoma (A549) and bronchial 16HBE14o- cells primary human bronchial (hAECB) and nasal (hAECN) cells | CI-Isobologram method derived from the median-effect according to Chou at $IC_{10,30,50}$ (1:1) | Cytotoxicity (MTT test):<br>in A549 cells synergism of DON + NIV and DON + FX at $IC_{10}$ and additive effect at $IC_{30}$; antagonism of NIV + FX at $IC_{30}$ and DON + NIV or FX at $IC_{50}$<br>in 16HBE14o- cells synergism of DON + FX and NIV + FX at $IC_{10\text{-}50}$; antagonism of DON + NIV at $IC_{10\text{-}50}$<br>in hAECB cells synergism of binary mixtures at $IC_{10.30}$ and NIV + FX at $IC_{50}$; additive effects of DON + NIV and DON + FX at $IC_{50}$<br>in hAECN cells of binary mixtures at $IC_{30,50}$ and DON + NIV and NIV + FX at $IC_{10}$; antagonism of DON + FX at $IC_{10}$ | [54] |
| DON + ZEN (1:7.5)<br>NIV + T-2 (1:0.067)<br>(ratio of $IC_{50}$) | HepaRG cells | CI-Isobologram according to Chou-Talalay method | Cytotoxicity (MTS):<br>synergism of DON + ZEN at all applied concentrations<br>- synergism of NIV + T-2 at low concentrations<br>antagonism of NIV + T-2 at medium concentrations | [39] |
| $AFB_1$ + DON (1:1.44)<br>$AFB_1$ + ZEN (1:15.19)<br>DON + ZEN (1:10.56)<br>$AFB_1$ + DON + ZEN (1:1.44:15.19) | Fibroblast cell line BF-2 from the caudal fin of *Lepomis macrochirus* | CI-Isobologram according to Chou-Talalay method; CI at $IC_{10}$-$IC_{50}$ | Cytotoxicity (resazurin):<br>synergism of $AFB_1$ + DON and $AFB_1$ + ZEN and ternary mixture at $IC_{10\text{-}30}$<br>additive effect of ternary mixture at $IC_{40}$<br>antagonism of DON + ZEN and ternary mixture at $IC_{50}$ | [55] |
| BEA + STC (1:5)<br>BEA + PAT (3.2:1)<br>PAT + STC + (1:5)<br>BEA + PAT + STC (3.2:1:5) | Chinese hamster ovary CHO-K1 cells | CI-Isobologram according to Chou-Talalay method; CI at $IC_5$-$IC_{50}$ | Cytotoxicity (MTT test) upon 24, 48 and 72 h:<br>synergism of BEA + STC at $IC_{5,10}$ (24 h); BEA + PAT at $IC_5$ (24 h); PAT + STC at $IC_{5,10}$ (24-72 h); BEA + PAT + STC at $IC_{5,10}$ (24 h) and $IC_{10\text{-}50}$ (72 h)<br>additive effect of BEA + STC at $IC_{25,50}$ (24 h), $IC_{50}$ (48 h) and $IC_{10\text{-}50}$ (72 h); BEA + PAT at $IC_{10\text{-}50}$ (24 h) and $IC_{25,50}$ (72 h); PAT + STC at $IC_{25}$ (24-72 h) and $IC_{50}$ (24, 48 h); BEA + PAT + STC at $IC_5$ (72 h) and $IC_{25,50}$ (24, 48h)<br>antagonism of BEA + STC at $IC_{5\text{-}25}$ (48 h); BEA +PAT at $IC_{5\text{-}50}$ (48 h) and $IC_{5,10}$ (72 h); PAT + STC at $IC_{50}$ (72 h); BEA + PAT + STC at $IC_{5,10}$ (48 h) | [56] |

**Table 2.** *Cont.*

| Mycotoxin Combination | *In Vitro* Model | Mathematical Model Applied for the Endpoint | Endpoint Combined Effect | Reference |
|---|---|---|---|---|
| BEA + OTA | HepG2 cells | CI-Isobologram according to Chou-Talalay method; CI at $IC_{25}$-$IC_{90}$ (1:1) and equimolar ration (1:10) | Cytotoxicity (MTT test) upon 24, 48 and 72 h:<br>synergism upon 72 h at $IC_{25}$-$IC_{90}$; 48 h at $IC_{25}$-$IC_{75}$; and 1:10 upon 48 and 72 h<br>additive effects upon 24 h at $IC_{25}$-$IC_{90}$; 48 h at $IC_{90}$; and 1:10 upon 24 h | [57] |
| CIT + STC<br>CIT + M-STC | Human adenocarcinoma lung A549 cells | CI-Isobologram with correction for unparalleled dose-response curves, developed by Anastasiadi et al. [50]; "ray" desing with 1:1, 1:2 and 2:1 concentration ratios | Cytotoxicity (MTT test)<br>additive effect<br>antagonism exceptionally in low affected areas for CIT + 5-MSTC and 2:1 CIT + STC, also between $IC_{25}$ and $IC_{50}$ for CIT + STC | Personal unpublished data shown in Figure 2. |
| DON + T2 | Human C-28/I2 and newborn rat primary costal chondrocytes (RC) | MixLow method; combination ratios of DON and T-2 toxin (R1=1:1 R10= 10:1, R100=100:1 and R1000=1000:1). | Cytotoxicity (MTT test):<br>synergism at fraction affected 0.5, 0.75, 0.9 of R10 concentrations in RC<br>antagonism at fraction affected 0.25 of R100 in both cell types; fraction affected 0.5 of R100 in C-28/12; fraction 0.5 of R1000 in RC | [67] |

$AFB_1$ and $AFM_1$: aflatoxin $B_1$ and $M_1$, DON: deoxynivalenol, ZEN: zearalenone, OTA: ochratoxin A, $FB_1$: fumonisn $B_1$, PAT: patulin, BEA: beauvericin, CIT: citrinin, MPA: mycophenolic acid, PA: penicillic acid, 15-ADON: 15-acetyldeoxynivalenol, FX: fusarenon-X, NIV: nivalenol, AOH: alternariol, ATX II: altertoxin II, α and β-ZEL: α and β-Zearalenol, STC: sterigmatocystin, 5-M-STC: 5-Methoxysterigmatocystin; $IC_{10-90}$: inhibitory concentration 10–90%, CI: combination index, AIP: alkaline phosphatase, MTT: (3-(4,5-dimethylthiazol-2-yl)-2,5-diphenyltetrazolium bromide) tetrazolium, OD: optical density, SRB: sulforhodamine B assay, NR: neutral red assay.

### 2.9. MixLow Method

Compared to the Chou-Talalay method, the MixLow method (Table 2) used by Lin et al. [67] improves model fitting and removes bias by fitting the log-logistic curve without prior linearization, similarly to the CISNE method (discussed in Section 2.10). However, another improvement of the MixLow method is the inclusion of random effects in a model that can account for different batches (trays) in the experiment and fit the model for both toxins and combination simultaneously [31]. Mixed modelling enables a more precise estimation of the combination index's (CI, here called Loewe's index) and more reliable confidence intervals or standard errors by accounting for both the error of single applied mycotoxins and combinations.

The MixLow method comes with the *mixlow* R package, which also includes functions for straigthforward data import and minimal data preprocessing, especially if the pattern suggested on the tray is followed during experimental design [68].

### 2.10. CISNE (Code for the Identification of Synergism Numerically Efficient)

Even though Chou-Talalay's method exceeded two and a half thousand citations in relevant article databases, it does possess some technical problems in model fitting leading to bias inclusion in parameter estimation. By Chou-Talalay's protocol Equation (17) is rearranged and transformed to linear form (Equation (18)):

$$\log[E/(1-E)] = m \times \log(D) - m \times \log(D_M), \quad (18)$$

where y is $\log[E/(1-E)]$, the intercept is $-m \times \log(D_M)$, the slope is m, and x is the log(D) of the linear equation form. Estimating slope and intercept by least squares fit, and calculating $D_m$ as presented by Equation (19):

$$D_M = e^{-\text{intercept/slope}} \quad (19)$$

This leads to bias, along with the exclusion of data points with effects smaller than 0% or larger than 100% (i.e., stimulation) which could not be used in the logarithm on the left side of Equation (18). García-Fuente et al. [33] showed that these biases can lead to significant false positive or false negative errors, depending on the slope of the dose-response curve. They also found that fitting the same equation as a non-linear regression model estimates model parameters better and reduces the rate of false positives or negatives, especially when the slope (m) deviates from 1. This non-linear regression can be easily applied using the free CISNE software [69]. In contrast, it has not yet been applied in mycotoxicology combination testing.

### 2.11. Other methods

Most of the recent studies used mathematical modelling according to Bliss or/and Loewe (or some modified Loewe's method) for assessing the nature of the effect of combination of mycotoxins. However several in vitro studies assed mycotoxin combined effects comparing the effect of combination to the effect of single mycotoxin [70–72] or only to negative controls [73–76] without estimating the theoretical (expected) effect of the combination (Table 3). Conclusions based on those studies are unreliable because the question of the nature of interaction of combination has not even been asked in a scientific manner to get a clear and exact answer. For example, Smith et al. [75] did not define the nature DON + ZEN interaction in HepRG cells; since the cytotoxic effect of a single DON was similar to the effect of DON + ZEN, it was concluded that a combined effect could not be classified as antagonistic nor synergistic. Any conclusion about an antagonistic or synergistic effect should include the effect of ZEN too, since it is a part of the mycotoxin combination.

**Table 3.** Interactions between mycotoxin combinations in vitro without applying a mathematical model.

| Mycotoxin Combination | *In Vitro* Model | Statistical Analysis Applied for the Endpoint | Endpoint Combined Effect | Reference |
|---|---|---|---|---|
| DON + ZEN | Porcine splenic lymphocytes | ANOVA followed by the Tukey post hoc test ($p < 0.05$) | Antioxidant parameters (MDA, GSH, CAT, SOD, Gpx): synergism<br>Apoptotic rate: synergism<br>Expression of p53, Bcl-2, Bax, caspase-3, and caspase-8: synergism | [70] |
| DON + ZEN (at concentrations corresponding to the AED, TDI and ML) | HepaRG cells | Student's t-test ($p <$ 0.05) | Cytotoxicity (MTS test) upon 14, 28 and 42 days:<br>at ML no antagonistic or synergistic effect<br>Gene expression of CYP4F3B, CYP3A4, C/EBPα, HNF4α, aldolase B, transferrin, albumin and claudin-1 (qPCR):<br>at AED majority of genes were ↑↑ after 14 days and ↓↓ after 28 days<br>at TDI the gene expression upon 14 and 28 days were less different but more ↑↑ after 28 days<br>at ML DON and DON+ZEA reduced the cell viability by more than 90%, no sufficient amounts of RNA<br>DON + ZEN affected different genes than single DON and ZEA | [75] |
| DON + 3ADON (3:1)<br>DON + 15-ADON (3:1)<br>3-ADON + 15-ADON (1:1)<br>DON + 3-ADON + 15-ADON (3:1:1)<br>(ratios of $IC_{50}$) | HepG2 cells | ANOVA followed by the Tukey post hoc test ($p \leq 0.05$) | Oxidative stress (ROS and MDA):<br>binary mixtures significantly increased ROS vs. control and initial time<br>binary and tertiary mixtures increased MDA vs. control (24, 48 and 72 h)<br>Cell cycle distribution upon 48 h (flow cytometry):<br>DON + 3-ADON ↓ G0/G1 and S, G0/G1 and S, G2/M phase ↑ at lower and ↓ at higher concentrations in respect to control<br>DON + 15-ADON ↑ G0/G1 and G2/M at lower and ↓ at higher concentrations in respect to control<br>3-ADON + 15-ADON ↓ G0/G1 and S at all concentrations vs. control<br>tertiary combination ↓ G0/G1, S and G2/M vs. control<br>Micronuclei (MN):<br>binary mixtures ↑ in MN at lower concentrations vs. control<br>tertiary mixtures ↑ in MN at all concentrations vs. control | [73,74] |

**Table 3.** *Cont.*

| Mycotoxin Combination | *In Vitro* Model | Statistical Analysis Applied for the Endpoint | Endpoint Combined Effect | Reference |
|---|---|---|---|---|
| ENN A + $A_1$ + B + $B_1$ (1.5 or 3 µM)<br>ENN A + $A_1$ + B + $B_1$ + DON (1.5 or 3 µM)<br>BEA (2.5 µM) + DON (1.5 or 3 µM)<br>Apicidin (0.438 µM) + DON (1.5 or 3 µM)<br>AURO (5 µM) + DON (1.5 or 3 µM) | Porcine epithelial cells IPEC-J2 | ANOVA followed by the Dunnett's t-test or Kruskall-Wallis test ($p < 0.05$) | TEER upon 24, 48 and 72 h:<br>dominant additive effect<br>DON had no effect on enniatin-induced TEER decrease<br>BEA + DON did not significantly reduce TEER | [76] |
| OTA + CIT | Multiple organ co-culture (IdMOC) of HepG2 and 3T3 cells | Paired sample *t*-test ($p < 0.05$) | Luciferin-IPA metabolism assay:<br>synergism at 20% $IC_{50}$ (CTN forms a reactive metabolite that diffuses out of HepG2 to cause cytotoxicity to 3T3 cells synergistically with OTA) | [71] |
| OTA + CIT (equimolar concentrations 0–30 µM) | Human embryonic kidney HEK293 cells | No statistical analysis indicated/ effect of combination was compared to the effects of mycotoxins acting alone | Cytotoxicity (MTT test):<br>synergism based on $IC_{50}$ of single OTA (16 µM) and CIT (189 µM) vs. combination (7 µM) | [72] |

DON: deoxynivalenol, ZEN: zearalenone, BEA: beauvericin, 3-ADON: 3-acetyldeoxynivalenol, 15-ADON: 15-acetyldeoxynivalenol, ENN A and B: enniatins A and B, AURO: aurofusarin, OTA: ochratoxin A, CIT: citrinin, $IC_{50}$: inhibitory concentration 50%, MDA: malondyaldehide, GSH: glutathione, Gpx: glutathione peroxidase, CAT: catalase, SOD: superoxide dismutase, ROS: reactive oxygen species, MTT: (3-(4,5-dimethylthiazol-2-yl)-2,5-diphenyltetrazolium bromide) tetrazolium, TEER: transepithelial/transendothelial electrical resistanceAED: average exposure dose of French adult population, TDI: Tolerable daily intake established by the JECFA, ML: maximum level permitted in cereals by the European regulation, ↑↑: up-regulated, ↓↓: down-regulated, ↑: increased, ↓: decreased.

## 3. Conclusions

Some of the methods found in studies assessing the effects of mycotoxins combination have been incorrectly based on the assumption that mycotoxin dose-effect curves are linear (simple addition of effects, factorial analysis of variance). For that reason, many conclusions have been derived incorrectly in published articles or review articles based on published data. There are many articles reviewing methods and discussing the problem of the misuse of some method, but it seems that the problem persists. The only appropriate approach to assess the nature of an interaction is to correctly estimate the dose-effect curves of each mycotoxin and combination and apply a well-defined model (based on Bliss or Loewe's theory) with respecting the model's assumptions and fitting the model by a direct estimation of all model parameters from a nonlinear least squares fitting. Results should be presented in a simple and clearly defined way (i.e., isobologram or combination index) with some of the most expected (mean) values accompanied by uncertainty bounds, where a 95% confidence interval should have priority over the standard error due to asymmetrical distributions.

Improvements to the presented methods are continuously being made but are not readily applied in the field of mycotoxicology.

**Author Contributions:** Conceptualization, D.K. and M.Š.K.; methodology, D.K.; investigation, D.K., D.J. and M.Š.K.; writing—original draft preparation, D.K., D.J. and M.Š.K. All authors have read and agreed to the published version of the manuscript.

**Funding:** This research was funded by Croatian Science Foundation, grant number IP-09-2014-5982.

**Acknowledgments:** The authors want to thank Makso Herman, MA for English language editing.

**Conflicts of Interest:** The authors declare no conflict of interest.

## References

1. Pitt, J.I.; David Miller, J. A Concise History of Mycotoxin Research. *J. Agric. Food Chem.* **2017**, *65*, 7021–7033. [CrossRef] [PubMed]
2. Venkatesh, N.; Keller, N.P. Mycotoxins in conversation with bacteria and fungi. *Front. Microbiol.* **2019**, *10*, 403. [CrossRef]
3. Fox, E.M.; Howlett, B.J. Secondary metabolism: Regulation and role in fungal biology. *Curr. Opin. Microbiol.* **2008**, *11*, 481–487. [CrossRef]
4. Van Egmond, H.P.; Schothorst, R.C.; Jonker, M.A. Regulations relating to mycotoxins in food. *Anal. Bioanal. Chem.* **2007**, *389*, 147–157. [CrossRef] [PubMed]
5. Assunção, R.; Silva, M.J.; Alvito, P. Challenges in risk assessment of multiple mycotoxins in food. *World Mycotoxin J.* **2016**, *9*, 791–811. [CrossRef]
6. Abdallah, M.F.; Girgin, G.; Baydar, T.; Krska, R.; Sulyok, M. Occurrence of multiple mycotoxins and other fungal metabolites in animal feed and maize samples from Egypt using LC-MS/MS. *J. Sci. Food Agric.* **2017**, *97*, 4419–4428. [CrossRef] [PubMed]
7. Malachová, A.; Sulyok, M.; Beltrán, E.; Berthiller, F.; Krska, R. Optimization and validation of a quantitative liquid chromatography-tandem mass spectrometric method covering 295 bacterial and fungal metabolites including all regulated mycotoxins in four model food matrices. *J. Chromatogr. A* **2014**, *1362*, 145–156. [CrossRef]
8. Gruber-Dorninger, C.; Novak, B.; Nagl, V.; Berthiller, F. Emerging Mycotoxins: Beyond Traditionally Determined Food Contaminants. *J. Agric. Food Chem.* **2017**, *65*, 7052–7070. [CrossRef]
9. Kovač, M.; Šubarić, D.; Bulaić, M.; Kovač, T.; Šarkanj, B. Yesterday masked, today modified; what do mycotoxins bring next? *Arh. Hig. Rada Toksikol.* **2018**, *69*, 196–214. [CrossRef]
10. Ibáñez-Vea, M.; González-Peñas, E.; Lizarraga, E.; López de Cerain, A. Co-occurrence of aflatoxins, ochratoxin A and zearalenone in barley from a northern region of Spain. *Food Chem.* **2012**, *132*, 35–42. [CrossRef]
11. Santini, A.; Meca, G.; Uhlig, S.; Ritieni, A. Fusaproliferin, beauvericin and enniatins: Occurrence in food-A review. *World Mycotoxin J.* **2012**, *5*, 71–81. [CrossRef]

12. Streit, E.; Schatzmayr, G.; Tassis, P.; Tzika, E.; Marin, D.; Taranu, I.; Tabuc, C.; Nicolau, A.; Aprodu, I.; Puel, O.; et al. Current situation of mycotoxin contamination and co-occurrence in animal feed focus on Europe. *Toxins* **2012**, *4*, 788–809. [CrossRef] [PubMed]
13. Vaclavikova, M.; Malachova, A.; Veprikova, Z.; Dzuman, Z.; Zachariasova, M.; Hajslova, J. "Emerging" mycotoxins in cereals processing chains: Changes of enniatins during beer and bread making. *Food Chem.* **2013**, *136*, 750–757. [CrossRef]
14. Kademi, H.I.; Baba, I.A.; Saad, F.T. Modelling the dynamics of toxicity associated with aflatoxins in foods and feeds. *Toxicol. Rep.* **2017**, *4*, 358–363. [CrossRef] [PubMed]
15. Garcia, D.; Ramos, A.J.; Sanchis, V.; Marín, S. Predicting mycotoxins in foods: A review. *Food Microbiol.* **2009**, *26*, 757–769. [CrossRef] [PubMed]
16. Lee, S.; Yoon, Y.; Kim, D.M.; Kim, D.S.; Park, K.H.; Chun, H.S. Mathematical models to predict kinetic behavior and aflatoxin production of Aspergillus flavus under various temperature and water activity conditions. *Food Sci. Biotechnol.* **2014**, *23*, 975–982. [CrossRef]
17. Smith, M.C.; Madec, S.; Coton, E.; Hymery, N. Natural Co-occurrence of mycotoxins in foods and feeds and their in vitro combined toxicological effects. *Toxins* **2016**, *8*, 94. [CrossRef]
18. Alassane-Kpembi, I.; Schatzmayr, G.; Taranu, I.; Marin, D.; Puel, O.; Oswald, I.P. Mycotoxins co-contamination: Methodological aspects and biological relevance of combined toxicity studies. *Crit. Rev. Food Sci. Nutr.* **2017**, *57*, 3489–3507. [CrossRef]
19. Grenier, B.; Oswald, I. Mycotoxin co-contamination of food and feed: Meta-analysis of publications describing toxicological interactions. *World Mycotoxin J.* **2011**, *4*, 285–313. [CrossRef]
20. Šegvić Klarić, M. Adverse effects of combined mycotoxins. *Arh. Hig. Rada Toksikol.* **2012**, *63*, 519–530. [CrossRef]
21. Šegvić Klarić, M.; Rašić, D.; Peraica, M. Deleterious effects of mycotoxin combinations involving ochratoxin A. *Toxins* **2013**, *5*, 1965–1987.
22. Tekin, E.; Beppler, C.; White, C.; Mao, Z.; Savage, V.M.; Yeh, P.J. Enhanced identification of synergistic and antagonistic emergent interactions among three or more drugs. *J. R. Soc. Interface* **2016**, *13*, 18–20. [CrossRef] [PubMed]
23. Foucquier, J.; Guedj, M. Analysis of drug combinations: Current methodological landscape. *Pharmacol. Res. Perspect.* **2015**, *3*. [CrossRef] [PubMed]
24. Weber, F.; Freudinger, R.; Schwerdt, G.; Gekle, M. A rapid screening method to test apoptotic synergisms of ochratoxin A with other nephrotoxic substances. *Toxicol. Vitr.* **2005**, *19*, 135–143. [CrossRef] [PubMed]
25. Caudle, R.M.; Williams, G.M. The misuse of analysis of variance to detect synergy in combination drug studies. *Pain* **1993**, *55*, 313–317. [CrossRef]
26. Bliss, C.I. The toxicity of poisons applied jointly. *Ann. Appl. Biol.* **1939**, *26*, 585–615. [CrossRef]
27. Loewe, S.; Muischnek, H. Über Kombinationswirkungen. *Arch. Für Exp. Pathol. Und Pharmakologie* **1926**, *114*, 313–326. [CrossRef]
28. Jonker, M.J.; Svendsen, C.; Bedaux, J.J.M.; Bongers, M.; Kammenga, J.E. Significance testing of synergistic/antagonistic, dose level–dependent, or dose ratio–dependent effects in mixture dose–response analysis. *Environ. Toxicol. Chem.* **2005**, *24*, 2701. [CrossRef]
29. Berenbaum, M.C. Criteria for analyzing interactions between biologically active agents. *Adv. Cancer Res.* **1981**, *35*, 269–335.
30. Chou, T.-C. Theoretical basis, experimental design, and computerized simulation of synergism and antagonism in drug combination studies. *Pharmacol. Rev.* **2006**, *58*, 621–681. [CrossRef]
31. Boik, J.C.; Newman, R.A.; Boik, R.J. Quantifying synergism/antagonism using nonlinear mixed-effects modeling: A simulation study. *Stat. Med.* **2008**, *27*, 1040–1061. [CrossRef] [PubMed]
32. Berenbaum, M.C. What is synergy? *Pharmacol. Rev.* **1989**, *41*, 93–141.
33. García-Fuente, A.; Vázquez, F.; Viéitez, J.M.; García Alonso, F.J.; Martín, J.I.; Ferrer, J. CISNE: An accurate description of dose-effect and synergism in combination therapies. *Sci. Rep.* **2018**, *8*, 1–9. [CrossRef] [PubMed]
34. Šegvić Klarić, M.; Daraboš, D.; Rozgaj, R.; Kašuba, V.; Pepeljnjak, S. Beauvericin and ochratoxin A genotoxicity evaluated using the alkaline comet assay: Single and combined genotoxic action. *Arch. Toxicol.* **2010**, *84*, 641–650. [CrossRef]

35. Huang, X.; Gao, Y.; Li, S.; Wu, C.; Wang, J.; Zheng, N. Modulation of Mucin (MUC2, MUC5AC AND MUC5B) mRNA expression and protein production and secretion in Caco-2/HT29-MTX co-cultures following exposure to individual and combined aflatoxin M1 and ochratoxin A. *Toxins* **2019**, *11*, 132. [CrossRef] [PubMed]
36. Du, M.; Liu, Y.; Zhang, G. Interaction of aflatoxin B1 and fumonisin B1 in HepG2 cell apoptosis. *Food Biosci.* **2017**, *20*, 131–140. [CrossRef]
37. Zheng, N.; Gao, Y.N.; Liu, J.; Wang, H.W.; Wang, J.Q. Individual and combined cytotoxicity assessment of zearalenone with ochratoxin A or α-zearalenol by full factorial design. *Food Sci. Biotechnol.* **2018**, *27*, 251–259. [CrossRef]
38. Smith, M.-C.; Gheux, A.; Coton, M.; Madec, S.; Hymery, N.; Coton, E. In vitro co-culture models to evaluate acute cytotoxicity of individual and combined mycotoxin exposures on Caco-2, THP-1 and HepaRG human cell lines. *Chem. Biol. Interact.* **2018**, *281*, 51–59. [CrossRef]
39. Smith, M.C.; Hymery, N.; Troadec, S.; Pawtowski, A.; Coton, E.; Madec, S. Hepatotoxicity of fusariotoxins, alone and in combination, towards the HepaRG human hepatocyte cell line. *Food Chem. Toxicol.* **2017**, *109*, 439–451. [CrossRef]
40. Li, Y.; Wang, T.Q.; Wu, J.; Zhang, X.L.; Xu, Y.Y.; Qian, Y.Z. Multi-parameter analysis of combined hepatotoxicity induced by mycotoxin mixtures in HepG2 cells. *World Mycotoxin J.* **2018**, *11*, 225–235. [CrossRef]
41. Vejdovszky, K.; Warth, B.; Sulyok, M.; Marko, D. Non-synergistic cytotoxic effects of Fusarium and Alternaria toxin combinations in Caco-2 cells. *Toxicol. Lett.* **2016**, *241*, 1–8. [CrossRef] [PubMed]
42. Tallarida, R.J. Quantitative methods for assessing drug synergism. *Genes Cancer* **2011**, *2*, 1003–1008. [CrossRef] [PubMed]
43. Geary, N. Understanding synergy. *Am. J. Physiol. Metab.* **2013**, *304*, E237–E253. [CrossRef] [PubMed]
44. Li, Y.; Zhang, B.; He, X.; Cheng, W.H.; Xu, W.; Luo, Y.; Liang, R.; Luo, H.; Huang, K. Analysis of individual and combined effects of ochratoxin a and zearalenone on HepG2 and KK-1 cells with mathematical models. *Toxins* **2014**, *6*, 1177–1192. [CrossRef] [PubMed]
45. Oh, S.Y.; Cedergreen, N.; Yiannikouris, A.; Swamy, H.V.L.N.; Karrow, N.A. Assessing interactions of binary mixtures of Penicillium mycotoxins (PMs) by using a bovine macrophage cell line (BoMacs). *Toxicol. Appl. Pharmacol.* **2017**, *318*, 33–40. [CrossRef] [PubMed]
46. Assunção, R.; Pinhão, M.; Loureiro, S.; Alvito, P.; Silva, M.J. A multi-endpoint approach to the combined toxic effects of patulin and ochratoxin a in human intestinal cells. *Toxicol. Lett.* **2019**, *313*, 120–129. [CrossRef]
47. Vejdovszky, K.; Sack, M.; Jarolim, K.; Aichinger, G.; Somoza, M.M.; Marko, D. In vitro combinatory effects of the Alternaria mycotoxins alternariol and altertoxin II and potentially involved miRNAs. *Toxicol. Lett.* **2017**, *267*, 45–52. [CrossRef]
48. Solhaug, A.; Karlsøen, L.M.; Holme, J.A.; Kristoffersen, A.B.; Eriksen, G.S. Immunomodulatory effects of individual and combined mycotoxins in the THP-1 cell line. *Toxicol. Vitr.* **2016**, *36*, 120–132. [CrossRef]
49. Tallarida, R.J. Revisiting the isobole and related quantitative methods for assessing drug synergism. *J. Pharmacol. Exp. Ther.* **2012**, *342*, 2–8. [CrossRef]
50. Anastasiadi, M.; Polizzi, K.; Lambert, R.J.W. An improved model for the analysis of combined antimicrobials: A replacement for the Chou-Talalay combination index method. *J. Appl. Microbiol.* **2018**, *124*, 97–107. [CrossRef]
51. Vejdovszky, K.; Hahn, K.; Braun, D.; Warth, B.; Marko, D. Synergistic estrogenic effects of Fusarium and Alternaria mycotoxins in vitro. *Arch. Toxicol.* **2017**, *91*, 1447–1460. [CrossRef] [PubMed]
52. Aupanun, S.; Phuektes, P.; Poapolathep, S.; Alassane-Kpembi, I.; Oswald, I.P.; Poapolathep, A. Individual and combined cytotoxicity of major trichothecenes type B, deoxynivalenol, nivalenol, and fusarenon-X on Jurkat human T cells. *Toxicon* **2019**, *160*, 29–37. [CrossRef] [PubMed]
53. Alassane-Kpembi, I.; Puel, O.; Pinton, P.; Cossalter, A.M.; Chou, T.C.; Oswald, I.P. Co-exposure to low doses of the food contaminants deoxynivalenol and nivalenol has a synergistic inflammatory effect on intestinal explants. *Arch. Toxicol.* **2017**, *91*, 2677–2687. [CrossRef] [PubMed]
54. Ferreira Lopes, S.; Vacher, G.; Ciarlo, E.; Savova-Bianchi, D.; Roger, T.; Niculita-Hirzel, H. Primary and Immortalized Human Respiratory Cells Display Different Patterns of Cytotoxicity and Cytokine Release upon Exposure to Deoxynivalenol, Nivalenol and Fusarenon-X. *Toxins* **2017**, *9*, 337. [CrossRef]
55. Zhou, H.; George, S.; Li, C.; Gurusamy, S.; Sun, X.; Gong, Z.; Qian, H. Combined toxicity of prevalent mycotoxins studied in fish cell line and zebrafish larvae revealed that type of interactions is dose-dependent. *Aquat. Toxicol.* **2017**, *193*, 60–71. [CrossRef]

56. Zouaoui, N.; Mallebrera, B.; Berrada, H.; Abid-Essefi, S.; Bacha, H.; Ruiz, M.J. Cytotoxic effects induced by patulin, sterigmatocystin and beauvericin on CHO-K1 cells. *Food Chem. Toxicol.* **2016**, *89*, 92–103. [CrossRef]
57. Juan-García, A.; Tolosa, J.; Juan, C.; Ruiz, M.-J. Cytotoxicity, genotoxicity and disturbance of cell cycle in HepG2 Cells exposed to OTA and BEA: Single and combined actions. *Toxins* **2019**, *11*, 341. [CrossRef]
58. Lei, Y.; Guanghui, Z.; Xi, W.; Yingting, W.; Xialu, L.; Fangfang, Y.; Goldring, M.B.; Xiong, G.; Lammi, M.J. Cellular responses to T-2 toxin and/or deoxynivalenol that induce cartilage damage are not specific to chondrocytes. *Sci. Rep.* **2017**, *7*, 1–14. [CrossRef]
59. Yang, Y.; Yu, S.; Tan, Y.; Liu, N.; Wu, A. Individual and combined cytotoxic effects of co-occurring deoxynivalenol family mycotoxins on human gastric epithelial cells. *Toxins* **2017**, *9*, 96. [CrossRef]
60. Zhou, H.; George, S.; Hay, C.; Lee, J.; Qian, H.; Sun, X. Individual and combined effects of aflatoxin B1, deoxynivalenol and zearalenone on HepG2 and RAW 264.7 cell lines. *Food Chem. Toxicol.* **2017**, *103*, 18–27. [CrossRef]
61. Gao, Y.N.; Wang, J.Q.; Li, S.L.; Zhang, Y.D.; Zheng, N. Aflatoxin M1 cytotoxicity against human intestinal Caco-2 cells is enhanced in the presence of other mycotoxins. *Food Chem. Toxicol.* **2016**, *96*, 79–89. [CrossRef] [PubMed]
62. Marin, D.E.; Pistol, G.C.; Bulgaru, C.V.; Taranu, I. Cytotoxic and inflammatory effects of individual and combined exposure of HepG2 cells to zearalenone and its metabolites. *Naunyn. Schmiedebergs. Arch. Pharmacol.* **2019**, *392*, 937–947. [CrossRef] [PubMed]
63. Juan-García, A.; Juan, C.; Manyes, L.; Ruiz, M.J. Binary and tertiary combination of alternariol, 3-acetyl-deoxynivalenol and 15-acetyl-deoxynivalenol on HepG2 cells: Toxic effects and evaluation of degradation products. *Toxicol. Vitr.* **2016**, *34*, 264–273. [CrossRef]
64. Sobral, M.M.C.; Faria, M.A.; Cunha, S.C.; Ferreira, I.M.P.L.V.O. Toxicological interactions between mycotoxins from ubiquitous fungi: Impact on hepatic and intestinal human epithelial cells. *Chemosphere* **2018**, *202*, 538–548. [CrossRef] [PubMed]
65. Fernández-Blanco, C.; Elmo, L.; Waldner, T.; Ruiz, M.J. Cytotoxic effects induced by patulin, deoxynivalenol and toxin T2 individually and in combination in hepatic cells (HepG2). *Food Chem. Toxicol.* **2018**, *120*, 12–23. [CrossRef] [PubMed]
66. Lee, J.J.; Kong, M. Confidence Intervals of Interaction Index for Assessing Multiple Drug Interaction. *Stat. Biopharm. Res.* **2009**, *1*, 4–17. [CrossRef] [PubMed]
67. Lin, X.; Shao, W.; Yu, F.; Xing, K.; Liu, H.; Zhang, F.; Goldring, M.B.; Lammi, M.J.; Guo, X. Individual and combined toxicity of T-2 toxin and deoxynivalenol on human C-28/I2 and rat primary chondrocytes. *J. Appl. Toxicol.* **2019**, *39*, 343–353. [CrossRef]
68. Boik, J.C.; Narasimhan, B. An R package for assessing drug synergism/antagonism. *J. Stat. Softw.* **2010**, *34*, 1–18. [CrossRef]
69. CISNE Code for the Identification of Synergism Numerically Efficient. Available online: https://cisnecode.github.io (accessed on 29 February 2020).
70. Ren, Z.; Deng, H.; Deng, Y.; Liang, Z.; Deng, J.; Zuo, Z.; Hu, Y.; Shen, L.; Yu, S.; Cao, S. Combined effects of deoxynivalenol and zearalenone on oxidative injury and apoptosis in porcine splenic lymphocytes in vitro. *Exp. Toxicol. Pathol.* **2017**, *69*, 612–617. [CrossRef]
71. Gayathri, L.; Karthikeyan, B.S.; Rajalakshmi, M.; Dhanasekaran, D.; Li, A.P.; Akbarsha, M.A. Metabolism-dependent cytotoxicity of citrinin and ochratoxin A alone and in combination as assessed adopting integrated discrete multiple organ co-culture (IdMOC). *Toxicol. Vitr.* **2018**, *46*, 166–177. [CrossRef]
72. Gong, L.; Zhu, H.; Li, T.; Ming, G.; Duan, X.; Wang, J.; Jiang, Y. Molecular signatures of cytotoxic effects in human embryonic kidney 293 cells treated with single and mixture of ochratoxin A and citrinin. *Food Chem. Toxicol.* **2019**, *123*, 374–384. [CrossRef] [PubMed]
73. Juan-García, A.; Juan, C.; Tolosa, J.; Ruiz, M.J. Effects of deoxynivalenol, 3-acetyl-deoxynivalenol and 15-acetyl-deoxynivalenol on parameters associated with oxidative stress in HepG2 cells. *Mycotoxin Res.* **2019**, *35*, 197–205. [CrossRef] [PubMed]
74. Juan-García, A.; Taroncher, M.; Font, G.; Ruiz, M.J. Micronucleus induction and cell cycle alterations produced by deoxynivalenol and its acetylated derivatives in individual and combined exposure on HepG2 cells. *Food Chem. Toxicol.* **2018**, *118*, 719–725. [CrossRef] [PubMed]

75. Smith, M.C.; Madec, S.; Pawtowski, A.; Coton, E.; Hymery, N. Individual and combined toxicological effects of deoxynivalenol and zearalenone on human hepatocytes in in vitro chronic exposure conditions. *Toxicol. Lett.* **2017**, *280*, 238–246. [CrossRef]
76. Springler, A.; Vrubel, G.J.; Mayer, E.; Schatzmayr, G.; Novak, B. Effect of Fusarium-derived metabolites on the barrier integrity of differentiated intestinal porcine epithelial cells (IPEC-J2). *Toxins* **2016**, *8*, 345. [CrossRef]

*toxins*

MDPI

*Article*

# Cytotoxicity, Genotoxicity and Disturbance of Cell Cycle in HepG2 Cells Exposed to OTA and BEA: Single and Combined Actions

**Ana Juan-García [1,*], Josefa Tolosa [1,2], Cristina Juan [1] and María-José Ruiz [1]**

1 Laboratory of Food Chemistry and Toxicology, Faculty of Pharmacy, University of Valencia, Av. Vicent Andrés Estellés s/n, Burjassot, 46100 València, Spain; josefa.tolosa@uv.es (J.T.); cristina.juan@uv.es (C.J.); m.jose.ruiz@uv.es (M.-J.R.)

2 ProtoQSAR, CEEI, Avda. Benjamin Franklin 12, Paterna, 46980 Valencia, Spain

* Correspondence: ana.juan@uv.es

Received: 21 March 2019; Accepted: 13 June 2019; Published: 14 June 2019

**Abstract:** Mycotoxins are produced by a number of fungal genera spp., for example, *Aspergillus*, *Penicillium*, *Alternaria*, *Fusarium*, and *Claviceps*. Beauvericin (BEA) and Ochratoxin A (OTA) are present in various cereal crops and processed grains. This goal of this study was to determine their combination effect in HepG2 cells, presented for the first time. In this study, the type of interaction among BEA and OTA through an isobologram method, cell cycle disturbance by flow cytometry, and genotoxic potential by in vitro micronucleus (MN) assay following the TG 487 (OECD, 2016) of BEA and OTA individually and combined in HepG2 cells are presented. Cytotoxic concentration ranges studied by the MTT assay over 24, 48, and 72 h were from 0 to 25 μM for BEA and from 0 to 100 μM for OTA, while BEA + OTA combinations were at a 1:10 ratio from 3.4 to 27.5 μM. The toxicity observed for BEA was higher than for OTA at all times assayed; additive and synergistic effects were detected for their mixtures. Cell cycle arrest in the G0/G1 phase was detected for OTA and BEA + OTA treatments in HepG2 cells. Genotoxicity revealed significant effects for BEA, OTA, and in combinations underlining the importance of studying real exposure scenarios of chronic exposure to mycotoxins.

**Keywords:** ochratoxin A; beauvericin; mixtures; HepG2 cells; genotoxicity; cell cycle

**Key Contribution:** Single mycotoxins OTA and BEA and their mixtures produce cytotoxicity, genotoxicity, and cell cycle disturbance in HepG2 cells.

## 1. Introduction

The presence of mycotoxins in food and feed have associated toxicological effects in consumers such as nephrotoxicity, hepatotoxicity, teratogenicity, etc., or potential effects such as synergism, additive or antagonism when a combination of more than one mycotoxin occurs [1–5]. The overall evidence on mixture effects indicates that combined effects can arise when each mixture component is present at doses around or above its no-effect level and provides a strong basis for developing robust approaches to assess the risk of chemical mixtures to support decision making [6].

Studies of mixtures of mycotoxins are directed to find whether there is an interaction between them, and if so, whether this interaction potentiates or diminishes the toxic effects of mycotoxins tested individually. When there is no interaction of mycotoxins between them, their effect is described as additive; while if the combination increases or decreases, the effect expected is described as a synergistic or antagonistic interaction, respectively. For this purpose, several models can be used to study such interactions. The mathematical model "*Loewe Additivity*" uses the isobologram equation proposed by Chou and Talalay et al. [7,8], which involves plotting the dose–effect curves (defined to a certain inhibition level) for each compound and their combinations in multiple diluted concentrations as described elsewhere [1–3,9].

The presence and co-presence of more than one mycotoxin in food and feed due to the ability of most *Fusarium* to simultaneously produce different mycotoxins is very common; thus, exposure to multi-mycotoxins often occurs [10–12]. Mixtures found worldwide have started to increase and become more diverse over the last decade due to the climatic changes and favorable growth conditions of different fungi spp. [12].

The EFSA has recently published a Draft Guidance document where a harmonized risk assessment methodology for combined exposure to multiple chemicals for all relevant areas is described (EFSA Journal 2018). There are specific requirements for chemical mixture risk assessment on the use of pesticides and food and feed additives [13,14], while for some mycotoxins, the sum of T-2 and HT-2 and the sum of aflatoxin B1 (AFB1), aflatoxin B2 (AFB2), aflatoxin G1 (AFG1), and aflatoxin G2 (AFG2) are underpinned in Regulation (EC) 1881/2006 [15]; however, neither beauvericin (BEA) nor ochratoxin A (OTA) are included.

For detecting genotoxicity, micronuclei (MN) induction assay has been accepted, validated, and recently updated in the Test Guideline 487 (TG 487) by the OECD [16]; and the inclusion of flow cytometry in the new TG 487 is a novelty which allows to determine cell cycle effect and MN-induction simultaneously [17,18]. Most of the articles published perform in vitro detection of MN through cytokinesis-block micronucleus (CBMN) assay for genotoxicity studies of mycotoxins produced by different fungal genera (*Fusarium*, *Penicillium*, and *Aspergillus*). Studies for Ochratoxin A (OTA), citrinin (CTN), patulin (PAT), beauvericin (BEA) [19–26], and aflatoxin B1 (AFB1) [27] can be found.

The new findings from cytotoxicity induced by binary mixtures of BEA + OTA in PK-15 cells and human leukocytes reveal that combined toxicity is higher than predicted from individuals; in fact, synergism and additive effects have been reported [28].

The in vitro system HepG2 cells are commonly used in toxicological studies. Effects reported for BEA, OTA, and its combination are diverse and it depends on different factors such as intake dose, exposure frequency, and timing of functional assays; in fact, their combination effect in HepG2 cells is here presented for the first time. In this study, the type of interaction between BEA and OTA through an isobologram method was studied. It is also presented the results of studying cell cycle disturbance by flow cytometry and genotoxic potential by in vitro micronucleus (MN) assay following the TG 487 [16] for BEA and OTA individually and in different mixtures in HepG2 cells.

## 2. Results

### 2.1. Cytotoxicity of Individual and Combined Mycotoxins

Ceauvericin and OTA mycotoxins and their combination on HepG2 cells during 24, 48, and 72 h were studied through the MTT assay to evaluate the cytotoxicity. The assay was driven to determine the $IC_{50}$ (inhibition of cell population to 50%) value. The $IC_{50}$ values denoted that BEA was above OTA (BEA > OTA) in toxicity potential when individual treatment was evaluated (Figure 1a,b and Table 1); however, a dose-dependent manner (Figure 1c) of toxicity in $IC_{50}$ values was achieved for mixtures of both mycotoxins. The highest toxic effect belonged to BEA at 72 h expressed by an $IC_{50}$ level of 5.5 ± 0.071 μM. The $IC_{50}$ values for each mycotoxin at different times of exposure are shown in Table 1.

For the BEA represented in Figure 1a, a concentration range of 2.5 to 25 μM viability values decreased in a time-dependent manner. At 24 h, reduction of viability was from 54 to 43%, whereas the reduction of viability was from 60 to 82% and from 90 to 73% for 48 h and 72 h, respectively. Figure 1b shows the concentration-dependent decrease of viability of HepG2 cells after OTA treatment. It produced a reduction of viability from 70 to 30% and from 65 to 47% at 24 and 48 h, respectively, whereas the reduction of viability for 72 h varied from 93 to 82%.

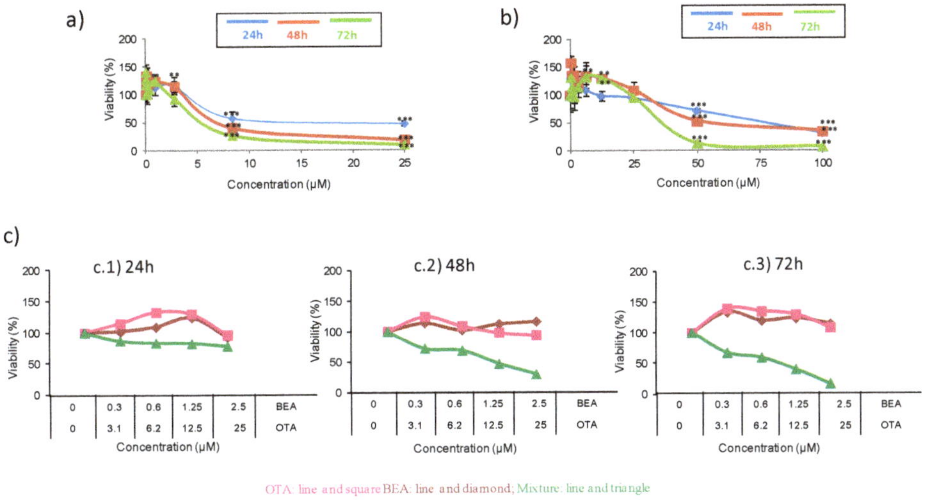


**Figure 1.** Cytotoxicity of BEA (**a**), OTA (**b**), and BEA + OTA (**c**) on HepG2 cells at mycotoxin exposures of 24, 48, and 72 h. The concentration for OTA mycotoxin was 0–100 μM (1:2 dilution), for BEA 0–25 μM (1:3 dilution), while for BEA + OTA at 1:10 ratio. * $p \leq 0.05$.

**Table 1.** The medium inhibitory concentration ($IC_{50}$) of beauvericin (BEA) and Ochratoxin A (OTA) in HepG2 cells after 24, 48, and 72 h of exposure by MTT assay.

| **Mycotoxins** | **$IC_{50}$ (μM)** | | |
|---|---|---|---|
| | **24 h** | **48 h** | **72 h** |
| OTA | 75 ± 0.04 | 52.62 ± 0.06 | 36 ± 0.09 |
| BEA | 12.5 ± 0.04 | 7.01 ± 0.05 | 5.5 ± 0.07 |

Figure 1c shows the concentration-dependent decrease in the HepG2 cell viability with combined treatment of BEA + OTA (1:10) at exposure times of 24, 48, and 72 h. The $IC_{50}$ values were obtained for 24 and 48 h comprised in a concentration mixture range of BEA + OTA from 0.6 + 6.2 to 1.25 + 12.5 μM for both exposure times. The reduction of viability caused by the mycotoxin combination BEA + OTA (1:10) was different according to the exposure time: (i) at 24 h it oscillated between 6–49% and 3–26% for BEA and OTA, respectively, compared to the individual mycotoxin exposure; (ii) at 48 h, the reduction oscillated between 25–84% and 40–78% for BEA and OTA, respectively, compared to the individual mycotoxin exposure. Finally, at 72 h, reduction of viability oscillated between 19–77% and 31–83% for BEA and OTA, respectively, compared to the individual mycotoxin exposure.

The isobologram analysis was used to determine the type of interaction between BEA and OTA. The parameters *Dm*, *m*, and *r* of the binary and tertiary combinations, as well as mean combination index (CI) values are shown in Table 2. The CI versus fractional effect (*fa*) curves for BEA and OTA combinations in HepG2 cells are shown in Figure 2. Both Table 2 and Figure 2 demonstrated that the main effect caused by binary mixtures of BEA and OTA is synergism; however, for BEA + OTA mixture at 24 h, additive effect was observed as well as at 48 h for the highest CI evaluated (Figure 2 and Table 2).

**Table 2.** The parameters *Dm*, *m*, and *r* are the antilog of x-intercept, the slope, and the linear correlation of the median-effect plot, which signifies the shape of the dose–effect curve, the potency ($IC_{50}$), and the conformity of the data to the mass action law, respectively [7,8]. *Dm* and *m* values are used for calculating the CI value (CI < 1, =1 and >1 indicates synergism (Syn), additive (Add), and antagonism (Ant) effects, respectively. $IC_{25}$, $IC_{50}$, $IC_{75}$, and $IC_{90}$ are the doses required to inhibit proliferation at 25, 50, 75, and 90%, respectively. CalcuSyn Software provide automatically these values.

| Mycotoxin | Time (h) | *Dm* (μM) | *m* | *r* | CI Values | | | | | | | |
|---|---|---|---|---|---|---|---|---|---|---|---|---|
| | | | | | $CI_{25}$ | | $CI_{50}$ | | $CI_{75}$ | | $CI_{90}$ | |
| BEA | 24 | 19.12 | 2.51 | 0.907 | | | | | | | | |
| | 48 | 13.13 | 2.94 | 0.920 | | | | | | | | |
| | 72 | 8.19 | 2.37 | 0.967 | | | | | | | | |
| OTA | 24 | 86.73 | 2.02 | 0.960 | | | | | | | | |
| | 48 | 77.57 | 4.24 | 0.915 | | | | | | | | |
| | 72 | 46.64 | 4.01 | 0.956 | | | | | | | | |
| BEA + OTA | 24 | 6.95 | 2.15 | 0.636 | 1.17 ± 2.48 | Add | 1.17 ± 3.8 | Add | 1.17 ± 5.8 | Add | 1.17 ± 8.9 | Add |
| | 48 | 1.79 | 1.86 | 0.948 | 0.27 ± 0.08 | Syn | 0.37 ± 0.14 | Syn | 0.49 ± 0.24 | Syn | 0.65 ± 0.42 | Add |
| | 72 | 0.95 | 1.57 | 0.987 | 0.22 ± 0.04 | Syn | 0.32 ± 0.06 | Syn | 0.46 ± 0.10 | Syn | 0.66 ± 0.19 | Syn |

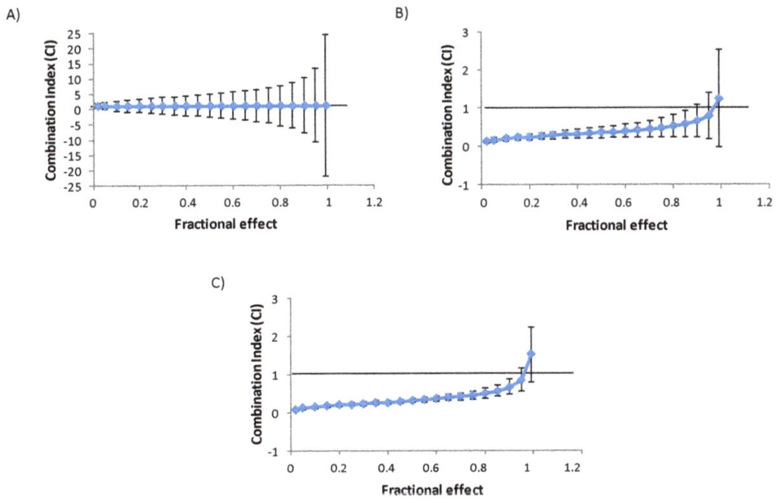


**Figure 2.** Combination index (CI) versus fractional effect curve as described by Chou and Talalay [7] model on HepG2 cells exposed to BEA + OTA (1:10) in binary combination. Each point represents the CI ± SD at a fractional effect as determined in our experiments. The line (CI = 1) indicates additivity, the area under this line synergism, and the area above the line antagonism. HepG2 cells were exposed during 24 (**A**), 48 (**B**), and 72 h (**C**) to BEA + OTA at a molar ratio of 1:10 (equimolar proportion).

### 2.2. Cell Cycle Distribution in Individual Mycotoxin Exposure

Analysis of DNA content by flow cytometry provides a measure of cell cycle perturbation in HepG2 cells following exposure to BEA, OTA, and BEA + OTA (Figure 3).

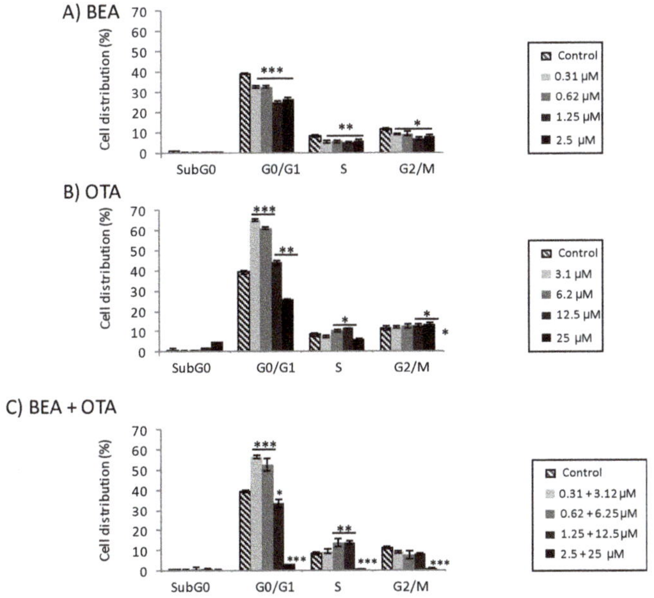


**Figure 3.** Cell cycle distribution in HepG2 cells exposed after 48 h to BEA (**A**), OTA (**B**), and BEA + OTA (1:10 molar proportion) (**C**). Data are expressed as mean ± SEM ($n$ = 3). * $p \leq 0.05$, ** $p \leq 0.01$, and *** $p \leq 0.001$ indicates significant differences compared to control.

Results for BEA exposure to all concentrations assayed resulted in statistically significant differences with respect to the control for all phases: G0/G1 ($p \leq 0.001$), S ($p \leq 0.01$), and G2/M ($p \leq 0.05$) (Figure 3A). Effects observed correspond to a statistically significant decrease in the percentage of the number of cells compared to the control. For OTA exposure to all concentrations assayed, the results were a statistically significant increase with respect to the control for the G0/G1 phase ($p \leq 0.001$ and $p \leq 0.01$ for both higher and lower concentrations, respectively) (Figure 3B). Similarly, this happened for the S and G2/M phases for doses of 6.2 and 12.5 μM (S phase), and 12.5 and 25 μM (G2/M phase). The sub-G0 phase reported an increase of HepG2 cells at the highest concentration assayed (25 μM, $p \leq 0.01$).

Regarding binary mixture BEA + OTA, a statistically significant increase was observed for the G0/G1 phase at concentrations of 0.31 + 3.12 and 0.62 + 6.25 μM and in the S phase for 1.25 + 12.5 and 2.5 + 25 μM compared to the control (Figure 3C).

### 2.3. Micronuclei Induction in Individual and Combined Mycotoxin Exposure

Figure 4 collects MN frequencies in HepG2 cells exposed to BEA, OTA, and BEA + OTA. Among all two individual treatments, the increase effect on MN frequency was detected for BEA at a concentration of 1.25 μM (14.2 ± 1.1%, $p \leq 0.01$). OTA revealed decreasing differences in respect to the no-treatment control for all concentrations except at 25 μM where statistically significant increases were detected ($p \leq 0.05$). Regarding BEA + OTA combined treatments, increases in MN frequency at the lowest concentrations assayed were detected as follows: 28.3 ± 1.32% and 24.0 ± 0.97% for 0.31 + 3.12 and 0.62 + 6.25 μM ($p \leq 0.01$), respectively.

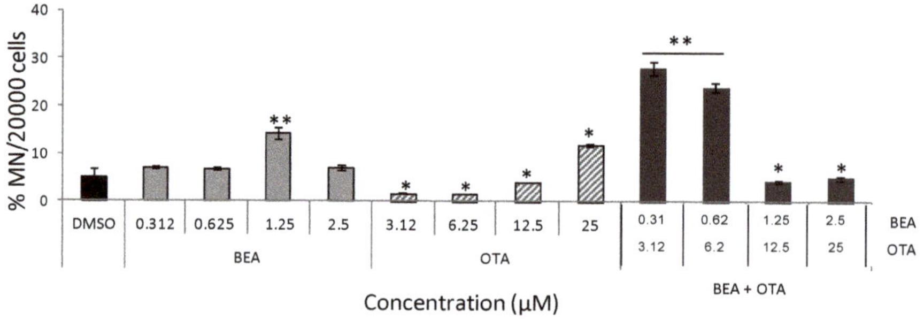


**Figure 4.** Induction of micronuclei in HepG2 cells treated by BEA, OTA, and BEA + OTA at several concentrations for 48 h. Results are expressed as a percentage of MN per 20,000 cells ± SEM ($n = 3$). $p \leq 0.05$ (*) and $p \leq 0.001$ (**), significantly different from the control.

## 3. Discussion

Cytotoxicity of BEA and OTA in HepG2 cells either in single or combined treatment was detected; subsequently, cell cycle alterations and micronuclei induction either individually or combined were assayed.

Among both mycotoxins, literature of OTA is wider than that compared to BEA; therefore, several studies performed in in vitro or in vivo models can be found. OTA has been classified as group 2B by the International Agency of Research in Cancer (IARC) and appears in the regulation EC No 1881/2006 [15] and recommendations [29] by the EC in respect to maximum levels in food and feed; in contrast, BEA is not classified as a carcinogen to humans and is not included in the Commission Regulation (EC) No 1881/2006 [15], which established maximum levels for specific contaminants to protect public health. However, efforts are focused in this mycotoxin, since in 2018 the EFSA published a Scientific Report related to in vivo toxicity and genotoxicity of BEA based on the fact that there are insufficient data to establish its reference values.

Regarding cytotoxicity, several authors studied OTA (0–200 μM at 4–24 h) in primary rat PT and LLC-PK1 cells [30], and $IC_{50}$ values were of 1.1-fold higher and 0.3-fold lower, respectively, to each cell line compared to those obtained for HepG2 cells at 24 h in this study. In BME-UV1 and MDCK cells, OTA $IC_{50}$ values were 0.8 and 1 μg/mL, respectively, showing a high sensitivity in this cell type compared with other cell models [31]. The HepG2 cells exposed to OTA (10–50 μM) reached an $IC_{50}$ value 0.6-fold lower than that obtained in this study for the same period of time (24 h). This can be related with the type of cells used; in this study, HepG2 were used, which are characterized by containing high enzymatic activity. Several studies have revealed alterations in different enzyme activities after OTA exposure, indicating such effect as a potential target for OTA mycotoxin [32].

On the other hand, cytotoxic studies of BEA can also be found. CCRF-CEM cells exposed to BEA (1–10 μM) for 24 h [33] revealed an $IC_{50}$ value 9.8-fold smaller than that of the HepG2 cells in this study. In HT-29 cells, $IC_{50}$ values were closer to those reported here differing 0.8- and 0.7-fold lower for 24 and 48 h, respectively; while for Caco-2 cells, it was 0.6- and 0.5-fold lower for 24 and 48 h, respectively [34,35]. In general terms, comparing data from the literature with the results of this work, BEA $IC_{50}$ values of HepG2 cells were smaller than those obtained with other cell lines; however, for the cell line CHO-K1, higher cytotoxicity was revealed since $IC_{50}$ values were lower than those obtained in this study (1.2- and 3.18-fold lower for 24 and 72 h, respectively) [36]. An explanation for HepG2 sensitivity might be related to the high enzyme activity of these cells and the possibility that BEA exerts cytotoxicity associated to its hexadepsipeptide structure which is able to affect DNA migration, intracellular calcium levels, and apoptosis, as reported [28].

A study on PK-15 cells at fixed doses of BEA and OTA revealed decreases in viability for BEA at 35% (5 μg/mL, 24 h) and 26% (0.5 μg/mL, 48 h); while for OTA at 32% (5 μg/mL, 24 h) and 23% (0.5 μg/mL, 48 h) but no $IC_{50}$ values were reached for any mycotoxin [37]. However, human leukocytes exposed to BEA, OTA, and BEA + OTA after 24 h, reached $IC_{50}$ values 2.5- and 4.74-fold lower for BEA and OTA, respectively, compared to those for HepG2 cells reported in this study [28], which coincides with our results of OTA being less toxic than BEA. When studying BEA + OTA (at a 1:10 ratio) (24 h) additive and synergism effects were observed in PK-15 cells [28]; at short times (24 h) in our study, only the additive effect was observed (see Table 2 and Figure 2). Differences in such combination effects could be associated to cell type but also to the concentration assayed. Klaric et al. [28] assayed from 3- to 5-times lower than the concentration of BEA and OTA, respectively, when combined, compared to the ones presented here where the effect was measured with the isobologram analysis, while Klaric et al. [28] reported effects comparing prediction between expected and measured values.

Cytotoxicity observed in HepG2 cells after exposure to mycotoxins BEA and OTA can interfere in cell proliferation; so, the study of phases in cell cycle distribution (Figure 3) and its association with MN induction were studied (Figure 4). In general terms, cell cycle accumulation in the G0/G1 phase was detected for OTA (all concentrations except at 25 μM) and its combination with BEA (at the lowest concentrations assayed), while for BEA a decrease in G0/G1 was detected, revealing induction of cell death at the concentrations assayed. The HepG2 cells need 48 h to occur 1.5–2 times more than the normal cell cycle division, which is the condition needed to perform the MN assay according to OCDE TG 487. Cell cycle and MN assays were performed in the same conditions to associate alterations in cell cycle and MN induction as described by Juan-García et al. [18]. Among that, although there are few studies carried out in evaluating genotoxicity for BEA and OTA, to our knowledge, this is the first report on BEA, OTA, and BEA + OTA genotoxicity determined by flow cytometry, as approved in the reviewed version of OCDE TG 487 from July 2016.

Results for BEA in the cell cycle disturbed the distribution of phases compared to the control as described in Section 2.2; however, BEA 1.25 μM reported differences in all cell cycle phases in respect to the control (Figure 3A) and the strongest MN induction (Figure 4). Positive results have been reported for genotoxicity of BEA through cytokinesis-block micronucleus (CBMN) assay [26] and the COMET assay [28] as well as negatives [38]. Our results coincide with those positives which for all concentrations BEA MN-induction (here through flow cytometry) in HepG2 cells was observed but it was only statistically significant at 1.25 μM.

For OTA, a marked arrest in the G0/G1 phase at the lowest concentration assayed was detected (Figure 3B), which reveals that the HepG2 cells had everything in the cells ready for DNA synthesis but no DNA division happened. This point is associated with the fact that no increase in MN induction was detected unless OTA-high doses were tested (Figure 4), coinciding with other authors [20]. Other authors have compared genotoxic assays (COMET and CBMN) in HepG2 cells exposed to OTA revealing formation of MN and associating this at least partly to clastogenic effects; although no additional assay to contrast the results were performed [19]. In the present study, MN formation was measured simultaneously with cell cycle and the results were linked (Figures 3 and 4). Previously, we performed this procedure for DON, 3-ADON and 15-ADON in the same cell line, and arrest in the G0/G1 phase was associated with MN induction and the procedure followed was the same as here (OECD TG487 reviewed in 2016 for cytoplasma MN detection in interphase cells) [18]. Several cell models, experimental conditions, and procedures have been used to study OTA-MN induction [21,39]. A recent study has been published using in Vero cells where OTA (25 μM, 30 min) produced a significant increase in the MN total number through CBMN assay [20]. It is important to mention that OTA is known as a DNA adducts-inductor [20]. Those chromosome breaks may point to a clastogenic mode of action if unrepaired. Thus, it is important to refer to the basis of each method and procedure followed; since MN generated through clastogenic or aneugenic events, are irreversible and persistent, and time that approximates a 1.5–2 normal cell cycle of the cell line is crucial.

Finally, the mycotoxin mixture OTA + BEA in HepG2 cells showed an arrest in the G0/G1 and S phases (Figure 3C) correlated with the MN induction detected (Figure 4). Mixture tested resulted in a stable solution (see Section 4.3). The natural occurrence of both mycotoxins has been reported in many maize fields and maize-based products worldwide [9,40]. According to the literature, BEA is not an inducer of the deletion of a DNA excision repair system gene [38], while oppositely, OTA has been reported as a DNA adducts-inductor [20]; therefore, this could support our results. DNA strand breaks through a COMET assay have been detected using a different in vitro system (PK-15 cells and human leukocytes) and exposure time for this combination and at doses lower than those presented in here (BEA: 0.1 and 0.5 μM; OTA: 1 and 5 μM). Coinciding with our results, a positive genotoxic effect was obtained.

In conclusion, individual and combined BEA and OTA cytotoxicity in HepG2 cells was studied. In binary mixtures, synergism and additive effect prevailed. Both OTA and BEA and their combinations provoked disturbance in the cell cycle and affected MN induction, thus underlining the importance of studying real exposure scenarios of chronic exposure to these toxins.

## 4. Materials and Methods

### 4.1. Reagents

All reagents and cell culture components were standard laboratory grade from Sigma–Aldrich (St. Louis, MO, USA). The standard of OTA (MW: 403.815 g/mol) and BEA (MW: 783.95 g/mol) was purchased from Sigma–Aldrich (St. Louis, MO, USA). Methanol (MeOH) was obtained from Fisher Scientific (Madrid, Spain). For MTT assay, thiazolyl blue tetrazolium bromide (approx. 98%; M2128-10G) was purchased from Sigma–Aldrich. A Milli-Q water purification system (Millipore, Bedford, MA, USA) permitted the obtainment of the deionized water (<18 MΩ cm resistivity). Stock solutions of mycotoxins were prepared in MeOH (OTA and BEA) and maintained at −20 °C in the dark. The final concentration of MeOH in the medium was ≤1% (*v*/*v*) as per established for performing this in vitro assays.

### 4.2. Cell Culture

Growth of HepG2 cells (ATCC HB-8065) was possible using Dulbecco's Modified Eagle's Medium (DMEM, Sigma–Aldrich) supplemented with antibiotic-free 10% newborn calf serum (NCS; Invitrogen, Christchurch, New Zealand), 100 U/mL penicillin, and 100 mg/mL streptomycin (Sigma–Aldrich). Cells were used between passages 12 and 19. The cells were trypsinized (Trypsin-EDTA, Sigma–Aldrich) and resuspended in complete medium in a 1:3 split ratio to perform the sub-cultivation. The procedure was repeated once or twice a week according to the monolayer confluence in flasks with filter screw caps (TPP, Trasadingen, Switzerland) at 37 °C in a humidified atmosphere and 5% $CO_2$.

### 4.3. Mycotoxin Exposure

In this study, concentration of mycotoxins and exposure time were two important factors to consider. Twenty-four, 48, and 72 h were the exposure times assayed in HepG2 cells for BEA and OTA either individually and combined. The situation of 72 h was considered due to the accumulation process possibly occurring because of the physicochemical properties of these compounds. Individual treatment was assayed at a concentration range of 0 to 25 μM for BEA (1:3 dilution), and at a range of 0 to 100 μM for OTA (1:2 dilution). For combination mixtures, individual treatment data were crucial for selecting starting concentration. Nevertheless, parallel assays of individual and combinations were performed for exact evaluation of combinatory effects. Concentration for combinations of both mycotoxins at a dilution ratio 1:10 (BEA + OTA) was from 3.3 to 27.5 μM, including four dilutions of each mycotoxin combination for BEA (0.3, 0.6, 1.25, and 2.5 μM) and OTA (3.1, 6.2, 12.5, and 25 μM).

### 4.4. In Vitro Cytotoxicity

The protocol published by Ruiz et al. [41], with slight modification, was followed to evaluate the cytotoxicity. It describes the MTT assay which consists of measuring the viability of cells by determining the reduction of the yellow, soluble tetrazolium salt only in cells that are metabolically active via a mitochondrial reaction to an insoluble, purple formazan crystal. The concentration of cells per well was $2 \times 10^4$ cells/well for culture plates of 96-wells. Cells adhered to the plates after 18–24 h, which was the elapsed time before proceeding with mycotoxin additions. Section 4.3 details the dilutions and combinations of mycotoxins tested for BEA and OTA. Fresh supplemented medium was used for preparing serial dilutions in the designed plate, while controls were prepared with culture medium with <1% methanol. After passing 24, 48 or 72 h, the medium containing the mycotoxin was removed and 200 μL of fresh medium containing 50 μL of MTT solution was added (5 mg/mL; MTT powder dissolved in phosphate buffered saline). Plates were kept for 4 h at 37 °C in darkness and afterwards the MTT was removed and 200 μL of DMSO and 25 μL of Soerensen's solution (composition: glycine 0.4 μM + 0.1 μM NaCl, pH 10.5) was added to each well. Plates were brought to read at 570 nm with the ELISA plate reader Multiskan EX (Thermo Scientific, Waltham, MA, USA). Replicates consisted of each mycotoxin combination plus a control tested in three independent experiments. Mean inhibition concentration ($IC_{50}$) values were calculated from full dose–response curves using the four parameter logistic equation with the SigmaPlot program. Three independent experiments were performed with eight replicates each.

### 4.5. Experimental Design and Combination Index

The isobologram analysis (Chou-Talalay model) was used to determine the type of interaction (synergism or antagonism effect) that occurs when mycotoxins studied were in combination. Chou-Talalay's model allows characterizing the interactions induced by combinations of mycotoxins, but no mechanisms associated can be elucidated. Combination effects are possible to analyze by the median-effect/combination index (CI)-isobologram equation by Chou [42] and Chou and Talalay [7]. The model involves plotting the dose–effect curves for each mycotoxin and its combinations in multiple diluted concentrations. There are several parameters included in the equation as *Dm* (the median-effect dose), *fa* (fraction affected by concentration), and *m* (coefficient signifying the shape of the dose–effect relationship) [7]. Therefore, both the potency (*Dm*) and shape (*m*) parameters are crucial for the evaluation.

The term combination index (CI) is included in Chou and Talalay's [42] method. According to the CI synergism, additive, and antagonism are, respectively, correlated as follows: CI < 1, =1, and >1. CalcuSyn software version 2.1. (Biosoft, Cambridge, UK, 1996–2007) was used to study the types of interactions assessed by isobologram analysis. It was decided to report $CI_{25}$, $CI_{50}$, $CI_{75}$, and $CI_{90}$ doses to produce toxicity at 25%, 50%, 75%, and 90%, respectively.

### 4.6. Cell Cycle Analysis by Flow Cytometry

Vindelov's PI staining solution previously described [43] was used. PI is a DNA intercalating agent that only stains stoichiometrically the DNA of cells in the late phases of cell death, when the integrity of both cellular and nuclear membranes is lost. Cell proliferation and cell cycle distribution was performed using BD FACSCanto™ Flow Cytometer (Beckton–Dickinson, Italy) with FACSDiva software version 6.1.3 (BD Biosciences, San José, CA, USA, 2007).

For this assay, plates of 6 wells were used and the concentration of cells was $4.8 \times 10^5$. Cells were seeded for 24 h and exposed for 48 h to BEA at 0.31, 0.62, 1.25, and 2.5 μM for 48 h; and OTA at 3.12, 6.25, 12.5, and 25 μM for individual treatment. For combinations, range doses went from 3.43 to 27.5 μM including four dilutions of each combination. Then, cells were trypsinized and incubated at 37 °C for 30 min with 860 μL of fresh medium containing 29 ng/mL of Vindelov's PI staining solution. Cell cycle analysis was carried out as described by Minervini et al. [44], by rectangular fitting (CYLCHRED software, Beckton–Dickinson, Milan, Italy) using 1024 channels, which produced histograms with a single G0/G1 peak at channel 200 when DNA was diploid, an S-peak between channels 200 and 400 when DNA was replicating, a G2/M peak at channels 400 when DNA was tetraploid, and a Sub-G0 peak (debris peak), between 100 and 200 when DNA was hypodiploid or damaged. The reduced coefficient of variation (CV) obtained in this study was the result of the high resolution reached by proper alignment. The positive control used was cicloheximide (CLX) (40 μg/mL), known as synthesis of proteins inhibitor that leads to cellular quiescence and cell death by apoptosis. Three independent experiments were performed for OTA and BEA and at least 10,000 cells were analyzed for each sample.

### 4.7. Genotoxic Evaluation by Micronucleus Detection through Flow Cytometry

Litron In Vitro Microflow Kit (Litron Laboratories, Rochester, NY, USA) was used for the micronucleus assay on HepG2 cells exposed to mycotoxins by flow cytometry following the OECD TG487. Conditions set for this assay point that it must be carried out after exposure of cells to the toxic during a time that approximates a 1.5–2-times normal cell cycle. For HepG2 cells, this time was set to 48 h; which doubled the time period necessary for this type of cell (2 normal cycles). Concentrations were maintained as per those detailed in Section 4.5 and were also used in the cell cycle assay. Previous reports [18,45–48] and manufacturer's instructions (Litron Laboratories, 2009) were followed, all according to the framework of the OECD Guideline [16].

Briefly, in 24-well plates, HepG2 cells ($2 \times 10^6$ cells/mL) were seeded and treated with BEA and OTA as detailed in Section 4.5 for 48 h. The day of the experiment Nucleic Acid Dye A Solution was added to the cells, placed on ice, and exposed to light for 30 min for photoactivation of the EMA flurorochrome dye. Afterwards, cells were washed and lysed with the Litron Lysis kit solution and preserved from light for 60 min. Afterwards, cells were gently resuspended and a lysis solution 2 containing Nucleic Acid Dye B (SYTOX flurorochrome) was added, incubated for 30 min at room temperature in the dark, and analyzed by flow cytometry. Gating cell population and analysis strategies were performed with the FACS Fortesa 7.1 software following the instructions and template provided with the in vitro microflow kit manual and as described by Bryce et al. [46,47]. The control cells received equal volume of the vehicle (cell culture medium). Etoposide was used as the positive control [45,47,49]. The percentage of micronucleus was determined after acquiring a total of 20,000 gated nuclei events per sample as indicated in OECD TG 487 for MN evaluation through flow cytometry.

### 4.8. Statistical Analysis

Statistical analysis of data was carried out using the IBM SPSS Statistic version 24.0 (SPSS, Chicago, IL, USA, 2017) statistical software package. Data were expressed as the mean ± SEM of four independent experiments. The statistical analysis of the results was performed by student's *t*-test for paired samples. Differences between groups were statistically analyzed using ANOVA followed by the Tukey HDS post-hoc test for multiple comparisons. $p \leq 0.05$ was considered statistically significant.

**Author Contributions:** Conceptualization: A.J.-G.; Methodology: A.J.-G.; Software: A.J.-G.; Validation: A.J.-G.; Formal analysis: A.J.-G.; Investigation: A.J.-G. and M.-J.R.; Resources: A.J.-G., C.J., J.T. and M.-J.R.; Data curation: A.J.-G.; Writing—Original Draft Preparation: A.J.-G. and C.J.; Writing—Review & Editing: A.J.-G. and M.-J.R.; Visualization: A.J.-G.; Supervision: M.-J.R.; Project Administration: M.-J.R.; Funding Acquisition: M.-J.R., C.J. and A.J.-G.

**Funding:** This research was funded by Spanish Ministry of Economy and Competitiveness grant number AGL2016-77610-R.

**Acknowledgments:** This work has been funded by the Spanish Ministry of Economy and Competitiveness AGL2016-77610-R.

**Conflicts of Interest:** The authors declare no conflict of interest.

## References

1. Juan-García, A.; Juan, C.; Manyes, L.; Ruiz, M.J. Binary and tertiary combination of alternariol, 3-acetyl-deoxynivalenol and 15-acetyl-deoxynivalenol on HepG2 cells: Toxic effects and evaluation of degradation products. *Toxicol. In Vitro* **2016**, *34*, 264–273. [CrossRef] [PubMed]
2. Juan-García, A.; Juan, C.; Tolosa, J.; Ruiz, M.J. Effects of deoxynivalenol, 3-acetyl-deoxynivalenol and 15-acetyl-deoxynivalenol on parameters associated with oxidative stress in HepG2 cells. *Mycotoxin Res.* **2019**, 1–9. [CrossRef] [PubMed]
3. Ruiz, M.J.; Franzova, P.; Juan-García, A.; Font, G. Toxicological interactions between the mycotoxins beauvericin, deoxynivalenol and T-2 toxin in CHO-K1 cells in vitro. *Toxicon* **2011**, *58*, 315–326. [CrossRef] [PubMed]
4. Ruiz, M.J.; Macáková, P.; Juan-García, A.; Font, G. Cytotoxic effects of mycotoxin combinations in mammalian kidney cells. *Food Chem. Toxicol.* **2011**, *49*, 2718–2724. [CrossRef] [PubMed]
5. Ferrer, E.; Juan-García, A.; Font, G.; Ruiz, M.J. Reactive oxygen species induced by beauvericin, patulin and zearalenone in CHO-K1 cells. *Toxicol. In Vitro* **2009**, *23*, 1504–1509. [CrossRef] [PubMed]
6. Maranghi, F.; Tassinari, R.; Narcis, L.; Tait, S.; La Rocca, C.; Di Felice, G.; Butteroni, C.; Corinti, S.; Barletta, B.; Cordelli, E.; et al. In vivo toxicity and genotoxicity of beauvericin and enniatins. Combined approach to study in vivo toxicity and genotoxicity of mycotoxins beauvericin (BEA) and enniatin B (ENNB). *EFSA Support. Publ.* **2018**, *15*, 1406E. [CrossRef]
7. Chou, T.C.; Talalay, P. Quantitative analysis of dose-effect relationships: The combined effects of multiple drugs or enzyme inhibitors. *Adv. Enzym. Regul.* **1984**, *22*, 27–55. [CrossRef]
8. Chou, T.C.; Hayball, M.P. *CalcuSyn for Windows: Multiple-drug Dose-effect Analyzer and Manual*; Biosoft: Cambridge, UK, 1997.
9. Juan-García, A.; Juan, C.; König, B.; Ruiz, M.J. Cytotoxic effects and degradation products of three mycotoxins: Alternariol, 3-acetyl-deoxynivalenol and 15-acetyl-deoxynivalenol in liver hepatocellular carcinoma cells. *Toxicol. Lett.* **2015**, *235*, 8–16. [CrossRef]
10. Juan, C.; Berrada, H.; Mañes, J.; Oueslati, S. Multi-mycotoxin determination in barley and derived products from Tunisia and estimation of their dietary intake. *Food Chem. Toxicol.* **2017**, *103*, 148–156. [CrossRef]
11. Oueslati, S.; Berrada, H.; Mañes, J.; Juan, C. Presence of mycotoxins in Tunisian infant foods samples and subsequent risk assessment. *Food Control* **2017**, *84*, 362–369. [CrossRef]
12. Stanciu, O.; Juan, C.; Miere, D.; Loghin, F.; Mañes, J. Occurrence and co-occurrence of Fusarium mycotoxins in wheat grains and wheat flour from Romania. *Food Control* **2017**, *73*, 147–155. [CrossRef]

13. Regulation (EC) No 1107/2009 of the European Parliament and of the Council of 21 October 2009 Concerning the Placing of Plant Protection Products on the Market and Repealing Council Directives 79/117/EEC and 91/414/EEC. Official Journal of the European Union. Available online: http://data.europa.eu/eli/reg/2009/1107/oj (accessed on 8 November 2018).
14. Commission Regulation (EC) No 429/2008 of 25 April 2008 on Detailed Rules for the Implementation of Regulation (EC) No 1831/2003 of the European Parliament and of the Council as Regards the Preparation and the Presentation of Applications and the Assessment and the Authorisation of Feed Additives. Available online: http://data.europa.eu/eli/reg/2008/429/oj (accessed on 8 November 2018).
15. Commission Regulation (EC) No 1881/2006 of 19 December 2006 Setting Maximum Levels for Certain Contaminants in Foodstuffs. Available online: https://eur-lex.europa.eu/LexUriServ/LexUriServ.do?uri=OJ:L:2006:364:0005:0024:EN:PDF (accessed on 8 November 2018).
16. OECD. Test No. 487: In Vitro Mammalian Cell Micronucleus Test. *Series OECD Guidelines for the Testing of Chemicals, Section 4: Health Effects*. Available online: https://read.oecd-ilibrary.org/environment/test-no-487-in-vitro-mammalian-cell-micronucleus-test_9789264264861-en#page1 (accessed on 8 November 2018).
17. Shi, J.; Bezabhie, R.; Szkudlinska, A. Further evaluation of a flow cytometric in vitro micronuclei assay in CHO-K1 cells: A reliable platform that detects micronuclei and discriminates apoptotic bodies. *Mutagenesis* **2010**, *25*, 33–40. [CrossRef] [PubMed]
18. Juan-García, A.; Taroncher, M.; Font, G.; Ruiz, M.J. Micronucleus induction and cell cycle alterations produced by deoxynivalenol and its acetylated derivatives in individual and combined exposure on HepG2 cells. *Food Chem. Toxicol.* **2018**, *118*, 719–725.
19. Ehrlich, V.; Darroudi, F.; Uhl, M.; Steinkellner, H.; Gann, M.; Majer, B.J.; Eisenbauer, M.; Knasmüller, S. Genotoxic effects of ochratoxin A in human-derived hepatoma (HepG2) cells. *Food Chem. Toxicol.* **2002**, *40*, 1085–1090. [CrossRef]
20. Costa, J.; Saraiva, N.; Guerreiro, P.; Louro, H.; Silva, M.J.; Miranda, J.P.; Castro, M.; Batinic-Haberle, I.; Fernandes, A.S.; Oliveira, N.G. Ochratoxin A-induced cytotoxicity, genotoxicity and reactive oxygen species in kidney cells: An integrative approach of complementary endpoints. *Food Chem. Toxicol.* **2016**, *87*, 65–76. [CrossRef] [PubMed]
21. Ali, R.; Mittelstaedt, R.A.; Shaddock, J.G.; Ding, W.; Bhalli, J.A.; Khan, Q.M.; Heflich, R.H. Comparative analysis of micronuclei and DNA damage induced by Ochratoxin A in two mammalian cell lines. *Mutat. Res.* **2011**, *723*, 58–64. [CrossRef] [PubMed]
22. Knasmüller, S.; Cavin, C.; Chakraborty, A.; Darroudi, F.; Majer, B.J.; Huber, W.W.; Ehrlich, V.A. Structurally related mycotoxins ochratoxin A, ochratoxin B, and citrinin differ in their genotoxic activities and in their mode of action in human-derived liver (HepG2) cells: Implications for risk assessment. *Nutr. Cancer* **2004**, *50*, 190–197.
23. González-Arias, C.A.; Trinidad-Benitez, A.B.; Sordo, M.; Robledo-Marenco, L.; Medina-Día, I.M.; Barrón-Vivanco, B.S.; Marín, S.; Sanchis, V.; Ramos, A.J.; Rojas-García, A.E. Low doses of ochratoxin A induce micronucleus formation and delay DNA repair in human lymphocytes. *Food Chem. Toxicol.* **2014**, *74*, 249–254.
24. Dönmez-Altuntas, H.; Dumlupinar, G.; Imamoglu, N.; Hamurcu, Z.; Cem Liman, B. Effects of the mycotoxin citrinin on micronucleus formation in a cytokinesis-block genotoxicity assay in cultured human lymphocytes. *J. Appl. Toxicol.* **2006**, *27*, 337–341. [CrossRef]
25. Alves, I.; Oliveira, N.G.; Laires, A.; Rodrigues, A.S.; Rueff, J. Induction of micronuclei and chromosomal aberrations by the mycotoxin patulin in mammalian cells: Role of ascorbic acid as a modulator of patulin clastogenicity. *Mutagenesis* **2000**, *15*, 229–234. [CrossRef]
26. Celik, M.; Aksoy, H.; Yılmaz, S. Evaluation of beauvericin genotoxicity with the chromosomal aberrations, sister-chromatid exchanges and micronucleus assays. *Ecotoxicol. Environ. Saf.* **2010**, *73*, 1553–1557. [CrossRef] [PubMed]
27. Corcuera, L.A.; Vettorazzi, A.; Arbillaga, L.; Pérez, N.; Gil, A.G.; Azqueta, A.; González-Peñas, E.; García-Jalón, J.A.; López de Cerain, A. Genotoxicity of Aflatoxin B1 and Ochratoxin A after simultaneous application of the in vivo micronucleus and comet assay. *Food Chem. Toxicol.* **2015**, *76*, 116–224. [CrossRef] [PubMed]

28. Klaric, M.S.; Darabos, D.; Rozgaj, R.; Kasuba, V.; Pepeljnjak, S. Beauvericin and ochratoxin A genotoxicity evaluated using the alkaline comet assay: Single and combined genotoxic action. *Arch. Toxicol.* **2010**, *84*, 641–650. [CrossRef] [PubMed]
29. Commission Recommendation of 17 August 2006 on the Prevention and Reduction of Fusarium Toxins in Cereals and Cereal Products. Available online: http://data.europa.eu/eli/reco/2006/583/oj (accessed on 8 November 2018).
30. Schaaf, G.J.; Nijmeijer, S.M.; Maas, R.F.; Roestenberg, P.; de Groene, E.M.; Fink-Gremmels, J. The role of oxidative stress in the ochratoxin A-mediated toxicity in proximal tubular cells. *BBA- Mol. Basis Dis.* **2002**, *1588*, 149–158. [CrossRef]
31. Giromini, C.; Rebucci, R.; Fusi, E.; Rossi, L.; Saccone, F.; Baldi, A. Cytotoxicity, apoptosis, DNA damage and methylation in mammary and kidney epithelial cell lines exposed to ochratoxin A. *Cell Biol. Toxicol.* **2016**, *32*, 249–258. [CrossRef] [PubMed]
32. Ramyaa, P.; Krishnasamy, R.; Padma, V.V. Quercetin modulates OTA-induced oxidative stress and redox signaling in HepG2 cells—Up regulation of Nrf2 expression and downregulation of NF-jB and COX-2. *BBA-Gen. Subj.* **2014**, *1840*, 681–692. [CrossRef] [PubMed]
33. Jow, G.M.; Chou, C.J.; Chen, B.F.; Tsai, J.H. Beauvericin induces cytotoxic effects in human acute lymphoblastic leukemia cells through cytochrome c release, caspase 3 activation: The causative role of calcium. *Cancer Lett.* **2004**, *216*, 165–173. [CrossRef]
34. Prosperini, A.; Meca, G.; Font, G.; Ruiz, M.J. Study of the cytotoxic activity of beauvericin and fusaproliferin and bioavailability in vitro on Caco-2 cells. *Food Chem. Toxicol.* **2012**, *50*, 2356–2361. [CrossRef]
35. Prosperini, A.; Juan-García, A.; Font, G.; Ruiz, M.J. Reactive oxygen species involment in apoptosis and mitochondrial damage in Caco-2 cells induced by enniatins A, A1, B and B1. *Toxicol. Lett.* **2013**, *222*, 36–44. [CrossRef]
36. Zouaoui, N.; Mallebrera, B.; Berrada, H.; Abid-Essefi, S.; Bacha, H.; Ruiz, M.J. Cytotoxic effects induced by patulin, sterigmatocystin and beauvericin on CHO-K1 cells. *Food Chem. Toxicol.* **2016**, *89*, 92–103. [CrossRef]
37. Klaric, M.S.; Papeljnjak, S.; Domijan, A.M.; Petrik, J. Lipid peroxidation and glutathione levels in porcine kidney PK15 cells after individual and combined treatment with fumonisin B1, beauvericin and ochratoxin a. *Basic Clin. Pharmacol. Toxicol.* **2006**, *100*, 157–164. [CrossRef] [PubMed]
38. Fotso, J.; Smith, J.S. Evaluation of beauvericin toxicity with the bacterial bioluminescence assay and the AMES mutagenicity bioassay. *J. Food Sci.* **2003**, *68*, 1938–1941. [CrossRef]
39. Follman, W.; Behn, C.; Degen, G.H. Toxicity of the mycotoxin citrinin and its metabolite dihydrocitrinone and of mixtures of citrinin and ochratoxin A in vitro. *Arch. Toxicol.* **2014**, *88*, 1097–1107. [CrossRef] [PubMed]
40. Domijan, A.; Peraica, M.; Cvjetkovic, B.; Turcin, S.; Jurjevic, Z.; Ivic, D. Mould contamination and co-occurrence of mycotoxins in maize grain in Croatia. *Acta Pharm.* **2005**, *55*, 349–356. [PubMed]
41. Ruiz, M.J.; Festila, L.E.; Fernández, M. Comparison of basal cytotoxicity of seven carbamates in CHO-K1 cells. *Toxicol. Environ. Chem.* **2006**, *88*, 345–354. [CrossRef]
42. Chou, T.C. Theoretical basis, experimental design, and computerized simulation of synergism and antagonism in drug combination studies. *Pharmacol. Rev.* **2006**, *58*, 621–681. [CrossRef] [PubMed]
43. Juan-García, A.; Manyes, L.; Ruiz, M.J.; Font, G. Involvement of enniatins-induced cytotoxicity in human HepG2 cells. *Toxicol. Lett.* **2013**, *218*, 166–173.
44. Minervini, F.; Fornelli, F.; Flynn, K.M. Toxicity and apoptosis induced by the mycotoxins nivalenol, deoxynivalenol and fumonisin B-1 in a human erythroleukemia cell line. *Toxicol. In Vitro* **2004**, *18*, 21–28. [CrossRef]
45. Bazin, E.; Mourot, A.; Humpage, A.R.; Fessard, V. Genotoxicity of a freshwater cyanotoxin, cylindrospermopsin, in two human cell lines: Caco-2 and HepaRG. Environ. *Mol. Mutagen.* **2010**, *51*, 251–259. [CrossRef]
46. Bryce, S.M.; Bemis, J.C.; Avlasevich, S.L.; Dertinger, S.D. In vitromicronucleus assay scored by flow cytometry provides a comprehensive evaluation of cytogenetic damage and cytotoxicity. *Mutat. Res.* **2007**, *630*, 78–91. [CrossRef]
47. Bryce, S.M.; Avlasevich, S.L.; Bemis, J.C.; Lukamowicz, M.; Elhajouji, A.; Van Goethem, F.; De Boeck, M.; Beerens, D.; Aerts, H.; Van Gompel, J.; et al. Interlaboratory evaluation of a flow cytometric high content in vitro micronucleus assay. *Mutat. Res.* **2008**, *650*, 181–195. [CrossRef] [PubMed]

48. Bryce, S.M.; Shi, J.; Nicolette, J.; Diehl, S.P.; Avlasevich, S.; Raja, S.; Bemis, J.C.; Dertinger, S.D. High content flocytometric micronucleus scoring method is applicable to attachment cells lines. *Environ. Mol. Mutagen.* **2010**, *51*, 260–266.
49. Sahu, S.C.; O'Donnel, M.W.; Wiesenfeld, P.L. Comparative hepatotoxicity of deoxynivalenol in rat, mouse and human liver cells in culture. *J. Appl. Toxicol.* **2010**, *30*, 566–573. [CrossRef] [PubMed]

*toxins*

MDPI

*Article*

# In Silico and In Vitro Studies of Mycotoxins and Their Cocktails; Their Toxicity and Its Mitigation by Silibinin Pre-Treatment

**Van Nguyen Tran [1], Jitka Viktorova [1], Katerina Augustynkova [1], Nikola Jelenova [1], Simona Dobiasova [1], Katerina Rehorova [1], Marie Fenclova [2], Milena Stranska-Zachariasova [2], Libor Vitek [3,4], Jana Hajslova [2] and Tomas Ruml [1,*]**

1 Department of Biochemistry and Microbiology, University of Chemistry and Technology, Technicka 3, 16628 Prague 6, Czech Republic
2 Department of Food Analysis and Nutrition, University of Chemistry and Technology, Technicka 3, 16628 Prague 6, Czech Republic
3 First Faculty of Medicine, Charles University, Katerinska 32, 12108 Prague 2, Czech Republic
4 Faculty General Hospital, U Nemocnice 2, 12808 Praha 2, Czech Republic
* Correspondence: rumlt@vscht.cz; Tel.: +420-220-443-021

Received: 30 December 2019; Accepted: 25 February 2020; Published: 28 February 2020

**Abstract:** Mycotoxins found in randomly selected commercial milk thistle dietary supplement were evaluated for their toxicity in silico and in vitro. Using in silico methods, the basic physicochemical, pharmacological, and toxicological properties of the mycotoxins were predicted using ACD/Percepta. The in vitro cytotoxicity of individual mycotoxins was determined in mouse macrophage (RAW 264.7), human hepatoblastoma (HepG2), and human embryonic kidney (HEK 293T) cells. In addition, we studied the bioavailability potential of mycotoxins and silibinin utilizing an in vitro transwell system with differentiated human colon adenocarcinoma cells (Caco-2) simulating mycotoxin transfer through the intestinal epithelial barrier. The $IC_{50}$ values for individual mycotoxins in studied cells were in the biologically relevant ranges as follows: 3.57–13.37 nM (T-2 toxin), 5.07–47.44 nM (HT-2 toxin), 3.66–17.74 nM (diacetoxyscirpenol). Furthermore, no acute toxicity was obtained for deoxynivalenol, beauvericin, zearalenone, enniatinENN-A, enniatin-A1, enniatin-B, enniatin-B1, alternariol, alternariol-9-methyl ether, tentoxin, and mycophenolic acid up to the 50 nM concentration. The acute toxicity of these mycotoxins in binary combinations exhibited antagonistic effects in the combinations of T-2 with DON, ENN-A1, or ENN-B, while the rest showed synergistic or additive effects. Silibinin had a significant protective effect against both the cytotoxicity of three mycotoxins (T-2 toxin, HT-2 toxin, DAS) and genotoxicity of AME, AOH, DON, and ENNs on HEK 293T. The bioavailability results confirmed that AME, DAS, ENN-B, TEN, T-2, and silibinin are transported through the epithelial cell layer and further metabolized. The bioavailability of silibinin is very similar to mycotoxins poor penetration.

**Keywords:** acute toxicity; combined toxicity; genotoxicity; cell protection; silibinin; in silico prediction; co-culture models

**Key Contribution:** Our data highlight the problem of mycotoxin cocktails, which usually occur in food and feed, whose effects are currently studied only simultaneously.

## 1. Introduction

Mycotoxins, toxic secondary metabolites produced by fungi, are contaminants that frequently occur in food and feed worldwide. The mycotoxigenic fungal genera involved in the human food chain are mainly *Fusarium*, *Aspergillus*, *Penicillium*, and *Alternaria* [1]. Trichothecenes and zearalenone (ZEA) belong to the most important classes of mycotoxins produced by *Fusarium* species [2]. Depending on their functional groups, trichothecenes have been divided into Groups A–D [3]. T-2 toxin (T-2), HT-2 toxin (HT-2), and diacetoxyscirpenol (DAS) are the main representatives of the Type A subgroup [4,5]. Deoxynivalenol (DON), also known as vomitoxin, is the most prevalent mycotoxin of the Type B trichothecenes [6]. Besides, Fusarium also produces emerging fusariotoxins such as beauvericin (BEA) and enniatins (ENNs) [7]. BEA and ENNs are cyclic depsipeptides, which consist of free electron pairs of oxygen carbonyl groups and tertiary amino groups of amide bonds giving these molecules the ability to act as nucleophiles [8]. Alternaria fungi contaminate a wide variety of food items such as cereals, fruits, wheat, barley, and sorghum, where it produces several toxins, with alternariol (AOH), alternariol-9-methyl ether (AME), and tentoxin (TEN) being the most important ones [9]. Penicillium species are known to produce mycophenolic acid (MPA) [10]. Despite their low acute cytotoxicity on human cell line compared to other mycotoxins, MPA has been shown to possess neurotoxic and immunosuppressive effects [11]. The effects of selected mycotoxins on cell functions are listed in Table 1.

**Table 1.** Toxicity of selected mycotoxins.

| Mycotoxins | Effects | References |
|---|---|---|
| T-2 and HT-2 | Inhibition of DNA, RNA, and protein synthesis.<br>Induction of mutations and apoptosis. | [12–15] |
| DAS | Inhibition of DNA and protein synthesis.<br>Suppression of macrophage phagocytic function. | [16,17] |
| DON | Inhibition of DNA, RNA, and protein synthesis.<br>Decrease of the cell proliferation. | [18,19] |
| ZEA | Activation of the estrogen receptor.<br>Inhibition of DNA and protein synthesis.<br>Triggering of lipid peroxidation and cell death. | [20–22] |
| BEA | Increase of the biological membrane.<br>Loss of ionic homeostasis.<br>Induction of lipid peroxidation. | [14,23,24] |
| ENNs | Increase of the membrane permeability for cations. | [25] |
| AOH and AME | Single and double strand DNA breaks.<br>Decrease of the cell proliferation. | [26–28] |
| TEN | ATP hydrolysis and inhibition of ATP synthesis. | [29] |
| MPA | Inhibition of inosine 5′-monophosphate dehydrogenase.<br>Blocking of the DNA synthesis and proliferation of both T and B lymphocytes. | [30,31] |

Although the main targets of mycotoxins are different, some of them have similar modes of actions and thus some additive effects of certain mycotoxins may be expected. Therefore, the presence of mycotoxins in plant products contaminated by several toxigenic fungi is an increasing health issue. Numerous studies have shown potential additive and even synergistic toxic effects of mycotoxins in vitro, summarized, e.g., in [32]. However, data on combined toxic effects of mycotoxins are generally limited and inconsistent. Most available publications in this field are dedicated to trichothecenes [33,34]. Moreover, reported studies focusing on the combined toxic effects of mycotoxins are incomparable to some extent due to the different experimental designs and conditions. For instance, the mixture of ZEA and DON showed a synergistic toxic effect in human hepatoblastoma HepG2 and RAW macrophage cells [18] but antagonistic effect in Bluegill fin fibroblast (BF-2 cells) [33]. Another study shows that, after 72 h of exposure, the combination of DON and T-2 toxins presented antagonistic effects in mammalian kidney epithelial (Vero) and Chinese hamster ovarian (CHO-K1) cells [14,23], while additive effects were observed in HepG2 cells [1]. In addition, the interaction between DON and T-2 varied from antagonism to synergism depending on the concentration and the ratio of mixtures. In general, in vitro studies of mycotoxin interactions have been mainly performed on single target cell lines. However, this does not fully mimic human metabolism or the complex interactions within the whole organism. Among other effects, such studies neglect intestinal epithelial transport and the first-pass hepatic metabolism [35].

Recently, the protective effects of silymarin or silibinin against mycotoxins have been reported in several publications. Silymarin extracted from seeds of *Silybum marianum* contains silibinin, isosilibinin, silydianin, and silychristin [36]. Silibinin, a major pharmacologically active compound, is a mixture of silybin A and silybin B. The studies of hepatoprotective effect of silymarin against fumonisin B1 (FB1) and aflatoxin B1 (AFB1) were performed in mice and bovine calves [37,38]. The FB1-induced hepatocyte damage was significantly diminished by the silymarin treatment. Silymarin decreased apoptosis rate, increased cell proliferation, and prevented the FB1-induced increase of TNF-$\alpha$ [37,39]. According to Naseer et al. [38], silymarin showed better results compared to choline chloride (liver tonics) in lowering the AFB1-induced serum aminotransferase, creatinine, and blood urea nitrogen. Silibinin has received much attention, but the negation of mycotoxins toxicity by silibinin has only been achieved on primary rat hepatocytes, isolated rat Kupffer cells, calves, and mice [37,38,40–42].

The in vitro co-culture system may offer suitable alternative to in vivo animal testing and it represents an indispensable tool to approximate the complex conditions in studies aimed at mycotoxin action mechanism in an organism [43]. There have been a few co-culture models used in vitro for studying the absorption of natural bioactive compounds and drug toxicity in hepatocytes [35,43–45]. However, this co-culture system was not used to test the efficacy of silibinin in preventing the effects of mycotoxins. In this context, we developed a simple in vitro co-culture model to investigate mycotoxin cytotoxicity on different cell lines. Then, this model was applied to evaluate potential protective effects of silibinin on mycotoxin toxicity.

The aim of this study was the complex evaluation of toxicity caused by mycotoxins and the possibility of using silibinin to prevent their cytotoxic effect. The toxicity of individual mycotoxins was predicted by in silico analysis and, after that, the data were verified in vitro. To show an additive and synergistic effects of mycotoxin mixtures, the binary mixture was formed by the addition of the second mycotoxin. Silibinin, the predominant compound of the *Silybum marianum*-based dietary supplement, was assessed for its potential protective capacity to prevent toxic effects of mycotoxins in tested cells.

## 2. Results and Discussion

As reported recently, milk thistle-based dietary supplements are usually a significant source of mycotoxins, especially those produced by *Fusarium* and *Alternaria* fungi [46,47]. For some of these mycotoxins, namely DON, HT2, T2, and ZEA, the human health risk has been assessed by European Food Safety Authority (EFSA) [48–53] and appropriate maximum limits exist for specific food commodities (1881/2006 EC). For other mycotoxins, such as DAS, ENNs, BEA, MPA, and *Alternaria* toxins, EFSA has not set the tolerable daily intake (TDI) values yet, especially because the relevant toxicity data are still missing, thus the risk assessment process has not been finished. Even though the scientific evidence for heightened toxicity from mycotoxins mixtures is mounting, the risk assessment process, thus the EU legislation, is based predominantly on assessments carried out on individual substances. In this paper, we report on toxicity of specific mycotoxins mixture typical for milk thistle-based preparations, and point to effects resulting from the co-occurrence of these toxins together with silymarin as the most abundant health positive component in this type of foods.

### 2.1. In Silico Prediction of Physicochemical, Pharmacological and Toxicological Properties

The basic physicochemical, pharmacological, and toxicological properties of the mycotoxins previously found in milk thistle-based dietary supplement were evaluated, as summarized in Table 2. Most of the found mycotoxins are soluble in octanol rather than in water. The only hydrophilic mycotoxin is DAS. On the opposite side, BEA is highly lipophilic with the logP value higher than five, which is the limit for bioavailability according to Lipinski's rule of five [54]. Besides BEA, the octanol–water partition coefficient corresponding to less than one per milliliter of water content was observed for AOH, AME, ENNs, MPA, and ZEA. The very low aqueous solubility of these compounds compromises bioavailability manifested by their poor penetration through the blood–brain barrier and sequestration by fatty tissues. Their poor passive diffusion through the barriers was confirmed by logBB and logPS values for AOH, AME, and MPA followed by high ability to plasma protein binding. In addition, DAS showed poor penetration through the barriers. On the opposite side, ENNs could penetrate and accumulate in CNS.

**Table 2.** In silico toxicity analysis of mycotoxins previously identified in milk thistle-based dietary supplement.

| **Parameters** | | ***Fusarium* Toxins** | | | | | | | | | | ***Alternaria* Toxins** | | | ***Penicillium* Toxin** | **Silibinin** |
|---|---|---|---|---|---|---|---|---|---|---|---|---|---|---|---|---|
| | | **trichothecenes** | | | | **others** | | | | | | | | | | |
| | | DON | HT-2 | T-2 | DAS | ZEA | ENN-A | ENN-A1 | ENN-B | ENN-B1 | BEA | AME | AOH | TEN | MPA | |
| **octanol–water partition coefficient** | logP | 1.5 | 1.2 | 2 | −0.4 | 4.1 | 4.7 * | 4.4 * | 3.9 * | 4.1 * | 5.9 * | 3.9 | 3.8 | 0.5 | 3.8 | 2.1 |
| **BBB (blood–brain barrier) permeability** | logPS | −2.2 | −2.0 | −2.0 | −3.8 | −1.4 | −1.3 | −1.4 | −1.8 | −1.6 | −1.4 | −1.6 | −1.9 | −2.5 | −2.9 | −2.9 |
| | logBB | 0.2 | 0.6 | 0.5 | −0.07 | 0.6 | 1.4 | 1.0 | 0.5 | 0.8 | 0.3 | −0.1 | −0.4 | −0.2 | −0.7 | −0.9 |
| **human serum affinity** | LogKa (HSA) | | | | | 4.0 * | | | | | | | | 3.4 * | 4.7 | |
| **plasma protein binding** | PPB (%) | | | | | 88.1 | | | | | | 97.0 * | 95.8 | 65.7 | 96.0 [a] | 98.0 |
| **estrogen receptor binding probability** | Log (RBA) > −3 | 0.0 * | 0.0 * | 0.0 | 0 | 0.9 | 0 [a] | 0 [a] | 0 [a] | 0 [a] | | 0.9 | 1.0 | 0 | | |
| **genotoxicity probability** | CHO/CHL all loci composite | 0.8 | 0.8 | 0.7 | 0.8 | 0.2 | 0.0 | 0.0 | 0.0 | 0.0 | 0.0 | 0.9 | 0.9 | 0.1 | 0.2 | 0.2 |
| | chromosomal aberration in vitro | 0.7 | 0.6 | 0.6 | 0.9 | 0.6 | 0.1 | 0.1 | 0.1 | 0.1 | 0.1 | 0.6 | 0.8 | 0.4 | 0.6 | 0.5 |
| | chromosomal aberration *in vivo* | 0.6 | 0.5 | 0.5 | 0.8 | 0.2 | 0.1 | 0.1 | 0.1 | 0.1 | 0.1 | 0.6 | 0.7 | 0.4 | 0.2 | 0.5 |
| | carcinogenicity in mice | 0.4 | 0.3 | 0.3 | 0.4 | 0.7 | 0.1 | 0.1 | 0.1 | 0.1 | 0.1 | 0.4 | 0.4 | 0.2 | 0.3 | 0.2 |
| **$LD_{50}$ for mouse** | (mg/kg) | 0.8 | 0.8 [a] | 0.9 | 1.2 | 3.3 * | 3.0 | 3.0 | 3.0 | 3.0 | 3.7 | | 3.4 * | 3.0 | 3.2 | |
| **P-gp substrate** | substrate probability | 0.8 | 0.9 | 0.9 | 0.8 * | 0.2 * | 1.0 | 1.0 | 0.9 | 0.9 | 1.0 * | | 0.1 | 0.8 * | 0.4 | 0.2 * |
| **Caco-2 permeability** | Pe ($10^{-4}$ cm/s) | 7.2 | 7.0 | 7.0 | 0.2 | 7.8 | 6.0 | 6.0 | 6.1 | 6.1 | 5.8 | 8.6 | 8.4 | 6.0 | 4.7 | 5.1 |
| **first pass metabolism** | | N | N | N | Y | N | N | N | Y/N | N | N | Y | Y | Y | Y | |

ACD/Percepta (ACD/Percepta Platform, version 2016, build 2911, Advanced Chemistry Development, Inc., Toronto, ON, Canada, www.acdlabs.com, 2016) was used to predict the most common physicochemical, pharmacokinetic, and toxicology properties. For ACD/Percepta data, a reliability index (RI) higher than 0.75 was considered as highly reliable (marked as [a]); RI < 0.5 was considered as borderline reliable (marked as *). AME, alternariol-9-methyl ether; AOH, alternariol; BEA, beauvericin; DAS, diacetoxyscirpenol; DON, deoxynivalenol; ENN A, enniatin A; ENN A1, enniatin A1; ENN B, enniatin B; ENN B1, enniatin B1; HT-2, HT-2 toxin; MPA, mycophenolic acid; T-2, T-2 toxin; TEN, tentoxin; ZEA, zearalenone.

Several mycotoxins (AOH, AME, and ZEA) showed ability to weakly bind to estrogen receptor (Table 2) and thus affect the endocrine system. From these mycotoxins, only ZEA is predicted to bind to the receptor strongly with the probability of 0.71 and high reliability (RI = 0.88). Genotoxicity was excluded for BEA, ENNs, MPA, TEN, and ZEA by the prediction tool. However, genotoxicity should be expected for AOH, AME, DAS, DON, HT-2, and T-2. The predicted lethal dose for mouse less than 1 ppm was observed for DON, HT-2, and T-2 followed by DAS. The highest lethal dose was found for BEA, which corresponds to its high logP value and low bioavailability. However, BEA is the only mycotoxin that is predicted as a good substrate of P-glycoprotein ($p = 0.9$, RI = 0.38), a transmembrane efflux pump comparable to classical P-gp substrates such as vinblastine, daunorubicin, or paclitaxel. This means that, even though BEA is not able to penetrate through barriers by passive absorption, it uses P-gp pump as the transporter-mediated penetration pathway. DAS, DON, ENNs, HT-2, T-2, and TEN are weaker substrates of P-gp than BEA. PepT1 (intestinal peptide transporter 1), ASBT (intestinal bile acid transporter), or other enzymes were not predicted to be actively involved in transport any of the tested compounds through the intestinal membrane.

In opposite to logP values, the high permeability via passive absorption across the Caco-2 layer was predicted for AOH, AME, DON, HT-2, and ZEA. The lowest permeability was predicted for DAS.

### 2.2. *Verification of the In Silico Prediction*

#### 2.2.1. Acute Toxicity of Pure Mycotoxins

The cytotoxic effect of T-2, HT-2, DAS, DON, BEA, ZEA, ENN-A, ENN-A1, ENN-B, ENN-B1, AOH, AME, TEN, and MPA on HepG2, Caco-2, RAW 264.7, and HEK 293T cells was evaluated by resazurin assay over 72 h to determine the mycotoxin concentration that halved the cellular viability ($IC_{50}$). The $IC_{50}$ (nM) values are demonstrated in Table 3. No $IC_{50}$ values were obtained for DON, BEA, ZEA, ENN-A, ENN-A1, ENN-B, ENN-B1, AOH, AME, TEN, and MPA because these toxins did not cause any acute cytotoxicity in a concertation range up to 50 nM. This concentration (50 nM) was chosen intentionally because it was equal to 5× exceeding the recommended daily dose under conditions of 100% bioavailability of the tested compounds. Therefore, this concentration covers absolutely the concentration which could be reached in human blood after oral administration of the supplement. These results are in accordance with observations of Fernández-Blanco et al. [55] studying the cytotoxicity of AME (0–100 μM) in Caco-2 cells. The same result for MPA was reported by Nielsen et al. [56] in human small intestinal cells, where no $IC_{50}$ values were achieved up to 156 nM concentration. Previous studies showed a statistically significant decrease in viability of cells treated at concentrations of BEA (3 μM), DON (1 μM), ZEA (25 μM), ENN-A (1 μM), A1 (1 μM), B (2 μM), B1 (2 μM), AOH (50 μM), and AME (25 μM) [14,19,57,58]. These results are in agreement with those presented in our study, which showed that mycotoxins including DON, BEA, ZEA, ENN-A, ENN-A1, ENN-B, ENN-B1, AOH, AME, TEN, and MPA did not decrease the viability at tested concentrations (up to 50 nM). The highest tested concentration is at least 5× higher than the possible concentration which can be reached by the chosen milk thistle-based dietary supplement (see Section 4.3). It means that even, if the recommended daily dose were exceeded, there would be no risk of acute toxicity of present mycotoxins.

**Table 3.** $IC_{50}$ of T-2, HT-2, and DAS on HepG2, Caco-2, HEK293T, and RAW 264.7 cell lines. Data are expressed as mean values ± SEM of independent experiments ($n = 3$), each with six technical replicates.

| **Mycotoxins (nM)** | **Cell lines** | | | |
|---|---|---|---|---|
| | **RAW 264.7** | **Caco-2** | **HepG2** | **HEK293T** |
| T-2 | 3.57 ± 0.27 | 13.37 ± 1.07 | 11.38 ± 0.37 | 3.87 ± 0.27 |
| HT-2 | 5.07 ± 0.46 | 44.23 ± 2.26 | 47.44 ± 1.29 | 21.22 ± 1.6 |
| DAS | 3.66 ± 0.37 | 17.74 ± 0.66 | 13.4 ± 1.79 | 6.58 ± 0.36 |

DAS, diacetoxyscirpenol; HT-2, HT-2 toxin; T-2, T-2 toxin.

Our results demonstrate that RAW 264.7 cells are extremely sensitive to T-2, HT-2, and DAS, and that T-2 was the most cytotoxic against all tested cell lines, consistent with Behm et al. [59]. These authors assessed the cytotoxicity of 14 mycotoxins in Chinese hamster lung fibroblast (V79 cells) and characterized T-2 as the most potent cytotoxic agent, followed by HT-2 and the other toxins tested. Similarly, previous studies also reported the $IC_{50}$ values for T-2 in the range of 3–500 nM in various mammalian cells [21,56,59,60]. The chemical analysis showed the following concentrations of acutely toxic mycotoxins expected to be in human blood after exposure to the recommended daily dose of milk thistle-based dietary supplement: 6.2 nM of T-2, 5.0 nM of HT-2, and 0.04 nM of DAS. It could be concluded that the doses of T-2 and HT-2 are in the range of $IC_{50}$; however, based on in silico prediction, their penetration through the cell membrane is really low. Therefore, it could be predicted that, after oral administration, neither T-2 nor HT-2 can reach the blood concentration causing the acute toxicity (see also Section 2.4).

The data of in silico and in vitro testing of acute toxicity are in good correlation. In both cases, T-2, HT-2, and DAS were found to be the most toxic mycotoxins. Based on in silico prediction, the doses of all other tested mycotoxins have to be 4-5× higher than those mentioned above, which is over the highest tested concentration as well as the concentration which can be reached in blood by milk thistle-based dietary supplement consumption. The only exception is DON, which was predicted to be as toxic as T-2 and HT-2 mycotoxins, but this was disproved by our in vitro measurements. The prediction was based on structural similarities of DON and T-2, HT-2, and DAS, belonging to the same group of trichothecenes characterized by the tetracyclic 12,13-epoxy trichothecene skeleton [61]. However, in contrast to the others, DON belongs to the Type B trichothecenes, which lack a carbonyl group at C-8 and hydroxyl group at C-7 [62]. Therefore, DON may be less toxic than other trichothecenes such as T-2 toxin. Sobrova et al. [63] published, in agreement with our results, that $LD_{50}$ for mice is several times higher (ranges from 46 to 78 mg/kg after oral administration) than the predicted value.

### 2.2.2. Genotoxicity of Single Mycotoxins

Comet assay, widely accepted to evaluate the genotoxic potential of many mycotoxins [64], was used also in our study, where DNA strand breaks in HEK293 cells exposed to mycotoxins (25 μM) were evaluated after 24 h treatment. The results demonstrate that incubation with AME, AOH, DON, and ENNs significantly increased the percentage of DNA in comet tail with respect to the negative control. However, no significant DNA damage was observed in the cells treated with BEA, MPA, TEN, and ZEA (Figure 1).

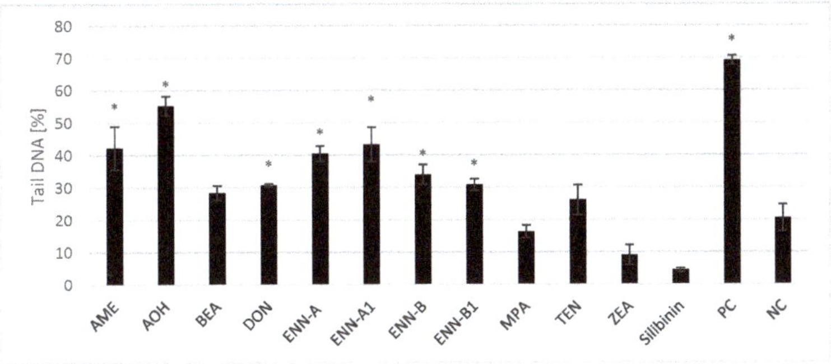


**Figure 1.** Percentage of DNA in comet tails measured by Comet assay in HEK 293T cells after the treatment with mycotoxins (25 μM) or silibinin (25 μM). Values are expressed as the mean ± SEM ($n$ = 4). * $p \leq 0.05$ indicates significant differences when compared to negative control (NC). AME, alternariol-9-methyl ether; AOH, alternariol; BEA, beauvericin; DON, deoxynivalenol; ENN A, enniatin A; ENN A1, enniatin A1; ENN B, enniatin B; ENN B1, enniatin B1; MPA, mycophenolic acid; TEN, tentoxin; ZEA, zearalenone.

Genotoxic properties of AOH and AME (25 μM) in HEK293T cells were confirmed by Comet assay where comet tails were about 55% and 42%, respectively. Previous work showed that AOH and AME significantly increased the rate of DNA breaks in human colon adenocarcinoma HT29 cells at concentrations ≥ 1 μM [65,66]. Fehr et al. [64] reported that AOH and AME potently bind to the minor groove of the DNA and act as topoisomerase inhibitors, which might also contribute to the DNA-damaging properties. Moreover, Tiessen et al. [66] indicated that oxidative stress does not play a predominant role in the induction of DNA damage by AOH and AME in HT29 cells.

The DON genotoxicity reported by Bonny et al. [67] in HepG2 and Caco-2 cells was consistent with our results. The DNA in comet tail increased significantly according to DON concentration ranging from 0.01 to 0.5 μM and the DNA breaks could be explained by DON genotoxicity partly related to the production of free radicals and ROS [67]. In contrast, in the study of Takakura et al. [68], DON (25 μM) failed to induce genotoxicity in human lymphoblast, thymidine kinase heterozygote TK6, and human hepatic HepaRG cells. This study showed that DON induced cytotoxicity without inducing primary DNA damage [68]. The differences may be due to variations among the used cell lines and lower sensitivity to oxidative stress of these cells compared to the HEK 293T cells [69].

Similar DNA damage was observed after 24 h exposure of PK15 and Caco-2 to BEA (0.5 and 12 μM, respectively) [70,71]. Nevertheless, no significant DNA damage was observed in the cells treated with BEA in our study. A similar result was obtained for BEA in the research of Dornetshuber et al. [72]. BEA significantly increased by 85% of DNA in tail with respect to the control at 1 μM but not at 5 μM after 24 h exposure. The reason is that, after 5 μM BEA exposure, antioxidant defense system activities were stimulated and therefore highly contributed to eliminate cell damage. Moreover, BEA inhibited the proliferation of damaged cells arresting them in G0/G1 phase and thus increased the apoptosis [73].

Regarding genotoxicity of ENNs, Prosperini et al. [74] reported significant DNA damage observed for ENN-A (1.5 μM), ENN-A1 (3 μM), and ENN-B1 (3 μM), whereas 3 μM ENN-B did not show genotoxic effect. This may be due to the lipophilicity of the ENNs with the most hydrophobic ENN-A and the least ENN-B (ENN-A > ENN-A1 > ENN-B1 > ENN-B). Moreover, increased ROS generation and lipid peroxidation was observed for all ENNs [74].

ZEA-induced oxidative effect on Chang liver cells was evaluated by Kang et al. [75], who found that growing concentrations of ZEA (50–200 μM) increased the DNA damage (from 7.43 ± 0.35% to 19.01 ± 0.42%) [75]. Other authors revealed that ZEA and its metabolites induced oxidative stress by increasing the level of ROS, which can cause damage to DNA [76]. Gao et al. [77] found that ZEA (2.5–20 μM, for 2 h) damaged DNA in HEK293 cells in a concentration-dependent manner. However, the results suggest lysosomes disruption rather than oxidative stress plays a key role in DNA strand breaks induced by ZEA. Therefore, the authors predicted the lysosomes as a primary target of ZEA [77]. On the contrary, we found that HEK 293T cells were resistant to the treatment with 25 μM of ZEA for 24 h. These results suggest activation of DNA repair mechanisms in the cells upon prolonged incubation [78].

#### 2.2.3. P-gp Substrate Probability of Single Mycotoxins

P-glycoprotein (P-gp), which is also known as multidrug resistance protein 1 (MDR1) or ATP-binding cassette sub-family member B 1 (ABCB1), is an ATP-dependent efflux pump transporting a wide range of hydrophobic compounds including drugs and other xenobiotics [79]. It limits the drug entry into the body, promotes drugs elimination into bile and urine, and decreases drug penetration into sensitive tissues [80]. For the in vitro evaluation of whether mycotoxins serve as P-gp substrates, an isolated fraction of the P-gp enriched membranes was used. As P-gp activation is coupled with ATP consumption, we measured the in vitro ATP consumption reflecting the transport activity [81]. From the whole spectrum of mycotoxins, only AOH, DON, T-2, and ZEA activated P-gp in dose-dependent manner. T-2 toxin caused the most significant increase in ATP consumption, suggesting its P-gp-mediated transport (Figure 2).

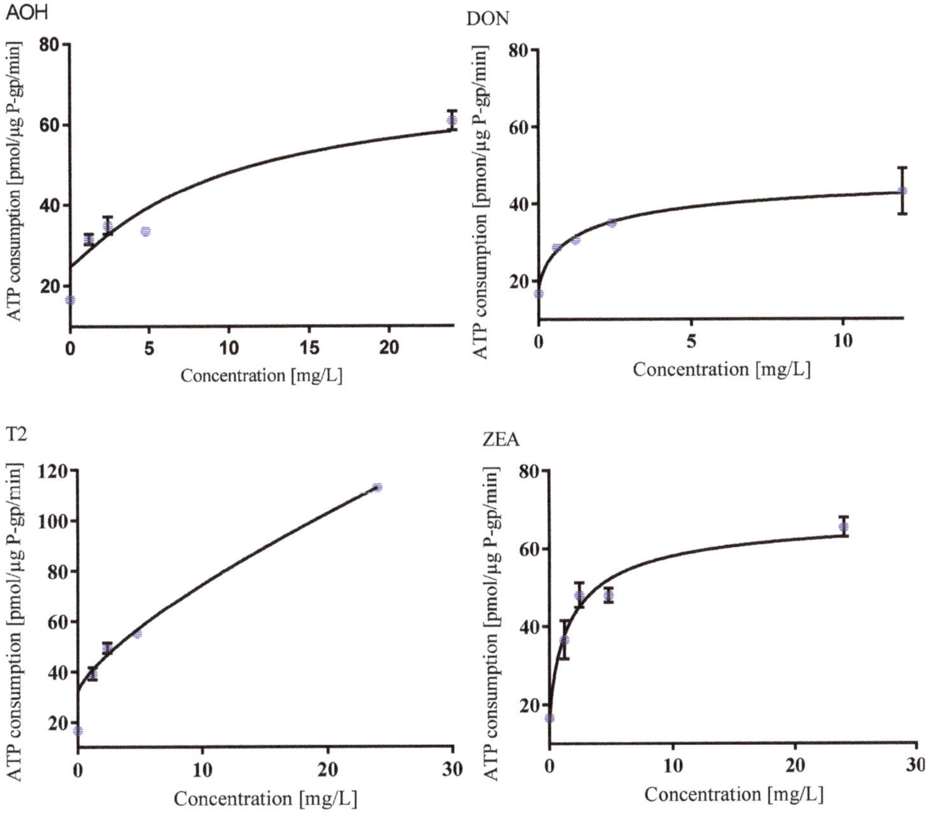


**Figure 2.** Mycotoxins as substrates of P-gp: AOH; DON; T2; and ZEA. Values are expressed as the mean ± SEM ($n = 3$). AOH, alternariol; DON, deoxynivalenol; T-2, T-2 toxin; ZEA, zearalenone.

Li et al. [82] and Videman et al. [83] proposed that P-gp is the foremost transporter of DON in Caco-2, HepG2, and MDCK cells. Different models indicate that P-gp is directly involved in the efflux of ZEA [84–86]. It was reported that T-2 is not a substrate of P-gp [87]. However, in our study, ATP consumption indicated the highest P-gp substrate probability of T-2 followed by ZEA, AOH, and DON. Even though T-2 and AOH are transported via isolated P-gp in our in vitro model, in the cells, the situation is more complex and P-gp efflux activity may be inhibited by various mechanisms or the mycotoxins could be metabolized or substituted.

### 2.3. Influence of the Mycotoxins Properties in Mixtures

In the above sections, we summarize the toxicity of single mycotoxins, but, in natural resources, they predominantly occur in mixtures. Mixtures of mycotoxins can be present in materials of natural origin (e.g., food, feed, and dietary supplements) because: (i) the material can be contaminated by several molds; (ii) some molds can produce several different mycotoxins; and (iii) the material is prepared from several contaminated plants or plant species [88]. Based on our analysis, the milk-thistle dietary supplement may be contaminated by up to 14 different mycotoxins originating from several molds. As the limits of detection were very low, we addressed the question whether the detected levels of mycotoxins are toxic to human cells.

2.3.1. Determination of Acute Toxicity of Milk Thistle-Based Dietary Supplement

Several mycotoxins model mixtures mimicking the milk thistle-based dietary supplement were prepared to determine their cytotoxic effects. These mixtures were mimicking: (i) the concentration and composition of mycotoxins in particular supplement; (ii) the concentration and composition of silymarin; and (iii) the concentration and composition of mycotoxins and silymarin in the supplement. The cytotoxicity of these model mixtures was compared with the cytotoxicity of milk thistle-based dietary supplement using human embryonal kidney cells (HEK 293T). As can be seen in Figure 3, all tested mixtures completely inhibited the cell viability at concentrations corresponding to 50–70% of recommended daily dose (100% recommended daily dose was equal to 8 nM of ALT, 4.5 nM of AME, 9.4 nM of DON, 6.2 nM of T-2, 5.0 nM of HT-2, 0.04 nM of DAS, 1.1 nM of ZEA, 3.7 nM of TEN, 3.5 nM of BEA, 0.7 nM of ENN-A, 1.7 nM of of ENN-A1, 2.7 nM ENN-B, 2.6 nM of ENN-B1, and 29 μM of silibinin). No toxic effect, manifested by zero effect on the cell viability, was observed at concentrations lower than 3% of recommended daily dose.

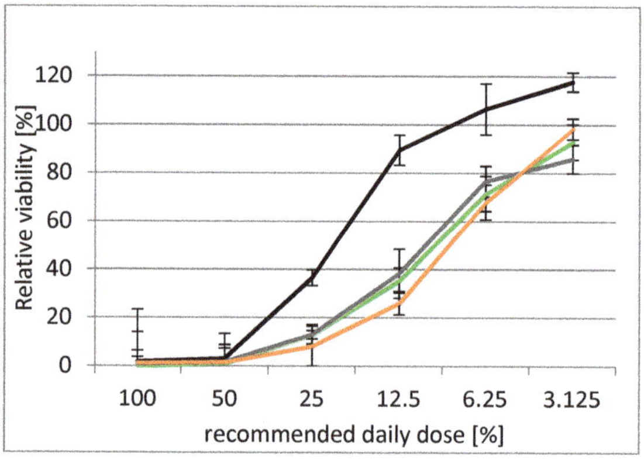


**Figure 3.** HEK 293T cytotoxicity of milk thistle-based dietary supplement and the model mixtures of toxins. The black line is a mixture mimicking the mycotoxins occurrence in the supplement, the green line is a mixture mimicking the silymarin composition, the grey line is a mixture mimicking the mycotoxins plus silymarin composition, and the orange line is a milk thistle-based dietary supplement.

The toxicity of silibinin, the main component of silymarin complex, has been previously published many times for such high doses as we tested (100% recommended daily dose was equal to 29 μM concentration of silibinin) [89]. The concentration of silymarin composition in recommended daily dose exceeds by one order of magnitude that of the mycotoxins occurring at considerably lower concentrations, which did not affect the acute cytotoxicity (Table 4). Even though fourteen different mycotoxins were present in the mixture, single mycotoxins can vary in their modes of action. Therefore, their combination may dramatically affect the cellular processes by an additive or synergistic effect.

**Table 4.** Cytotoxicity of the milk thistle-based dietary supplements and the model mixtures. Cytotoxicity was evaluated by the Duncan's post hoc analysis expressing the differences between the groups. Similar or sharing letters within one concentration (e.g., a and ab) show that there are no significant differences in cell viability of HEK 293T cells treated with milk thistle-based dietary supplements and the model mixtures. Different letters (e.g., a and b) show the statistical difference ($p \leq 0.05$) between milk thistle-based dietary supplements and the model mixtures within the tested concentration.

| Tested Mixtures | Recommended Daily Dose (%) | | | | | |
|---|---|---|---|---|---|---|
| | 100 | 50 | 25 | 12.5 | 6.25 | 3.13 |
| Silymarin | a | a | a | a | a | a |
| Mycotoxins plus silymarin | a | a | a | a | a | a |
| Milk thistle-based dietary supplement | a | a | a | a | a | a,b |
| Mycotoxins | a | a | b | b | b | b |

### 2.3.2. Acute Toxicity of Mycotoxins in Binary Mixtures

To investigate the type of interactions between selected mycotoxins in binary combinations, T-2, HT-2, and DAS were applied in $IC_{50}$ doses in a mixture with another mycotoxin in a 1:1 ratio. At these concentration, T-2, HT-2, and DAS caused 50% cell mortality, while the others did not significantly reduce the cell viability.

The binary combinations lowered cell viability compared to single compounds. The T-2 and DAS mixture (DAS+T-2) as well as their combination with HT-2 (HT-2+T-2 and HT-2+DAS) and some others (ENN A1+DAS and MPA+DAS) significantly reduced cell viability by about 31%, 33%, 24%, 16%, and 15%, respectively. In contrast, cell viability was not significantly reduced by other combinations of toxins (mixtures containing DON, ZEA, ENN-A, ENN-B, ENN-B1, TEN, BEA, AOH, and AME, as well as ENN-A1+T-2, ENN-A1+DAS, MPA+T-2, and MPA+DAS) (data not shown).

To determine the mode of action, the binary mycotoxin interactions were further assessed by the conceptual model called a "linear interaction effect". Table 5 indicates additive effect for the binary mixtures of T-2 with ZEA, BEA, AOH, or AME. Similarly, additive effect was demonstrated for the binary mixtures of DAS with TEN, BEA, AOH, or AME and also for the binary mixtures of HT-2 with ENN-A1, ENN-B1, TEN, MPA, BEA, AOH, or AME. Summarizing the results, each binary combination of T-2, DAS, and HT-2 with TEN, BEA, AOH, or AME had an additive effect. The binary mixture of BEA and T-2 has been previously demonstrated as antagonistic in Vero cells [23] while synergistic in CHO-K1 cells [14].

We found synergistic effects in the binary mixtures of T-2 with ENN-A, ENN-B1, MPA, HT-2, or DAS. A synergistic effect of DAS was also observed when mixed together with either HT-2, DON, ZEA, ENNs, or MPA and for HT-2 combined with DON, ZEA, ENN-A, or ENN-B in a binary mixture. Summarizing the results, ZEA, ENNs, and MPA caused either a synergistic or at least an additive effect except two combinations (T2 with ENN-A1 or ENN-B) where an antagonistic effect was observed.

The observed additive or synergistic effect for combinations with ENNs, MPA, BEA, AOH, or AME could be explained (based on Table 1) as follows: BEA and ENNs increase the cell permeability and thus make the cells more accessible for the other mycotoxins acting as ionophores. Similarly, MPA, AOH, and AME decrease the cell proliferation, which in general decreases cell viability.

A synergistic effect might be caused by the fact that mycotoxins influence different stages of the same toxicity pathway by increased absorption or decreased metabolic degradation of one mycotoxin at the presence of another one [90]. The synergistic effect of T-2 in combination with DAS demonstrated in this study is in agreement with the results of Thuvander et al. [91].

**Table 5.** The combination indexes of binary mycotoxin mixtures on HEK293T after 72 h exposure. The indexes report on mechanism of combined exposition. T-2, HT-2, and DAS were applied in $IC_{50}$ doses in a mixture with another mycotoxin in a 1:1 ratio.

| Mycotoxins | DAS | HT-2 | DON | ZEA | ENN A | ENN A1 | ENN B | ENN B1 | TEN | MPA | BEA | AOH | AME |
|---|---|---|---|---|---|---|---|---|---|---|---|---|---|
| Mixture of T-2 (3.87 nM) | 0.64 ± 0.01 Syn | 0.67 ± 0.04 Syn | 1.29 ± 0.13 Ant | 0.92 ± 0.01 Add | 0.86 ± 0.07 Syn | 1.27 ± 0.13 Ant | 1.11 ± 0.10 Ant | 0.88 ± 0.07 Syn | 0.92 ± 0.07 Add | 0.85 ± 0.05 Syn | 0.95 ± 0.07 Add | 1.00 ± 0.09 Add | 0.97 ± 0.07 Add |
| Mixture of DAS (6.58 nM) | | 0.54 ± 0.03 Syn | 0.88 ± 0.17 Syn | 0.85 ± 0.07 Syn | 0.83 ± 0.05 Syn | 0.79 ± 0.04 Syn | 0.79 ± 0.08 Syn | 0.82 ± 0.06 Syn | 0.92 ± 0.17 Add | 0.83 ± 0.07 Syn | 0.96 ± 0.04 Add | 0.91 ± 0.07 Add | 0.90 ± 0.05 Add |
| Mixture of HT-2 (21.22 nM) | | | 0.87 ± 0.04 Syn | 0.83 ± 0.03 Syn | 0.80 ± 0.06 Syn | 0.93 ± 0.01 Add | 0.87 ± 0.05 Syn | 0.90 ± 0.05 Add | 0.94 ± 0.04 Add | 0.90 ± 0.04 Add | 0.91 ± 0.04 Add | 0.92 ± 0.02 Add | 0.92 ± 0.06 Add |

Data are expressed as mean values ± SEM of independent experiment ($n = 3$), each with six technical replicates. Combination index (CI) < 0.9, 0.9 ≤ CI ≤ 1, and CI > 1 indicate synergism (Syn), additivity (Add), and antagonism (Ant), respectively. AME, alternariol-9-methyl ether; AOH, alternariol; BEA, beauvericin; DAS, diacetoxyscirpenol; DON, deoxynivalenol; ENN A, enniatin A; ENN A1, enniatin A1; ENN B, enniatin B; ENN B1, enniatin B1; HT-2, HT-2 toxin; MPA, mycophenolic acid; T-2, T-2 toxin; TEN, tentoxin; ZEA, zearalenone.

In contrast, an antagonistic effect was demonstrated in the combination of T-2 with DON, ENN-A1, or ENN-B. Several previous studies are consistent with our results describing the interaction between DON and T-2 in Vero cells [14], in CHO-K1 cells [14], and in human lymphocytes [91]. A similar result was obtained by Fernadez-Blanco et al. [14,19] who found that the combination of DON and ENN-B resulted in the antagonistic interaction. The authors explained this interaction by the competition between the mycotoxins for the same target/receptor site [14,19]. Lin et al. [92] suggested that the effect of DON and T-2 is additive/synergistic at middle and high concentrations but antagonistic at low concentrations in rat chondrocytes and C-28/I2 cells. Additionally, synergic effect was also detected when the individual levels were at nearly the same ratio and antagonistic effect when the concentration of DON was much higher (100-1000×) than T-2 [92].

In general, additive, antagonistic, and synergistic effects depend not only on the compounds in the mixture, but also on their mutual concentrations and exposure time [92,93].

### 2.3.3. Suppression of Mycotoxins' Acute Toxicity by Silibinin

The $IC_{50}$ of T-2, HT-2, and DAS halving the HEK293T cells viability after 24 h of incubation were determined as 7, 30, and 15 nM, respectively. At these concentrations, silibinin at the concentration range from 0.9 to 109 μM was added to evaluate its preventive effect in extended range of recommended daily dose of the supplement. As previously published, the co-treatment with both silibinin and mycotoxins did not improve the cell growth, but pretreatment of the cells by silibinin for 2 h before mycotoxins addition protected the cells against mycotoxins-mediated apoptosis [41,42]. Thus, we chose this approach to evaluate the protective effect of silibinin against mycotoxins-induced cytotoxicity.

The presence of silibinin alleviated the HEK 293T viability decrease caused by single mycotoxins (T-2, HT-2, and DAS) in a concentration-dependent manner. The pretreatment with silibinin at lower concentrations (below 54.5 μM) had almost no effect on the cell viability. The highest tested concentration of silibinin (109 μM) showed an additive toxic effect resulting in about 30% decrease of the cell viability when compared to viability of cells cultured with a single mycotoxin. Regarding the effect of the sole silibinin treatment on the cell viability, no toxicity was shown after 24 h of exposure, except for the highest concentration point (109 μM), which significantly reduced the cell viability by 45%. It has been already reported that silibinin had no significant cytotoxic effect on human fibroblasts at the 50 μM concentration for 24 h [94].

Due to the different effect of silibinin pretreatment on the HEK 293T cells cultivated with toxic doses of T-2, HT-2, and DAS, the type of interaction between silibinin and mycotoxins was evaluated by the "linear interaction effect" model (see Table 6). The strongest antagonism was found with the silibinin pretreatments at concentration of 13.6 μM for T-2 and 6.8 μM for HT-2 and DAS exposure,. The cytoprotective effect of silibinin, may be ascribed to its antioxidant and free-radical scavenger role [41]. Based on the results of Al-Anati et al. [40], low silibinin dose (0.2 μM) reduced OTA-induced TNF-α level to 70% while the higher doses (1–26 μM) completely blocked OTA-induced TNF-α within 24 h. Furthermore, the protective effect of 130 μM silibinin against OTA cytotoxicity in hepatocyte cells was reported [41,42]. The authors assumed that silibinin acts on the cell membranes to prevent the entry of toxic substances, stimulates protein synthesis, and accelerates regeneration processes. According to Fan et al. [95], silibinin activated p53 in a dose-dependent manner and thus induced ROS generation in HeLa cells. Therefore, there is evidence of silibinin's pro-oxidative action [36]. However, silibinin could not induce ROS generation in A431 cells without normally functioning p53 [95]. In this cell line, silibinin did not trigger ROS generation but scavenged ROS.

**Table 6.** Mechanism of action of combined exposition to mycotoxins and silibinin. Mechanism of action is evaluated by combination indexes of mycotoxins on HEK 293T cells pretreated with silibinin 2 h prior to exposure to T-2, HT-2 and DAS.

| Silibinin Concentration (μM) | 109.00 | 54.5 | 27.3 | 13.6 | 6.8 | 3.4 | 1.7 | 0.9 |
|---|---|---|---|---|---|---|---|---|
| T-2 exposure | 1.00 ± 0.08 Add | 0.91 ± 0.04 Add | 1.41 ± 0.11 Ant | 1.82 ± 0.06 Ant | 1.46 ± 0.14 Ant | 0.99 ± 0.02 Add | | |
| HT-2 exposure | 1.08 ± 0.03 Add | 1.03 ± 0.04 Add | 1.06 ± 0.07 Add | 1.25 ± 0.08 Ant | 1.57 ± 0.15 Ant | 1.27 ± 0.11 Ant | 1.10 ± 0.02 Add | |
| DAS exposure | 1.14 ± 0.01 Ant | 1.15 ± 0.02 Ant | 1.48 ± 0.08 Ant | 1.56 ± 0.13 Ant | 1.50 ± 0.04 Ant | 1.21 ± 0.05 Ant | 1.23 ± 0.06 Ant | 1.00 ± 0.04 Add |

Data are expressed as mean values ± SEM of independent experiment ($n = 3$), each with six technical replicates. Combination index (CI) < 0.9, 0.9 ≤ CI ≤ 1, and CI > 1 indicate synergism (Syn), additivity (Add), and antagonism (Ant), respectively. DAS, diacetoxyscirpenol; HT-2, HT-2 toxin; T-2, T-2 toxin.

Similarly, a silibinin-induced cell death in human breast cancer cell lines MCF7 and MDA-MB-231 was dependent on ROS generation [96]. Similar to silibinin, trichothecenes also generate free radicals resulting in lipid peroxidation with changes in the membrane integrity, cellular redox signaling, and overall redox status [97]. In this study, high doses of silibinin (55–109 μM) caused cytotoxic effect when HEK293T cells were exposed to T-2, HT-2, and DAS. In this case, it could be hypothesized that the additivity and slight antagonism are the sum of individual effects of silibinin and mycotoxins. Consequently, antioxidant and pro-oxidant effects of silibinin are largely related to its concentration in a given biological system. Duan et al. [98] suggested that silibinin can possess both survival and death effects depending on the dose and time of exposure.

#### 2.3.4. Protective Effects of Silibinin Against Mycotoxin Genotoxicity

The trend of DNA damage induced by AME, AOH, DON, or ENNs in HEK 293T cells was significantly decreased by the addition of 25 μM silibinin (Figure 4). Silibinin at the concentration of 25 μM did not induce genotoxic effects in HEK 293T cells and silibinin treatment attenuated the mycotoxin-induced DNA damage indicating its anticlastogenic potential. Abdel-Wahhab et al. [99] reported that treatment with silymarin nanoparticles protected the liver against hepatic oxidative stress, genotoxicity, and cytotoxicity of DON in rats. In the study of Togay et al. [100], DNA damage in rats with streptozotocin-induced diabetes symptoms were decreased after silibinin treatment. Similarly, Fernandes Veloso Borges et al. [101] showed that silibinin (5.2–15.5 mM) reduced the amount of DNA in the comet tail compared to positive control. Silibinin is known to exhibit strong antioxidant activities and its protective effects against ROS have been demonstrated in different cell lines [41,42]. Protective effects of silibinin on DNA can be explained by scavenging of ROS [102,103]. DON- and ENNs-induced genotoxicity may be associated with the oxidative stress [67,74], while oxidative stress does not play a predominant role in the induction of DNA damage by AOH and AME [66]. This could explain why the treatment with silibinin caused formation of smaller DNA tails induced by DON and ENNs compared to AOH and AME.

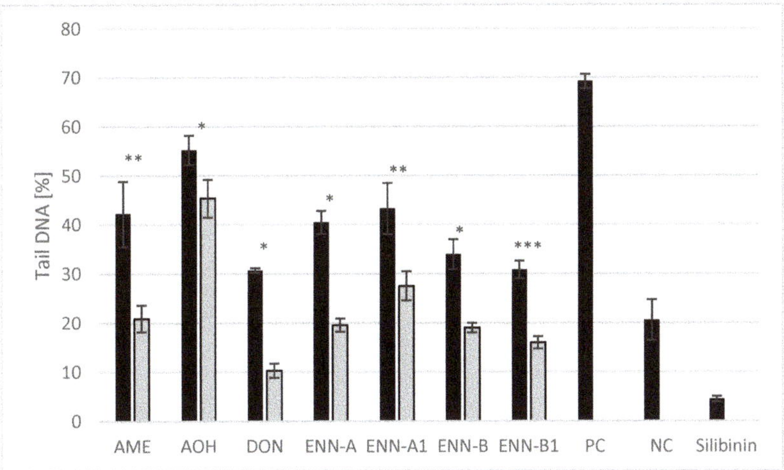


**Figure 4.** Inhibitory effect of silibinin on DNA damage induced by mycotoxins in HEK 293T cells. Values are expressed as the mean ± SEM ($n = 4$). Stars indicate significant differences between silibinin-treated (grey columns) and silibinin-untreated (black columns) comets caused by mycotoxins: * $p \leq 0.05$, ** $p \leq 0.005$, *** $p \leq 0.0005$. AME, alternariol-9-methyl ether; AOH, alternariol; DON, deoxynivalenol; ENN A, enniatin A; ENN A1, enniatin A1; ENN B, enniatin B; ENN B1, enniatin B1.

### 2.4. *Bioavailability of Mycotoxins and Silibinin*

Upon ingestion, mycotoxins can be degraded or modified by biotransformation in the intestinal mucosal wall and only a fraction of the initial content can be absorbed from the gut via intestinal cells [44,104,105]. In this sense, bioavailability is a term used to describe the portion of ingested contaminant that reaches the bloodstream [106]. In the present study, we evaluated the transport of mycotoxins and silibinin by using a two-compartment transwell system representing a co-culture of Caco-2 and RAW 264.7 cells.

Based on the results in Table 7, the bioavailability of silibinin and mycotoxins were not significantly different, especially in the systems treated with AME, DAS, and ZEA. For most of the mycotoxins and silibinin, low aqueous solubility was predicted, which could limit their bioavailability. Previous publications showed that DON, T-2, and HT-2 were transported efficiently through the epithelial cell layers with up to 38% after 24 h, 24% after 6 h, and 32% after 24 h, respectively [107]. ZEA was efficiently absorbed and α-ZEA and β-ZEA are the two major metabolites produced by Caco-2 cells (41% and 32% of total metabolites, respectively; after 3 h exposure to 10 μM ZEA) [108]. BEA bioavailability was 50% and 54% after 4 h exposure to 3 and 4.5 μM of this mycotoxin, respectively [71].

**Table 7.** Transepithelial transport of mycotoxins through Caco-2 cells (%)

| Mycotoxins | Apical Medium | Caco-2 Cells | Basolateral Medium | Raw 264.7 Cells | Total |
|---|---|---|---|---|---|
| AME | 35.92 ± 1.53 [c] | 0.49 ± 0.02 [ab] | 17.68 ± 0.86 [bcd] | 0.01 ± 0.00 [ab] | 53.94 ± 1.59 [bc] |
| AOH | 39.00 ± 22.02 [cd] | 0.04 ± 0.02 [a] | 59.97 ± 2.86 [h] | 0.07 ± 0.02 [h] | 99.08 ± 24.47 [e] |
| BEA | 10.40 ± 3.89 [a] | 10.36 ± 0.98 [d] | 2.31 ± 0.24 [a] | 0.57 ± 0.03 [c] | 23.65 ± 3.33 [a] |
| DAS | 29.61 ± 0.87 [abc] | 0.02 ± 0.00 [a] | 40.12 ± 0.50 [f] | 0.02 ± 0.00 [a] | 69.77 ± 0.99 [cd] |
| DON | 73.33 ± 2.90 [f] | 0.00 ± 0.00 [a] | 21.48 ± 0.91 [cde] | 0.01 ± 0.00 [a] | 94.83 ± 2.14 [e] |
| ENN-A | 15.08 ± 5.18 [ab] | 10.76 ± 0.43 [d] | 16.18 ± 3.17 [b] | 0.29 ± 0.04 [b] | 42.31 ± 5.00 [a] |
| ENN-A1 | 9.52 ± 3.02 [a] | 2.09 ± 0.28 [c] | 13.06 ± 0.45 [b] | 0.22 ± 0.03 [b] | 24.89 ± 3.24 [a] |
| ENN-B | 24.08 ± 3.20 [abc] | 1.15 ± 0.25 [b] | 25.49 ± 4.31 [e] | 0.31 ± 0.03 [b] | 51.02 ± 7.70 [bc] |
| ENN-B1 | 10.46 ± 2.43 [a] | 0.51 ± 0.03 [ab] | 28.16 ± 3.37 [e] | 0.60 ± 0.10 [c] | 39.72 ± 4.74 [ab] |
| HT-2 | 72.63±2.25 [f] | 0.01 ± 0.00 [a] | 49.18 ± 1.80 [g] | 0.01 ± 0.00 [a] | 121.83 ± 1.33 [f] |
| MPA | 57.27 ± 0.79 [ef] | 0.00 ± 0.00 [a] | 39.77 ± 0.52 [f] | 0.02 ± 0.00 [a] | 97.07 ± 0.27 [e] |
| T-2 | 11.63 ± 0.62 [a] | 0.01 ± 0.00 [a] | 28.13 ± 0.48 [e] | 0.01 ± 0.00 [a] | 39.77 ± 0.98 [b] |
| TEN | 28.07 ± 0.62 [abc] | 0.00 ± 0.00 [a] | 7.25 ± 0.72 [ab] | 0.00 ± 0.00 [a] | 35.33 ± 0.10 [ab] |
| ZEA | 32.23 ± 1.71 [bc] | 0.19 ± 0.01 [ab] | 54.24 ± 2.38 [gh] | 0.05 ± 0.01 [a] | 86.70 ± 0.67 [de] |
| Silibinin | 44.34 ± 1.96 [cd] | 0.00 ± 0.00 [a] | 23.24 ± 1.79 [de] | 0.00 ± 0.00 [a] | 67.58 ± 2.95 [cd] |

Values are expressed as the mean ± SEM ($n = 3$). The different letters (e.g., a and b) indicate the significant differences between the mycotoxins in one type of medium/cell based on post-hoc Duncan's test ($p \leq 0.05$). Similar or sharing letters (e.g., a and ab) show no significant differences between the mycotoxins in one type of medium/cell ($p \leq 0.05$). AME, alternariol-9-methyl ether; AOH, alternariol; BEA, beauvericin; DAS, diacetoxyscirpenol; DON, deoxynivalenol; ENN A, enniatin A; ENN A1, enniatin A1; ENN B, enniatin B; ENN B1, enniatin B1; HT-2, HT-2 toxin; MPA, mycophenolic acid; T-2, T-2 toxin; TEN, tentoxin; ZEA, zearalenone.

In our study, the bioavailability of ENNs was similar. However, ENN-A and A1 were detected in higher amount in cells while ENN-B and B1 had higher concentration in basolateral medium. A similar result was also obtained in study by Meca et al. [109]; ENN-B and B1 were more bioavailable from the lumen to blood in the Caco-2 cells compared to ENN-A and A1. Because the total amounts of mycotoxins AME, AOH, DAS, ENN-B, and TEN in the system were significantly lower than their original amounts added into the apical medium, we can presume their metabolization. This fact was also confirmed by our in silico prediction as well as by non-target U-HPLC-MS analysis. By this analysis, we confirmed the presence of AME metabolites (3-O-glucuronide, 7-O-glucuronide, and 3-O-sulfate), AOH metabolites (3-O-glucuronide and 9-O-glucuronide), DAS metabolites (15-monoacetoxyscirpenol, 4-monoacetoxyscirpenol, 7-hydroxy, 8β-hydroxy, and deepoxy-15- monoacetoxyscirpenol), ENN-B metabolite (metabolite M6), and TEN metabolites (metabolite M1, metabolite M2, and metabolite M3). These metabolites were previously described in several studies [110–113].

Based on the total amount of mycotoxins found in our transepithelial system, BEA, ENN-A, A1, B1, T-2, and silibinin should be metabolized as well. T-2 metabolites were detected in our system, namely 3′-hydroxy, 3-hydroxy-15-deacetyl as well as its main metabolite, and HT-2 derivatives (3′-hydroxy-HT-2, 4′-hydroxy-HT-2, deepoxy-3′,7-dihydroxy-HT-2 [111]). The main silibinin metabolite found was a sulfate derivative. In human cells, T-2 could mainly transform to HT-2 and nesolaniol or other products such as 3′-hydroxy-T-2, 4-deacetylnesolaniol, T-2 glucuronide, and HT-2-glucuronide [97].

HT-2 and DON were dominantly detected, mostly in apical medium. This might be because DON was not metabolized by intestinal cells and HT-2 was the main metabolite of T-2, which was previously observed [107]. Besides, BEA and enniatins were found in both RAW 264.7 and Caco-2 cell fractions. It seems that these mycotoxins interact with the membrane according to their in silico predicted lipophilicity.

In agreement with in silico prediction, MPA was unavailable to the cells thanks to its low solubility.

## 3. Conclusions

In the present study, ACD/Percepta was used to predict the properties of mycotoxins and silibinin. In comparison to in silico prediction, in vitro cytotoxicity studies confirmed that T-2, HT-2, and DAS exhibited the highest cytotoxicity of the fourteen mycotoxins tested. The binary combination results suggest that the co-occurrence of these mycotoxins may increase their cytotoxic effects compared to a single mycotoxin. The findings on protective effects of silibinin against both the acute cytotoxicity of mycotoxins (T-2, HT-2, and DAS) and genotoxicity of AME, AOH, DON, and ENNs on HEK 293T in a dose-dependent manner should be taken into account. Finally, the bioavailability of mycotoxins and silibinin does not differ too much and most of the them are metabolized during the transport through epithelial cell layer.

## 4. Materials and Methods

### 4.1. Reagents and Instrumentations

The following chemical reagents and cell culture components were purchased from Sigma-Aldrich (USA): Dulbecco's Modified Eagle's Medium (DMEM), Minimum Essential Medium (MEM), trypsin/EDTA solutions, antibiotic mixture (penicillin and streptomycin), phosphate buffer saline (PBS), resazurin sodium salt, silymarin, silibinin and mycotoxins. Stock solutions of T-2, HT-2, DAS, DON, BEA, ZEA, ENN-A, ENN-A1, ENN-B, ANN-B1, AOH, AME, TEN, and MPA were prepared in methanol and maintained at −20 °C in dark. The final concentrations of methanol in the solutions of mycotoxins in culture medium were $\leq 1\%$ (v/v).

### 4.2. Cell Lines and Cell Cultures

Human colon adenocarcinoma (Caco-2), mouse macrophage (RAW 264.7), human hepatoblastoma (HepG2), and embryonic kidney (HEK 293T) cell lines were obtained from ATCC (USA). Stock cultures of RAW 264.7 and HEK 293T cells were maintained in DMEM, while Caco-2 and HepG2 cells were cultured in EMEM. Both media were supplemented with fetal bovine serum (FBS) (10%) and 1% of antibiotic mixture (penicillin, 100 IU/mL and streptomycin, 100 g/mL) incubated at 37 °C in the atmosphere of 5% $CO_2$. For cell counting and subculture, the cells were dispersed with a solution of 0.05% trypsin and 0.02% EDTA. The medium was changed every third day, and the cells were passaged at approximately 80% confluence. At passages 9–29, the cells were seeded in 96-well plates for the cytotoxicity assays and, passages 30–50 of the Caco-2 cells were used for the co-culture system.

### 4.3. Milk Thistle-Based Dietary Supplement

The milk thistle-based dietary supplement (Ostropestřec plus, Farmax®, Ruakura, New Zealand) was purchased on the Czech market. Its characterization, as provided by manufacturers, was as follows: milk thistle extract (*Silybum marianum*, seed) 250 mg in one capsule—standardized to contain 80% silymarin. The internal content of twenty capsules was weighed separately and then mixed together to obtain the homogenized representative sample.

The quantitative analysis, which was published previously [46], showed total content of mycotoxins equal to 4 ng in one capsule. This content was recalculated according to recommended daily dose and the volume of blood in the human body (5 L) as follows: 8 nM AOH, 4.5 nM AME, 9.4 nM DON, 6.2 nM T-2, 5.0 nM HT-2, 0.04 nM DAS, 1.1 nM ZEA, 3.7 nM TEN, 3.5 nM BEA, 0.7 nM ENN-A, 1.7 nM ENN-A1, 2.7 nM ENN-B, and 2.6 nM ENN-B1. The concentrations of silibinin, the most abundant component of silymarin complex, was 29 μM in the supplement.

### 4.4. In Silico Toxicity Analysis

ACD/Percepta (ACD/Percepta Platform, version 2016, build 2911, Advanced Chemistry Development, Inc., Toronto, ON, Canada, www.acdlabs.com, 2016) was used to predict the most common physicochemical, pharmacokinetic and toxicology properties. For ACD/Percepta data, a reliability index (RI) higher than 0.75 was considered as highly reliable (marked as a), while RI < 0.5 was considered as borderline reliable (marked as *).

### 4.5. Cytotoxicity Assay

The cells were counted by Cellometer Auto T4 (Nexcelom Bioscience, Lawrence, MA) and the cell suspension containing cell density $10^5$ cells/mL was split into the 96-well plate. The plates were then incubated for 24 h at 37 °C in humidified atmosphere of 5% $CO_2$. Then, the tested compounds were added. To assess the effect of silibinin, cells were pre-treated with silibinin at the given concentrations 2 h prior to mycotoxin exposure. After 72 h incubation, the cell viability was tested by standard resazurin assay [114]. Briefly, the cells were washed three times with 100 µL of PBS and incubated with 100 µL of resazurin solution (0.025 mg/mL) for 3 h. Finally, the fluorescence was measured by a SpectraMax i3x microplate reader (Molecular Devices, UK) at a wavelength of 560 nm excitation/590 nm emission.

### 4.6. P-gp Substrate Determination

The in vitro P-gp activation was tested using the Pgp-Glo Assay System according to the standard procedure [79]. Briefly, the reaction mixture contained Pgp-Glo Assay buffer, P-gp containing membranes, and MgATP in a total volume of 50 µL. As the controls, $Na_3VO_4$ (P-gp inhibitor) and verapamil (P-gp substrate) were used. Mycotoxins were added and the reaction mixture was incubated for 1 h in 37 °C. The reaction was stopped by the addition of the detection reagent (50 µL). After 20 min of incubation, the luminescence was recorded.

The luminescence (ΔRLU samples) was calculated as the difference between the relative luminescence of $Na_3VO_4$ and that of the samples. For the P-gp substrates, the specific activity of P-gp was determined using the standard ATP curve and calculating the amount of nanomoles of ATP consumed per µg of P-gp per minute. The standard ATP curve was determined by linear regression and the concentrations of ATP consumed in the samples were recalculated by the subsequent standard interpolation of RLU ATP.

### 4.7. Caco-2/RAW 264.7 Co-Culture System

Caco-2 cells were re-seeded in polycarbonate membrane inserts (0.4 µm pore diameter, 12 mm insert 12-well plate; Corning, USA) at $2 \times 10^5$ cells/cm$^2$ [43]. The culture medium was changed three times a week. After 21 days post-seeding, the monolayers of differentiated Caco-2 cells were used for co-culture experiments. Only the monolayers expressing a transepithelial flux of phenol red to the basolateral compartment of approximately $10^{-7}$ cm/s [115] were used in subsequent experiments. For the co-culture system, RAW 264.7 cells were seeded in 12-wells plates at a density of $8.5 \times 10^5$ cells/well (at Day 20 of the Caco-2 cells differentiated monolayers) [116]. Twenty-four hours after seeding of RAW 264.7 cells, the co-cultures were performed (Day 21). Non-cytotoxic doses of mycotoxins were selected for 4 h treatment in transwell plates.

### 4.8. U-HPLC-MS Determination of Mycotoxins and Silibinin

All culture medium from apical, basolateral compartments, Caco-2 and RAW 264.7 cells were collected after treatments. Mycotoxins and silibinin were extracted by ethanol and the extracts were analyzed by U-HPLC-MS according to previously described instrumental method [46]. The concentration of mycotoxins and silibinin were determined by external calibration batch of analytical standards dissolved in ethanol to concentration range of 0.1–200 ng/mL for mycotoxins and 50–2500 ng/mL of silibinin. The repeatability of the method, expressed as relative standard deviation (RSD), was evaluated by repeated analysis ($n$ = 7) of control samples (both culture media and cell types) fortified before extraction by mycotoxins standard mixture and silibinin to final concentration in extract of 50 and 500 ng/mL, respectively. The RSD were in the range of 1.5–7.3% for all of the analyte/matrix combinations. The limits of quantitation (LOQ), evaluated for each of the analytes as the lowest level of calibration batch laying within linear concentration range, were 0.1–0.5 ng/mL for particular mycotoxins and 50 ng/mL for silibinin.

### 4.9. Combination Effect of Mycotoxins in Binary Mixtures

The "linear interaction effect", also called "response additivity", was used to evaluate the mycotoxins combined effects [43]. A combination index (CI) was calculated for each combination. This index is recognized as a standard measure of combination effect and CI < 0.9, 0.9 ≤ CI ≤ 1.1, and CI > 1.1 indicate synergism, additivity, and antagonism, respectively. The CI of "linear interaction effect" model can be calculated as:

$$CI = \frac{observed\ effect\ (mycotoxin\ 1) + observed\ effect\ (mycotoxin\ 2)}{observed\ effect\ (mycotoxin\ 1 + mycotoxin\ 2)} \quad (1)$$

### 4.10. Genotoxicity Assay

Genotoxicity was studied by standardized method known as a single cell gel electrophoresis (Comet assay) [117]. Briefly, HEK 293T cells were seeded in 12-well plates ($10^6$ cells/mL) and treated with mycotoxins (25 µM) or combination of mycotoxin (25 µM) and silibinin (25 µM) for 24 h.

DMSO was added to control cells in the concentration of 0.6%, which is identical to the concentration of the solvent in the tested samples. Cells for the positive control were treated with 100 µM $H_2O_2$ in PBS for 10 min in 37 °C.

The cells were detached using trypsin (EDTA) and frozen in freezing medium (10% DMSO, 40% serum, 50% DMEM) at −160 °C. For the Comet assay, the cell suspension was centrifuged at 1000 × *g* for 1 min. The pellet was resuspended in 0.5 mL of PBS. A 50-µL aliquot of the suspension was mixed with 150 µL of LMP agarose (0.01 g/mL). Then, 80 µL of resulting agarose–cell suspension were spread onto the slide pre-coated with 1% regular agarose. The slides were allowed to solidify followed by cell lysis, gel electrophoresis, and staining [118] Slides were scored using an image analysis software (ImageJ 1.51s, National Institutes of Health, WI, USA) connected to a fluorescence microscope (AX70 Provis, Olympus, Japan). All experiments were performed in tetraplicate, and in each parallel images of 100 randomly selected cells were evaluated. Comet parameters considered in this study were the tail length and the proportion of DNA in the comet tail (tail DNA or tail intensity).

### 4.11. Data Processing and Statistical Analysis

All experiments were independently repeated at least three times (biological replicates). In addition, each replicate included at least three replicated treatments (technical replicate). The relative activity was evaluated as a percentage according to the formula:

$$RA\ (\%) = 100 \times \frac{(\text{slope of sample} - \text{average slope of PC})}{(\text{average slope of NC} - \text{average slope of PC})} \quad (2)$$

The results are expressed as the average ± standard error of the mean (SEM). Values of $IC_{50}$ were obtained by using the software GraphPad Prism 8.0 (GraphPad Software Inc., San Diego, CA, USA) and nonlinear regression:

$$Y = \frac{\text{Bottom} + (\text{Top} - \text{Bottom})}{1 + 10^{(logIC_{50} - X) \times HillSlope}} \quad (3)$$

The significance was tested by one-way ANOVA followed by the t-test for multiple comparisons using Statgraphics software (Statgraphics Technologies, Inc., USA) and the Excel t-test function (two-tailed distribution, heteroscedastic type). $p$-values < 0.05 were considered statistically significant.

**Author Contributions:** Conceptualization, T.R., L.V., and M.S.-Z.; methodology, J.V., M.F., N.J., S.D., K.A., V.N.T., T.R., and J.H.; software, J.V., K.R., and M.F.; validation, J.V., N.J., K.A., V.N.T., S.D. and M.F.; formal analysis, J.V. and M.F.; investigation, J.V., M.F., M.S.-Z., T.R., and J.H.; resources, J.V., M.S.-Z., and L.V.; data curation, J.V. and M.F.; writing—original draft preparation, V.N.T., J.V.; writing—review and editing, M.S.-Z., T.R., L.V., and K.A.;

visualization, J.V.; supervision, T.R. and J.H.; project administration, M.S.-Z.; J.V.; funding acquisition, J.V., T.R., J.H., and L.V. All authors have read and agreed to the published version of the manuscript.

**Funding:** The financial support of the projects of the Czech Science Foundation, Nos. 16-06008S and 18-00150S; the European Union Horizon 2020 research and innovation program, No. 692195 ("MultiCoop"); and mobility project from the Czech Ministry of Education, Youth and Sports INTER-COST LTC19007 (COST Action CA17104 STRATAGEM) is gratefully acknowledged. The work was also supported by the Operational Programme Prague-Competitiveness (CZ.2.16/3.1.00/21537 and CZ.2.16/3.1.00/24503), by the Czech National Program of Sustainability NPU I (LO1601 and MSMT-43760/2015), and grants AZV 16-27317A and RVO-VFN64165/2019 from the Czech Ministry of Health.

**Acknowledgments:** The authors thank Pavel Drasar (UCT Prague, Czech Republic) for the in silico prediction analysis.

**Conflicts of Interest:** The authors declare no conflict of interest.

## Abbreviations

| | |
|---|---|
| ABCB1 | ATP-binding cassette sub family member 1 |
| AFB1 | aflatoxin B1 |
| AME | alternariol-9-methyl ether |
| AOH | alternariol |
| ASBT | intestinal bile acid transporter |
| BEA | beauvericin |
| BF-2 | a fibroblast cell line originally established from the caudal fin of *Lepomis macrochirus* (Bluegill) |
| C-28/I2 | immortalized human chondrocyte |
| Caco-2 | Caucasian colon adenocarcinoma |
| CI | combination index |
| CHO-K1 | Chinese hamster ovary |
| DAS | diacetoxyscirpenol |
| DMEM | Dulbecco's Modified Eagle's Medium |
| DON | deoxynivalenol |
| EMEM | Minimum Essential Medium |
| ENN A | enniatin A |
| ENN A1 | enniatin A1 |
| ENN B | enniatin B |
| ENN B1 | enniatin B1 |
| ENNs | enniatins |
| FB1 | fumonisin B1 |
| FBS | fetal bovine serum |
| HEK-293T | human embryonic kidney 293 |
| HepG2 | hepatocellular carcinoma epithelial |
| HT-2 | HT-2 toxin |
| HT29 | human Caucasian colon adenocarcinoma |
| $IC_{50}$ | the mycotoxin concentration that halved the cellular viability |
| LMP | low melting point |
| LogP | logarithmic values of octanol–water partition coefficient |
| LOQ | limit of quantitation |
| MCF7 | human Caucasian breast adenocarcinoma |
| MDA-MD-231 | human breast adenocarcinoma |
| MDCK | Madin–Darby canine kidney |
| MDR1 | multidrug resistance protein 1 |
| MPA | mycophenolic acid |
| NADH | 1,4-Dihydronicotinamide adenine dinucleotide |
| OTA | ochratoxin A |
| PBS | phosphate buffer saline |

| | |
|---|---|
| PepT1 | intestinal peptide transporter 1 |
| P-gp | P-glycoprotein |
| RAW | mouse macrophage |
| ROS | reactive oxygen species |
| RSD | relative standard deviation |
| SF-9 | the lepidopteran (*S. frugiperda*) cells obtained from the envelope of pupal ovaries |
| T-2 | T-2 toxin |
| TEN | tentoxin |
| TNF-α | tumor necrosis factor alpha |
| V79 | lung fibroblasts from male Chinese hamster |
| Vero | mammalian kidney epithelial |
| ZEA | zearalenone |

## References


1. Fernández-Blanco, C.; Elmo, L.; Waldner, T.; Ruiz, M.J. Cytotoxic Effects Induced by Patulin, Deoxynivalenol and Toxin T2 Individually and in Combination in Hepatic Cells (HepG2). *Food Chem. Toxicol.* **2018**, *120*, 12–23. [CrossRef] [PubMed]
2. Stanciu, O.; Loghin, F.; Filip, L.; Cozma, A.; Miere, D.; Mañes, J.; Banc, R. Occurence of Fusarium Mycotoxins in Wheat from Europe—A Review. *Acta Univ. Cibiniensis Ser. E Food Technol.* **2015**, *19*, 35–60. [CrossRef]
3. Pestka, J.J.; Zhou, H.R.; Moon, Y.; Chung, Y.J. Cellular and Molecular Mechanisms for Immune Modulation by Deoxynivalenol and Other Trichothecenes: Unraveling a Paradox. *Toxicol. Lett.* **2004**, *153*, 61–73. [CrossRef] [PubMed]
4. Zhang, J.; Zhang, H.; Liu, S.; Wu, W.; Zhang, H. Comparison of Anorectic Potencies of Type a Trichothecenes T-2 Toxin, HT-2 Toxin, Diacetoxyscirpenol, and Neosolaniol. *Toxins* **2018**, *10*, 179. [CrossRef]
5. Wang, X.; Wang, Y.; Qiu, M.; Sun, L.; Wang, X.; Li, C.; Xu, D.; Gooneratne, R. Cytotoxicity of T-2 and Modified T-2 Toxins: Induction of JAK/STAT Pathway in RAW264.7 Cells by Hepatopancreas and Muscle Extracts of Shrimp Fed with T-2 Toxin. *Toxicol. Res.* **2017**, *6*, 144–151. [CrossRef]
6. Creppy, E.E. Update of Survey, Regulation and Toxic Effects of Mycotoxins in Europe. *Toxicol. Lett.* **2002**, *127*, 19–28. [CrossRef]
7. Fraeyman, S.; Croubels, S.; Devreese, M.; Antonissen, G. Emerging Fusarium and Alternaria Mycotoxins: Occurrence, Toxicity and Toxicokinetics. *Toxins* **2017**, *9*, 228. [CrossRef]
8. Luz, C.; Saladino, F.; Luciano, F.B.; Mañes, J.; Meca, G. Occurrence, Toxicity, Bioaccessibility and Mitigation Strategies of Beauvericin, a Minor Fusarium Mycotoxin. *Food Chem. Toxicol.* **2017**, *107*, 430–439. [CrossRef]
9. Rodríguez-Carrasco, Y.; Mañes, J.; Berrada, H.; Juan, C. Development and Validation of a LC-ESI-MS/MS Method for the Determination of Alternaria Toxins Alternariol, Alternariol Methyl-Ether and Tentoxin in Tomato and Tomato-Based Products. *Toxins* **2016**, *8*, 328. [CrossRef]
10. Zambonin, C.G.; Monaci, L.; Aresta, A. Solid-Phase Microextraction-High Performance Liquid Chromatography and Diode Array Detection for the Determination of Mycophenolic Acid in Cheese. *Food Chem.* **2002**, *78*, 249–254. [CrossRef]
11. Fontaine, K.; Passeró, E.; Vallone, L.; Hymery, N.; Coton, M.; Jany, J.L.; Mounier, J.Ô.; Coton, E. Occurrence of Roquefortine C, Mycophenolic Acid and Aflatoxin M1 Mycotoxins in Blue-Veined Cheeses. *Food Control* **2015**, *47*, 634–640. [CrossRef]
12. De Angelis, E.; Monaci, L.; Mackie, A.; Salt, L.; Visconti, A. Reprint of "Bioaccessibility of T-2 and HT-2 Toxins in Mycotoxin Contaminated Bread Models Submitted to in Vitro Human Digestion". *Innov. Food Sci. Emerg. Technol.* **2013**, *25*, 88–96. [CrossRef]
13. Weidner, M.; Hüwel, S.; Ebert, F.; Schwerdtle, T.; Galla, H.J.; Humpf, H.U. Influence of T-2 and HT-2 Toxin on the Blood-Brain Barrier In Vitro: New Experimental Hints for Neurotoxic Effects. *PLoS ONE* **2013**, *8*, 1–10. [CrossRef]
14. Ruiz, M.J.; Franzova, P.; Juan-García, A.; Font, G. Toxicological Interactions between the Mycotoxins Beauvericin, Deoxynivalenol and T-2 Toxin in CHO-K1 Cells in Vitro. *Toxicon* **2011**, *58*, 315–326. [CrossRef] [PubMed]

15. Li, Y.; Wang, Z.; Beier, R.C.; Shen, J.; Smet, D.D.; De Saeger, S.; Zhang, S. T-2 Toxin, a Trichothecene Mycotoxin: Review of Toxicity, Metabolism, and Analytical Methods. *J. Agric. Food Chem.* **2011**, *59*, 3441–3453. [CrossRef] [PubMed]
16. Hassanane, M.; ESA, A.; S, E.-F.; MA, A.; A, H. Mutagenicity of the Mycotoxin Diacetoxyscirpenol on Somatic and Germ Cells of Mice. *Mycotoxin Res.* **2000**, *16*, 54–64. [CrossRef] [PubMed]
17. Qureshi, M.A.; Brundage, M.A.; Hamilton, P.B. 4β, 15-Diacetoxyscirpenol Induces Cytotoxicity and Alterations in Phagocytic and Fc-Receptor Expression Functions in Chicken Macrophages *In Vitro*. *Immunopharmacol. Immunotoxicol.* **1998**, *20*, 541–553. [CrossRef]
18. Zhou, H.; George, S.; Hay, C.; Lee, J.; Qian, H.; Sun, X. Individual and Combined Effects of Aflatoxin B1, Deoxynivalenol and Zearalenone on HepG2 and RAW 264.7 Cell Lines. *Food Chem. Toxicol.* **2017**, *103*, 18–27. [CrossRef]
19. Fernández-Blanco, C.; Font, G.; Ruiz, M.J. Interaction Effects of Enniatin B, Deoxinivalenol and Alternariol in Caco-2 Cells. *Toxicol. Lett.* **2016**, *241*, 38–48. [CrossRef]
20. Wang, H.W.; Wang, J.Q.; Zheng, B.Q.; Li, S.L.; Zhang, Y.D.; Li, F.D.; Zheng, N. Cytotoxicity Induced by Ochratoxin A, Zearalenone, and α-Zearalenol: Effects of Individual and Combined Treatment. *Food Chem. Toxicol.* **2014**, *71*, 217–224. [CrossRef]
21. Bouaziz, C.; Sharaf el dein, O.; El Golli, E.; Abid-Essefi, S.; Brenner, C.; Lemaire, C.; Bacha, H. Different Apoptotic Pathways Induced by Zearalenone, T-2 Toxin and Ochratoxin A in Human Hepatoma Cells. *Toxicology* **2008**, *254*, 19–28. [CrossRef] [PubMed]
22. Kouadio, J.H.; Mobio, T.A.; Baudrimont, I.; Moukha, S.; Dano, S.D.; Creppy, E.E. Comparative Study of Cytotoxicity and Oxidative Stress Induced by Deoxynivalenol, Zearalenone or Fumonisin B1 in Human Intestinal Cell Line Caco-2. *Toxicology* **2005**, *213*, 56–65. [CrossRef] [PubMed]
23. Ruiz, M.J.; Macáková, P.; Juan-García, A.; Font, G. Cytotoxic Effects of Mycotoxin Combinations in Mammalian Kidney Cells. *Food Chem. Toxicol.* **2011**, *49*, 2718–2724. [CrossRef] [PubMed]
24. Ferrer, E.; Juan-García, A.; Font, G.; Ruiz, M.J. Reactive Oxygen Species Induced by Beauvericin, Patulin and Zearalenone in CHO-K1 Cells. *Toxicol. Vitr.* **2009**, *23*, 1504–1509. [CrossRef]
25. Prosperini, A.; Berrada, H.; Ruiz, M.J.; Caloni, F.; Coccini, T.; Spicer, L.J.; Perego, M.C.; Lafranconi, A. A Review of the Mycotoxin Enniatin B. *Front. Public Health* **2017**, *5*, 304. [CrossRef]
26. Fernández-Blanco, C.; Juan-García, A.; Juan, C.; Font, G.; Ruiz, M.J. Alternariol Induce Toxicity via Cell Death and Mitochondrial Damage on Caco-2 Cells. *Food Chem. Toxicol.* **2016**, *88*, 32–39. [CrossRef]
27. Frizzell, C.; Ndossi, D.; Kalayou, S.; Eriksen, G.S.; Verhaegen, S.; Sørlie, M.; Elliott, C.T.; Ropstad, E.; Connolly, L. An in Vitro Investigation of Endocrine Disrupting Effects of the Mycotoxin Alternariol. *Toxicol. Appl. Pharmacol.* **2013**, *271*, 64–71. [CrossRef]
28. Pfeiffer, E.; Schmit, C.; Burkhardt, B.; Altemöller, M.; Podlech, J.; Metzler, M. Glucuronidation of the Mycotoxins Alternariol and Alternariol-9-Methyl Ether in Vitro: Chemical Structures of Glucuronides and Activities of Human UDP-Glucuronosyltransferase Isoforms. *Mycotoxin Res.* **2009**, *25*, 3–10. [CrossRef]
29. Gomis, J.-M.; Haraux, F.; Santolini, J.; André, F.; Sigalat, C.; Minoletti, C. An Insight into the Mechanism of Inhibition and Reactivation of the F 1 -ATPases by Tentoxin. *Biochemistry* **2002**, *41*, 6008–6018. [CrossRef]
30. Wu, T.Y.; Fridley, B.L.; Jenkins, G.D.; Batzler, A.; Wang, L.; Weinshilboum, R.M. Mycophenolic Acid Response Biomarkers: A Cell Line Model System-Based Genome-Wide Screen. *Int. Immunopharmacol.* **2011**, *11*, 1057–1064. [CrossRef]
31. Huang, Y.; Liu, Z.; Huang, H.; Liu, H.; Li, L. Effects of Mycophenolic Acid on Endothelial Cells. *Int. Immunopharmacol.* **2005**, *5*, 1029–1039. [CrossRef] [PubMed]
32. Fung, F.; Clark, R.F. Health Effects of Mycotoxins: A Toxicological Overview. *J. Toxicol. Clin. Toxicol.* **2004**, *42*, 217–234. [CrossRef] [PubMed]
33. Zhou, H.; George, S.; Li, C.; Gurusamy, S.; Sun, X.; Gong, Z.; Qian, H. Combined Toxicity of Prevalent Mycotoxins Studied in Fish Cell Line and Zebrafish Larvae Revealed That Type of Interactions Is Dose-Dependent. *Aquat. Toxicol.* **2017**, *193*, 60–71. [CrossRef] [PubMed]
34. Speijers, G.J.A.; Speijers, M.H.M. Combined Toxic Effects of Mycotoxins. *Toxicol. Lett.* **2004**, *153*, 91–98. [CrossRef] [PubMed]
35. Castell-Auví, A.; Motilva, M.J.; Macià, A.; Torrell, H.; Bladé, C.; Pinent, M.; Arola, L.; Ardévol, A. Organotypic Co-Culture System to Study Plant Extract Bioactivity on Hepatocytes. *Food Chem.* **2010**, *122*, 775–781. [CrossRef]

36. Surai, P. Silymarin as a Natural Antioxidant: An Overview of the Current Evidence and Perspectives. *Antioxidants* **2015**, *4*, 204–247. [CrossRef]
37. He, Q.; Kim, J.; Sharma, R.P. Silymarin Protects against Liver Damage in BALB/c Mice Exposed to Fumonisin B1despite Increasing Accumulation of Free Sphingoid Bases. *Toxicol. Sci.* **2004**, *80*, 335–342. [CrossRef]
38. Naseer, O.; Khan, J.A.; Khan, M.S.; Omer, M.O.; Chishti, G.A.; Sohail, M.L.; Saleem, M.U. Comparative Efficacy of Silymarin and Choline Chloride (Liver Tonics) in Preventing the Effects of Aflatoxin B1in Bovine Calves. *Pol. J. Vet. Sci.* **2016**, *19*, 545–551. [CrossRef]
39. Sozmen, M.; Devrim, A.K.; Tunca, R.; Bayezit, M.; Dag, S.; Essiz, D. Protective Effects of Silymarin on Fumonisin B1-Induced Hepatotoxicity in Mice. *J. Vet. Sci.* **2014**, *15*, 51–60. [CrossRef]
40. Al-Anati, L.; Essid, E.; Reinehr, R.; Petzinger, E. Silibinin Protects OTA-Mediated TNF-α Release from Perfused Rat Livers and Isolated Rat Kupffer Cells. *Mol. Nutr. Food Res.* **2009**, *53*, 460–466. [CrossRef]
41. Essid, E.; Dernawi, Y.; Petzinger, E. Apoptosis Induction by OTA and TNF-?? In Cultured Primary Rat Hepatocytes and Prevention by Silibinin. *Toxins* **2012**, *4*, 1139–1156. [CrossRef] [PubMed]
42. Essid, E.; Petzinger, E. Silibinin Pretreatment Protects against Ochratoxin A-Mediated Apoptosis in Primary Rat Hepatocytes. *Mycotoxin Res.* **2011**, *27*, 167–176. [CrossRef] [PubMed]
43. Duca, R.; Mabondzo, A.; Bravin, F.; Delaforge, M. In Vitro Co-Culture Models to Evaluate Acute Cytotoxicity of Individual and Combined Mycotoxin Exposures on Caco-2, THP-1 and HepaRG Human Cell Lines. *Chem. Biol. Interact.* **2018**, *281*, 51–59. [CrossRef]
44. González-Arias, C.A.; Marín, S.; Rojas-García, A.E.; Sanchis, V.; Ramos, A.J. UPLC-MS/MS Analysis of Ochratoxin A Metabolites Produced by Caco-2 and HepG2 Cells in a Co-Culture System. *Food Chem. Toxicol.* **2017**, *109*, 333–340. [CrossRef] [PubMed]
45. González-Arias, C.A.; Crespo-Sempere, A.; Marín, S.; Sanchis, V.; Ramos, A.J. Modulation of the Xenobiotic Transformation System and Inflammatory Response by Ochratoxin A Exposure Using a Co-Culture System of Caco-2 and HepG2 Cells. *Food Chem. Toxicol.* **2015**, *86*, 245–252. [CrossRef] [PubMed]
46. Fenclova, M.; Novakova, A.; Viktorova, J.; Jonatova, P.; Dzuman, Z.; Ruml, T.; Kren, V.; Hajslova, J.; Vitek, L.; Stranska-Zachariasova, M. Poor Chemical and Microbiological Quality of the Commercial Milk Thistle-Based Dietary Supplements May Account for Their Reported Unsatisfactory and Non-Reproducible Clinical Outcomes. *Sci. Rep.* **2019**, *9*, 1–12. [CrossRef]
47. Veprikova, Z.; Zachariasova, M.; Dzuman, Z.; Zachariasova, A.; Fenclova, M.; Slavikova, P.; Vaclavikova, M.; Mastovska, K.; Hengst, D.; Hajslova, J. Mycotoxins in Plant-Based Dietary Supplements: Hidden Health Risk for Consumers. *J. Agric. Food Chem.* **2015**, *63*, 6633–6643. [CrossRef]
48. EFSA Panel on Contaminants in the Food Chain (CONTAM). Scientific Opinion on the Risks for Animal and Public Health Related to the Presence of Alternaria Toxins in Feed and Food. *EFSA J.* **2011**, *9*, 2407. [CrossRef]
49. EFSA Panel on Contaminants in the Food Chain (CONTAM). Scientific Opinion on the Risks for Animal and Public Health Related to the Presence of T-2 and HT-2 Toxin in Food and Feed. *EFSA J.* **2011**, *9*, 2481. [CrossRef]
50. EFSA Panel on Contaminants in the Food Chain. Scientific Opinion on the Risks for Public Health Related to the Presence of Zearalenone in Food. *EFSA J.* **2011**, *9*, 2197. [CrossRef]
51. EFSA Panel on Contaminants in the Food Chain (CONTAM). Scientific Opinion on the Risks to Human and Animal Health Related to the Presence of Beauvericin and Enniatins in Food and Feed. *EFSA J.* **2014**, *12*, 3802. [CrossRef]
52. Knutsen, H.K.; Alexander, J.; Barregård, L.; Bignami, M.; Brüschweiler, B.; Ceccatelli, S.; Cottrill, B.; Dinovi, M.; Grasl-Kraupp, B.; Hogstrand, C.; et al. Risks to Human and Animal Health Related to the Presence of Deoxynivalenol and Its Acetylated and Modified Forms in Food and Feed. *EFSA J.* **2017**, *15*. [CrossRef]
53. Knutsen, H.K.; Alexander, J.; Barregård, L.; Bignami, M.; Brüschweiler, B.; Ceccatelli, S.; Cottrill, B.; Dinovi, M.; Grasl-Kraupp, B.; Hogstrand, C.; et al. Risk to Human and Animal Health Related to the Presence of 4,15-Diacetoxyscirpenol in Food and Feed. *EFSA J.* **2018**, *16*. [CrossRef]
54. Lipinski, C.A.; Lombardo, F.; Dominy, B.W.; Feeney, P.J. Experimental and Computational Approaches to Estimate Solubility and Permeability in Drug Discovery and Development Settings. *Adv. Drug Deliv. Rev.* **2012**, *64*, 4–17. [CrossRef]
55. Fernández-Blanco, C.; Font, G.; Ruiz, M.J. Role of Quercetin on Caco-2 Cells against Cytotoxic Effects of Alternariol and Alternariol Monomethyl Ether. *Food Chem. Toxicol.* **2016**, *89*, 60–66. [CrossRef]

56. Nielsen, T.S.; Sørensen, I.F.; Sørensen, J.L.; Søndergaard, T.E.; Purup, S. Cytotoxic and Apoptotic Effect of Mycotoxins in Human Small Intestinal Cells. *J. Anim. Sci.* **2016**, *94*. [CrossRef]
57. Tatay, E.; Meca, G.; Font, G.; Ruiz, M.J. Interactive Effects of Zearalenone and Its Metabolites on Cytotoxicity and Metabolization in Ovarian CHO-K1 Cells. *Toxicol. In Vitro* **2014**, *28*, 95–103. [CrossRef]
58. Prosperini, A.; Font, G.; Ruiz, M.J. Interaction Effects of Fusarium Enniatins (A, A1, B and B1) Combinations on in Vitro Cytotoxicity of Caco-2 Cells. *Toxicol. Vitr.* **2014**, *28*, 88–94. [CrossRef]
59. Behm, C.; Fllmann, W.; Degen, G.H. Cytotoxic Potency of Mycotoxins in Cultures of V79 Lung Fibroblast Cells. *J. Toxicol. Environ. Health Part Curr. Issues* **2012**, *75*, 1226–1231. [CrossRef]
60. Lautraite, S.; Rio, B.; Guinard, J.; Parent-Massin, D. In Vitro Effects of Diacetoxyscirpenol (DAS) on Human and Rat Granulo-Monocytic Progenitors. *Mycopathologia* **1997**, *140*, 59–64. [CrossRef]
61. Jha, S.N.; Jaiswal, P.; Grewal, M.K.; Gupta, M.; Bhardwaj, R. Detection of Adulterants and Contaminants in Liquid Foods—A Review. *Crit. Rev. Food Sci. Nutr.* **2016**, *56*, 1662–1684. [CrossRef] [PubMed]
62. Rychlik, M. *Mycotoxins Except Fusarium Toxins in Foods*; Elsevier Ltd.: Cambridge, UK, 2017. [CrossRef]
63. Sobrova, P.; Adam, V.; Vasatkova, A.; Beklova, M.; Zeman, L.; Kizek, R. Deoxynivalenol and Its Toxicity. *Interdiscip. Toxicol.* **2010**, *3*, 94–99. [CrossRef] [PubMed]
64. Tsuda, S.; Kosaka, Y.; Murakami, M.; Matsuo, H.; Matsusaka, N.; Taniguchi, K.; Sasaki, Y.F. Detection of Nivalenol Genotoxicity in Cultured Cells and Multiple Mouse Organs by the Alkaline Single-Cell Gel Electrophoresis Assay. *Mutat. Res. Genet. Toxicol. Environ. Mutagen.* **1998**, *415*, 191–200. [CrossRef]
65. Fehr, M.; Pahlke, G.; Fritz, J.; Christensen, M.O.; Boege, F.; Altemöller, M.; Podlech, J.; Marko, D. Alternariol Acts as a Topoisomerase Poison, Preferentially Affecting the IIα Isoform. *Mol. Nutr. Food Res.* **2009**, *53*, 441–451. [CrossRef] [PubMed]
66. Tiessen, C.; Fehr, M.; Schwarz, C.; Baechler, S.; Domnanich, K.; Böttler, U.; Pahlke, G.; Marko, D. Modulation of the Cellular Redox Status by the Alternaria Toxins Alternariol and Alternariol Monomethyl Ether. *Toxicol. Lett.* **2013**, *216*, 23–30. [CrossRef] [PubMed]
67. Bony, S.; Carcelen, M.; Olivier, L.; Devaux, A. Genotoxicity Assessment of Deoxynivalenol in the Caco-2 Cell Line Model Using the Comet Assay. *Toxicol. Lett.* **2006**, *166*, 67–76. [CrossRef]
68. Takakura, N.; Nesslany, F.; Fessard, V.; Le Hegarat, L. Absence of in Vitro Genotoxicity Potential of the Mycotoxin Deoxynivalenol in Bacteria and in Human TK6 and HepaRG Cell Lines. *Food Chem. Toxicol.* **2014**, *66*, 113–121. [CrossRef]
69. Ma, S.; Zhao, Y.; Sun, J.; Mu, P.; Deng, Y. MiR449a/SIRT1/PGC-1α Is Necessary for Mitochondrial Biogenesis Induced by T-2 Toxin. *Front. Pharmacol.* **2018**, *8*, 954. [CrossRef]
70. Klarić, M.Š.; Daraboš, D.; Rozgaj, R.; Kašuba, V.; Pepeljnjak, S. Beauvericin and Ochratoxin A Genotoxicity Evaluated Using the Alkaline Comet Assay: Single and Combined Genotoxic Action. *Arch. Toxicol.* **2010**, *84*, 641–650. [CrossRef]
71. Prosperini, A.; Juan-García, A.; Font, G.; Ruiz, M.J. Beauvericin-Induced Cytotoxicity via ROS Production and Mitochondrial Damage in Caco-2 Cells. *Toxicol. Lett.* **2013**, *222*, 204–211. [CrossRef]
72. Dornetshuber, R.; Heffeter, P.; Lemmens-Gruber, R.; Elbling, L.; Marko, D.; Micksche, M.; Berger, W. Oxidative Stress and DNA Interactions Are Not Involved in Enniatin- and Beauvericin-Mediated Apoptosis Induction. *Mol. Nutr. Food Res.* **2009**, *53*, 1112–1122. [CrossRef] [PubMed]
73. Mallebrera, B.; Juan-Garcia, A.; Font, G.; Ruiz, M.J. Mechanisms of Beauvericin Toxicity and Antioxidant Cellular Defense. *Toxicol. Lett.* **2016**, *246*, 28–34. [CrossRef] [PubMed]
74. Prosperini, A.; Juan-García, A.; Font, G.; Ruiz, M.J. Reactive Oxygen Species Involvement in Apoptosis and Mitochondrial Damage in Caco-2 Cells Induced by Enniatins A, A1, B and B1. *Toxicol. Lett.* **2013**, *222*, 36–44. [CrossRef] [PubMed]
75. Kang, C.; Lee, H.; Yoo, Y.S.; Hah, D.Y.; Kim, C.H.; Kim, E.; Kim, J.S. Evaluation of Oxidative DNA Damage Using an Alkaline Single Cell Gel Electrophoresis (SCGE) Comet Assay, and the Protective Effects of N-Acetylcysteine Amide on Zearalenone-Induced Cytotoxicity in Chang Liver Cells. *Toxicol. Res.* **2013**, *29*, 43–52. [CrossRef] [PubMed]
76. Tatay, E.; Font, G.; Ruiz, M.J. Cytotoxic Effects of Zearalenone and Its Metabolites and Antioxidant Cell Defense in CHO-K1 Cells. *Food Chem. Toxicol.* **2016**, *96*, 43–49. [CrossRef] [PubMed]
77. Gao, F.; Jiang, L.P.; Chen, M.; Geng, C.Y.; Yang, G.; Ji, F.; Zhong, L.F.; Liu, X.F. Genotoxic Effects Induced by Zearalenone in a Human Embryonic Kidney Cell Line. *Mutat. Res. Genet. Toxicol. Environ. Mutagen.* **2013**, *755*, 6–10. [CrossRef] [PubMed]

78. Tiessen, C.; Gehrke, H.; Kropat, C.; Schwarz, C.; Bächler, S.; Fehr, M.; Pahlke, G.; Marko, D. Role of Topoisomerase Inhibition and DNA Repair Mechanisms in the Genotoxicity of Alternariol and Altertoxin-II. *World Mycotoxin J.* **2013**, *6*, 233–244. [CrossRef]
79. Viktorová, J.; Dobiasová, S.; Řehořová, K.; Biedermann, D.; Káňová, K.; Šeborová, K.; Václavíková, R.; Valentová, K.; Ruml, T.; Křen, V.; et al. Antioxidant, Anti-Inflammatory, and Multidrug Resistance Modulation Activity of Silychristin Derivatives. *Antioxidants* **2019**, *8*, 303. [CrossRef]
80. Fromm, M.F. Importance of P-Glycoprotein at Blood-Tissue Barriers. *Trends Pharmacol. Sci.* **2004**, *25*, 423–429. [CrossRef]
81. Meyer, M.R.; Wagmann, L.; Schneider-Daum, N.; Loretz, B.; De Souza Carvalho, C.; Lehr, C.M.; Maurer, H.H. P-Glycoprotein Interactions of Novel Psychoactive Substances—Stimulation of ATP Consumption and Transport across Caco-2 Monolayers. *Biochem. Pharmacol.* **2015**, *94*, 220–226. [CrossRef]
82. Li, X.; Mu, P.; Wen, J.; Deng, Y. Carrier-Mediated and Energy-Dependent Uptake and Efflux of Deoxynivalenol in Mammalian Cells. *Sci. Rep.* **2017**, *7*, 1–10. [CrossRef] [PubMed]
83. Videmann, B.; Tep, J.; Cavret, S.; Lecoeur, S. Epithelial Transport of Deoxynivalenol: Involvement of Human P-Glycoprotein (ABCB1) and Multidrug Resistance-Associated Protein 2 (ABCC2). *Food Chem. Toxicol.* **2007**, *45*, 1938–1947. [CrossRef] [PubMed]
84. Prouillac, C.; Videmann, B.; Mazallon, M.; Lecoeur, S. Induction of Cells Differentiation and ABC Transporters Expression by a Myco-Estrogen, Zearalenone, in Human Choriocarcinoma Cell Line (BeWo). *Toxicology* **2009**, *263*, 100–107. [CrossRef] [PubMed]
85. Duca, R.-C.; Mabondzo, A.; Bravin, F.; Delaforge, M. In Vivo Effects of Zearalenone on the Expression of Proteins Involved in the Detoxification of Rat Xenobiotics. *Environ. Toxicol.* **2012**, *27*, 98–108. [CrossRef] [PubMed]
86. Koraichi, F.; Videmann, B.; Mazallon, M.; Benahmed, M.; Prouillac, C.; Lecoeur, S. Zearalenone Exposure Modulates the Expression of ABC Transporters and Nuclear Receptors in Pregnant Rats and Fetal Liver. *Toxicol. Lett.* **2012**, *211*, 246–256. [CrossRef] [PubMed]
87. Wang, X.; Wang, W.; Cheng, G.; Huang, L.; Chen, D.; Tao, Y.; Pan, Y.; Hao, H.; Wu, Q.; Wan, D.; et al. High Risk of Embryo-Fetal Toxicity: Placental Transfer of T-2 Toxin and Its Major Metabolite HT-2 Toxin in BeWo Cells. *Toxicol. Sci.* **2014**, *137*, 168–178. [CrossRef]
88. Smith, M.C.; Madec, S.; Coton, E.; Hymery, N. Natural Co-Occurrence of Mycotoxins in Foods and Feeds and Their in Vitro Combined Toxicological Effects. *Toxins* **2016**, *8*, 94. [CrossRef]
89. Entezari, M.; Mokhtari, M.J.; Hashemi, M. Evaluation of Silibinin on the Viability of MCF-7 Human Breast Adenocarcinoma and HUVEC ( Human Umbilical Vein Endothelial ) Cell Lines. *Breast* **2011**, *3*, 283–288.
90. Wan, L.Y.M.; Turner, P.C.; El-Nezami, H. Individual and Combined Cytotoxic Effects of Fusarium Toxins (Deoxynivalenol, Nivalenol, Zearalenone and Fumonisins B1) on Swine Jejunal Epithelial Cells. *Food Chem. Toxicol.* **2013**, *57*, 276–283. [CrossRef]
91. Thuvander, A.; Wikman, C.; Gadhasson, I. In Vitro Exposure of Human Lymphocytes to Trichothecenes: Individual Variation in Sensitivity and Effects of Combined Exposure on Lymphocyte Function. *Food Chem. Toxicol.* **1999**, *37*, 639–648. [CrossRef]
92. Lin, X.; Shao, W.; Yu, F.; Xing, K.; Liu, H.; Zhang, F.; Goldring, M.B.; Lammi, M.J.; Guo, X. Individual and Combined Toxicity of T-2 Toxin and Deoxynivalenol on Human C-28/I2 and Rat Primary Chondrocytes. *J. Appl. Toxicol.* **2019**, *39*, 343–353. [CrossRef] [PubMed]
93. Klarić, M.Š.; Rumora, L.; Ljubanović, D.; Pepeljnjak, S. Cytotoxicity and Apoptosis Induced by Fumonisin B1, Beauvericin and Ochratoxin a in Porcine Kidney PK15 Cells: Effects of Individual and Combined Treatment. *Arch. Toxicol.* **2008**, *82*, 247–255. [CrossRef] [PubMed]
94. Juranova, J.; Aury-Landas, J.; Boumediene, K.; Bauge, C.; Biedermann, D.; Ulrichova, J.; Frankova, J. Modulation of Skin Inflammatory Response by Active Components of Silymarin. *Mol. Basel Switz.* **2018**, *24*, 123. [CrossRef]
95. Fan, S.; Li, L.; Chen, S.; Yu, Y.; Qi, M.; Tashiro, S.I.; Onodera, S.; Ikejima, T. Silibinin Induced-Autophagic and Apoptotic Death Is Associated with an Increase in Reactive Oxygen and Nitrogen Species in HeLa Cells. *Free Radic. Res.* **2011**, *45*, 1307–1324. [CrossRef]
96. Kim, T.H.; Woo, J.S.; Kim, Y.K.; Kim, K.H. Silibinin Induces Cell Death through Reactive Oxygen Species-Dependent Downregulation of Notch-1/ERK/Akt Signaling in Human Breast Cancer Cells. *J. Pharmacol. Exp. Ther.* **2014**, *349*, 268–278. [CrossRef]

97. Wu, Q.H.; Wang, X.; Yang, W.; Nüssler, A.K.; Xiong, L.Y.; Kuča, K.; Dohnal, V.; Zhang, X.J.; Yuan, Z.H. Oxidative Stress-Mediated Cytotoxicity and Metabolism of T-2 Toxin and Deoxynivalenol in Animals and Humans: An Update. *Arch. Toxicol.* **2014**, *88*, 1309–1326. [CrossRef]
98. Duan, W.; Jin, X.; Li, Q.; Tashiro, S.; Onodera, S.; Ikejima, T. Silibinin Induced Autophagic and Apoptotic Cell Death in HT1080 Cells Through a Reactive Oxygen Species Pathway. *J. Pharmacol. Sci.* **2010**, *113*, 48–56. [CrossRef]
99. Abdel-Wahhab, M.A.; El-Nekeety, A.A.; Salman, A.S.; Abdel-Aziem, S.H.; Mehaya, F.M.; Hassan, N.S. Protective Capabilities of Silymarin and Inulin Nanoparticles against Hepatic Oxidative Stress, Genotoxicity and Cytotoxicity of Deoxynivalenol in Rats. *Toxicon* **2018**, *142*, 1–13. [CrossRef]
100. Toğay, V.A.; Sevimli, T.S.; Sevimli, M.; Çelik, D.A.; Özçelik, N. DNA Damage in Rats with Streptozotocin-Induced Diabetes; Protective Effect of Silibinin. *Mutat. Res. Genet. Toxicol. Environ. Mutagen.* **2018**, *825*, 15–18. [CrossRef]
101. Fernandes Veloso Borges, F.; Ribeiro E Silva, C.; Moreira Goes, W.; Ribeiro Godoy, F.; Craveiro Franco, F.; Hollanda Véras, J.; Luiz Cardoso Bailão, E.F.; De Melo E Silva, D.; Gomes Cardoso, C.; Divino Da Cruz, A.; et al. Protective Effects of Silymarin and Silibinin against DNA Damage in Human Blood Cells. *BioMed Res. Int.* **2018**, *2018*. [CrossRef]
102. Tiwari, P.; Kumar, A.; Ali, M.; Mishra, K.P. Radioprotection of Plasmid and Cellular DNA and Swiss Mice by Silibinin. *Mutat. Res. Genet. Toxicol. Environ. Mutagen.* **2010**, *695*, 55–60. [CrossRef] [PubMed]
103. Alcaraz-Contreras, Y.; Mendoza-Lozano, R.P.; Martínez-Alcaraz, E.R.; Martínez-Alfaro, M.; Gallegos-Corona, M.A.; Ramírez-Morales, M.A.; Vázquez-Guevara, M.A. Silymarin and Dimercaptosuccinic Acid Ameliorate Lead-Induced Nephrotoxicity and Genotoxicity in Rats. *Hum. Exp. Toxicol.* **2016**, *35*, 398–403. [CrossRef] [PubMed]
104. Bordin, K.; Saladino, F.; Fernández-Blanco, C.; Ruiz, M.J.; Mañes, J.; Fernández-Franzón, M.; Meca, G.; Luciano, F.B. Reaction of Zearalenone and α-Zearalenol with Allyl Isothiocyanate, Characterization of Reaction Products, Their Bioaccessibility and Bioavailability in Vitro. *Food Chem.* **2017**, *217*, 648–654. [CrossRef] [PubMed]
105. Gajęcka, M.; Jakimiuk, E.; Zielonka, Ł.; Obremski, K.; Gajęcki, M. The Biotransformation of Chosen Mycotoxins. *Pol Viet Sci.* **2009**, *12*, 293–303.
106. Kabak, B.; Ozbey, F. Assessment of the Bioaccessibility of Aflatoxins from Various Food Matrices Using an in Vitro Digestion Model, and the Efficacy of Probiotic Bacteria in Reducing Bioaccessibility. *J. Food Compos. Anal.* **2012**, *27*, 21–31. [CrossRef]
107. Gratz, S.W.; Dinesh, R.; Yoshinari, T.; Holtrop, G.; Richardson, A.J.; Duncan, G.; MacDonald, S.; Lloyd, A.; Tarbin, J. Masked Trichothecene and Zearalenone Mycotoxins Withstand Digestion and Absorption in the Upper GI Tract but Are Efficiently Hydrolyzed by Human Gut Microbiota in Vitro. *Mol. Nutr. Food Res.* **2017**, *61*, 1600680. [CrossRef]
108. Videmann, B.; Mazallon, M.; Tep, J.; Lecoeur, S. Metabolism and Transfer of the Mycotoxin Zearalenone in Human Intestinal Caco-2 Cells. *Food Chem. Toxicol.* **2008**, *46*, 3279–3286. [CrossRef]
109. Meca, G.; Mañes, J.; Font, G.; Ruiz, M.J. Study of the potential toxicity of enniatins A, A 1, B, B 1 by evaluation of duodenal and colonic bioavailability applying an invitro method by Caco-2 cells. *Toxicon* **2012**, *59*, 1–11. [CrossRef]
110. Burkhardt, B.; Pfeiffer, E.; Metzler, M. Absorption and Metabolism of the Mycotoxins Alternariol and Alternariol-9-Methyl Ether in Caco-2 Cells in Vitro. *Mycotoxin Res.* **2009**, *25*, 149–157. [CrossRef]
111. Vidal, A.; Mengelers, M.; Yang, S.; De Saeger, S.; De Boevre, M. Mycotoxin Biomarkers of Exposure: A Comprehensive Review. *Compr. Rev. Food Sci. Food Saf.* **2018**, *17*, 1127–1155. [CrossRef]
112. Fæste, C.K.; Ivanova, L.; Uhlig, S. In vitro metabolism of the mycotoxin enniatin B in different species and cytochrome P450 enzyme phenotyping by chemical inhibitors. *Drug Metab. Dispos.* **2011**, *39*, 1768–1776. [CrossRef]
113. Delaforge, M.; Andre, F.; Jaouen, M.; Dolgos, H.; Benech, H.; Gomis, J.M.; Noel, J.P.; Cavelier, F.; Verducci, J.; Aubagnac, J.L.; et al. Metabolism of tentoxin by hepatic cytochrome P-450 3A isozymes. *Eur. J. Biochem.* **1997**, *250*, 150–157. [CrossRef] [PubMed]
114. Riss, T.L.; Moravec, R.A.; Niles, A.L.; Duellman, S.; Benink, H.A.; Worzella, T.J.; Minor, L. Cell Viability Assays. *Assay Guid. Man. Internet* **2013**, *114*, 785–796. [CrossRef]

115. Ferruzza, S.; Scarino, M.L.; Gambling, L.; Natella, F.; Sambuy, Y. Biphasic Effect of Iron on Human Intestinal Caco-2 Cells: Early Effect on Tight Junction Permeability with Delayed Onset of Oxidative Cytotoxic Damage. *Cell. Mol. Biol.* **2003**, *49*, 89–99. [PubMed]
116. Stukonis, V.; Armonienė, R.; Lemežienė, N.; Kemešytė, V.; Statkevičiūtė, G. Identification of Fine-Leaved Species of Genus Festuca by Molecular Methods. *Pak. J. Bot.* **2015**, *47*, 1137–1142. [CrossRef]
117. Singh, N.P.; McCoy, M.T.; Tice, R.R.; Schneider, E.L. A Simple Technique for Quantitation of Low Levels of DNA Damage in Individual Cells. *Exp. Cell Res.* **1988**, *175*, 184–191. [CrossRef]
118. McKelvey-Martin, V.J.; Green, M.H.L.; Schmezer, P.; Pool-Zobel, B.L.; De Meo, M.P.; Collins, A. The Single Cell Gelelectrophores is Assay (comet Assay): A European Review. *Mutat. Res.* **1993**, *288*, 47–63. [CrossRef]

toxins

MDPI

Article

# Transcriptome Analysis of Ochratoxin A-Induced Apoptosis in Differentiated Caco-2 Cells

**Xue Yang [1,2,3,4,†], Yanan Gao [1,2,3,4,†], Qiaoyan Yan [1,2,3,4,†], Xiaoyu Bao [1,2,3,4], Shengguo Zhao [1,2,3,4], Jiaqi Wang [1,2,3,4] and Nan Zheng [1,2,3,4,*]**

1 Key Laboratory of Quality & Safety Control for Milk and Dairy Products of Ministry of Agriculture and Rural Affairs, Institute of Animal Sciences, Chinese Academy of Agricultural Sciences, Beijing 100193, China; 82101182216@caas.cn (X.Y.); gyn758521@126.com (Y.G.); yeqiaoyan@caas.cn (Q.Y.); xbao@ualberta.ca (X.B.); zhaoshengguo@caas.cn (S.Z.); wangjiaqi@caas.cn (J.W.)

2 Laboratory of Quality and Safety Risk Assessment for Dairy Products of Ministry of Agriculture and Rural Affairs, Institute of Animal Sciences, Chinese Academy of Agricultural Sciences, Beijing 100193, China

3 Milk and Dairy Product Inspection Center of Ministry of Agriculture and Rural Affairs, Institute of Animal Sciences, Chinese Academy of Agricultural Sciences, Beijing 100193, China

4 State Key Laboratory of Animal Nutrition, Institute of Animal Sciences, Chinese Academy of Agricultural Sciences, Beijing 100193, China

* Correspondence: zhengnan@caas.cn; Tel.: +86-10-6281-6069; Fax: +86-10-6289-7587

† These authors contributed equally to this work.

Received: 4 November 2019; Accepted: 24 December 2019; Published: 31 December 2019

**Abstract:** Ochratoxin A (OTA), an important mycotoxin that occurs in food and animal feed, has aroused widespread concern in recent years. Previous studies have indicated that OTA causes nephrotoxicity, hepatotoxicity, genotoxicity, immunotoxicity, cytotoxicity, and neurotoxicity. The intestinal toxicity of OTA has gradually become a focus of research, but the mechanisms underlying this toxicity have not been described. Here, differentiated Caco-2 cells were incubated for 48 h with different concentrations of OTA and transcriptome analysis was used to estimate damage to the intestinal barrier. Gene expression profiling was used to compare the characteristics of differentially expressed genes (DEGs). There were altogether 10,090 DEGs, mainly clustered into two downregulation patterns. The Search Tool for Retrieval of Interacting Genes (STRING), which was used to analyze the protein–protein interaction network, indicated that 24 key enzymes were mostly responsible for regulating cell apoptosis. Quantitative reverse transcription-polymerase chain reaction (qRT-PCR) analysis was used to validate eight genes, three of which were key genes (*CASP3*, *CDC25B*, and *EGR1*). The results indicated that OTA dose-dependently induces apoptosis in differentiated Caco-2 cells. Transcriptome analysis showed that the impairment of intestinal function caused by OTA might be partly attributed to apoptosis, which is probably associated with downregulation of murine double minute 2 (MDM2) expression and upregulation of Noxa and caspase 3 (CASP3) expression. This study has highlighted the intestinal toxicity of OTA and provided a genome-wide view of biological responses, which provides a theoretical basis for enterotoxicity and should be useful in establishing a maximum residue limit for OTA.

**Keywords:** ochratoxin A; differentiated Caco-2 cells; cell apoptosis; transcriptome analysis

**Key Contribution:** Transcription analysis indicated that OTA-induced intestinal toxicity may be induced by apoptosis through the regulation of MDM2 and CASP3 which provide a theoretical basis for toxicological evaluation of OTA.

## 1. Introduction

Ochratoxin A (OTA) is a fungal secondary metabolite produced by certain *Penicillium* and *Aspergillus* species, including *Penicillium verrucosum*, *Aspergillus ochraceus*, and *Aspergillus niger* [1]. OTA was first isolated from *A. ochraceus* in 1965 and was found to contaminate the food chain worldwide [2]. It is widely found in various grains and vegetables [3–5], as well as in food products of animal origin, such as meat, eggs, and milk [6–9]. Milk, which has high bioavailability and is an abundant source of nutrients, is widely recognized to be an important component of the human diet. As the consumption of milk has increased over recent years, the mycotoxins found in milk have received increasing attention. A provisional tolerable weekly intake of 100 ng/kg.bw/week has been established for OTA by the Joint FAO/WHO Expert Committee on Food Additives (JECFA) [10], JECFA, 2001), although a maximum residue limit (MRL) for OTA in milk has not been agreed upon internationally. A study in Italy detected OTA concentrations of 70–110 ng/L in organic milk [11]. In China, Huang et al. [12] measured levels of OTA in raw, powdered, and liquid cow's milk, and found mean concentrations of 56.7, 27.0, and 26.8 ng/kg, respectively. In Sudan, the level of OTA in a contaminated milk sample was as high as 2730 ng/L [13]. OTA has been classified in Group 2B (possible carcinogens in humans) by The International Agency for Research on Cancer, because of evidence of carcinogenicity in animals, but not in humans [14].

The gastrointestinal tract (GIT) is essential for human health and provides a barrier between the external environment and the tightly regulated internal environment [15]. The GIT can be exposed to numerous contaminated foods and high doses of some mycotoxins [16]. Early studies on OTA focused mainly on the diversity of toxic effects in different animal species [17–19]. Recent studies, however, have reported the toxic effect of OTA on the intestine [20,21]. OTA-induced intestinal damage has been reported in both animals and in vitro intestinal models [22,23]. It has been shown to damage the intestinal epithelium in chickens and rats [24–26] and also shows toxicity in intestinal epithelial cells, including a porcine intestinal cell line (IPEC-J2) and human intestinal epithelial lines (HT-29-D4 cells and Caco-2 cells) [20,27,28]. Previously published studies have shown that cell apoptosis is one of the ways by which OTA exerts intestinal toxicity [20,26,29]. Wang et al. [20] suggested that apoptosis induced by OTA may play a major role in the intestinal toxicity of this mycotoxin, and Bouaziz et al. [30] also suggested that OTA causes toxicity through apoptosis. OTA has been shown to induce apoptosis in different cell lines [31–35], which may be one of the main cellular mechanisms underlying the toxic effects. However, the molecular mechanisms responsible for cell apoptosis, which leads to intestinal toxicity, are still inadequately understood. It is, therefore, important to investigate the mechanism of apoptosis of intestinal epithelial cells following exposure to OTA. In the present study, we used differentiated Caco-2 cells as they can form polarized apical/mucosal and basolateral/serosal membranes that are similar to those formed by epithelial cells in the small intestine [36]. Moreover, it has been acknowledged by the Food and Drug Administration that differentiated Caco-2 cells are a suitable model for evaluating the impact of toxins on intestinal barrier function [37,38].

With large-scale transcription approaches, a comprehensive overview, provided by high throughput data, can easily reveal biological pathways and processes that have not been found before [39]. Using whole-genome transcriptome profiling, RNA sequencing (RNA-seq), an unbiased sequencing tool, has been used to detect changes of gene expression in tissue samples or cells [40,41]. The aim of this study was to investigate the mechanism of OTA-induced apoptosis in differentiated Caco-2 cells and to use RNA-seq technology to evaluate changes in gene expression and profile to clarify the mechanism of OTA-induced apoptosis in differentiated Caco-2 cells.

## 2. Results

### 2.1. OTA Induces Apoptosis in Differentiated Caco-2 Cells in a Dose-Dependent Manner

After treatment with OTA (0.0005, 0.005, and 4 μg/mL) for 48 h, Annexin V-PI dual staining and flow cytometry were used to detect apoptosis of differentiated Caco-2 cells (Figure 1a). As depicted in the histogram (Figure 1b), the percentage of apoptotic cells was increased by treatment for 48 h with 0.0005 μg/mL (2.9% ± 0.67%), 0.005 μg/mL (5.23% ± 0.21%), and 4 μg/mL (20.9% ± 2.49%) OTA, compared with the control (2.3% ± 0.08%). The percentage of cell apoptosis was significantly increased in differentiated Caco-2 cells ($p < 0.05$) when the concentration of OTA was 4 μg/mL (Figure 1b). The number of living cells in the Q3 regions of the flow cytometry plots also decreased as the concentration of OTA increased (Figure 1a).

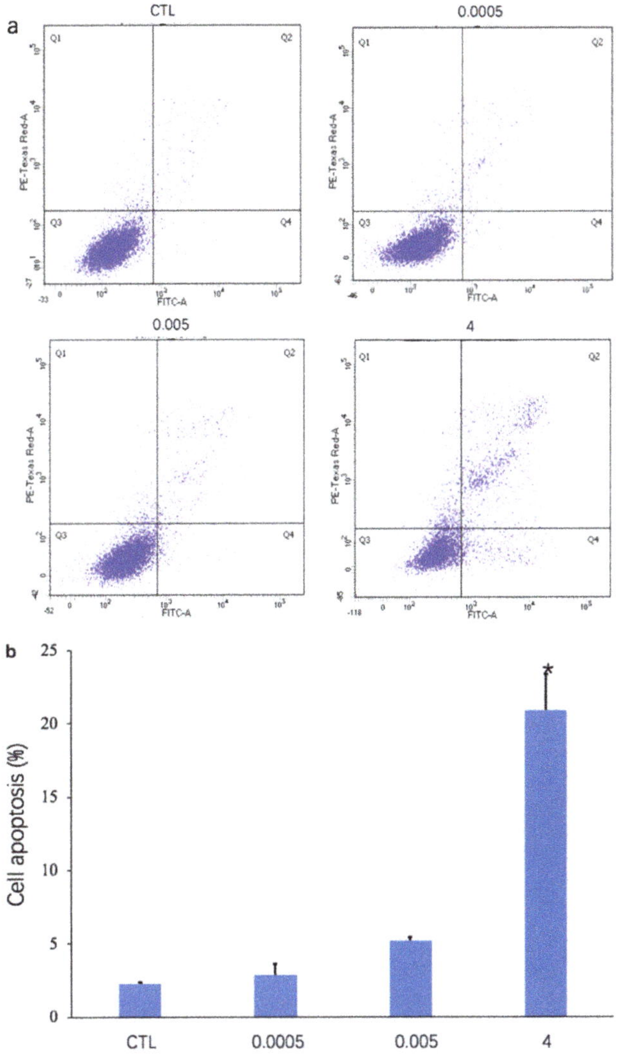


**Figure 1.** Effects of ochratoxin A (OTA) on apoptosis in differentiated Caco-2 cells. Incubation of cells for 48 h with OTA (0, 0.0005, 0.005, and 4 μg/mL) was followed by analysis using flow cytometry. (**a**) Representative flow cytometry plots are presented for the control group (CTL) and OTA groups (0.0005 μg/mL, 0.005 μg/mL, and 4 μg/mL). (**b**) Histogram showing number of differentially expressed genes after treatment with three concentrations of OTA compared with the control group. * represents a significant difference ($p < 0.05$).

*2.2. Effect of OTA on Gene Expression Patterns*

There were 18,654 unigene annotations in the control group (56.56% of all the 32,938 reference unigene sequences) and 18,475 (56.56%), 18,898 (57.30%), and 19,853 (55.61%) unigene annotations in the 0.0005, 0.005, and 4 μg/mL OTA groups., respectively. Using a *p*-value < 0.05 and a 2-fold change (FC) as the conditions for discrimination, we identified 503, 2139, and 9402 differentially expressed genes (DEGs) when the cells were incubated for 48 h with 0.0005, 0.005, and 4 μg/mL OTA, respectively. At these three concentrations of OTA, 35, 258, and 1437 genes were upregulated and 468, 1881, and 7965 genes were downregulated, respectively (Figure 2). At all concentrations of OTA, downregulation of genes was the main trend (93%, 88%, and 85% of the total DEGs, respectively). The number of DEGs in differentiated Caco-2 cells increased with increasing OTA concentration. Using a Venn diagram, we found that 3 upregulated DEGs and 169 downregulated DEGs were commonly modulated by all three concentrations of OTA (Figure 3a,b). Compared with the control, there were 257 overlapping DEGs between the 0.0005 and 0.005 μg/mL OTA groups and 1532 overlapping DEGs between the 0.005 and 4 μg/mL groups (Supplementary Figure S1), showing that the common DEGs were increased in a dose-dependent manner. To assess the expression patterns of mRNAs at different concentrations of OTA, we used heatmaps to analyze the overall transcriptome differences (Figure 3c). The same differently expressed transcripts were present in three separate runs of the control group (CTL1, CTL2, CTL3), the 0.0005 μg/mL treatment group (0.0005-1,2,3), the 0.005 μg/mL treatment group (0.005-1,2,3), and the 4 μg/mL treatment group (4-1,2,3) (Figure 3c). The heatmap (Figure 3c) shows accurate repeatability and high reliability.

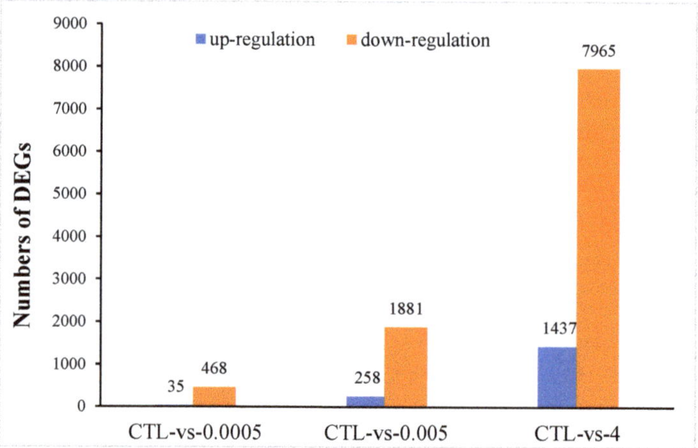


**Figure 2.** Differentially expressed genes (DEGs) identified in differentiated Caco-2 cells after exposure to 0.0005, 0.005, and 4 μg/mL OTA for 48 h. Histogram shows the number of DEGs compared with the control (CTL).

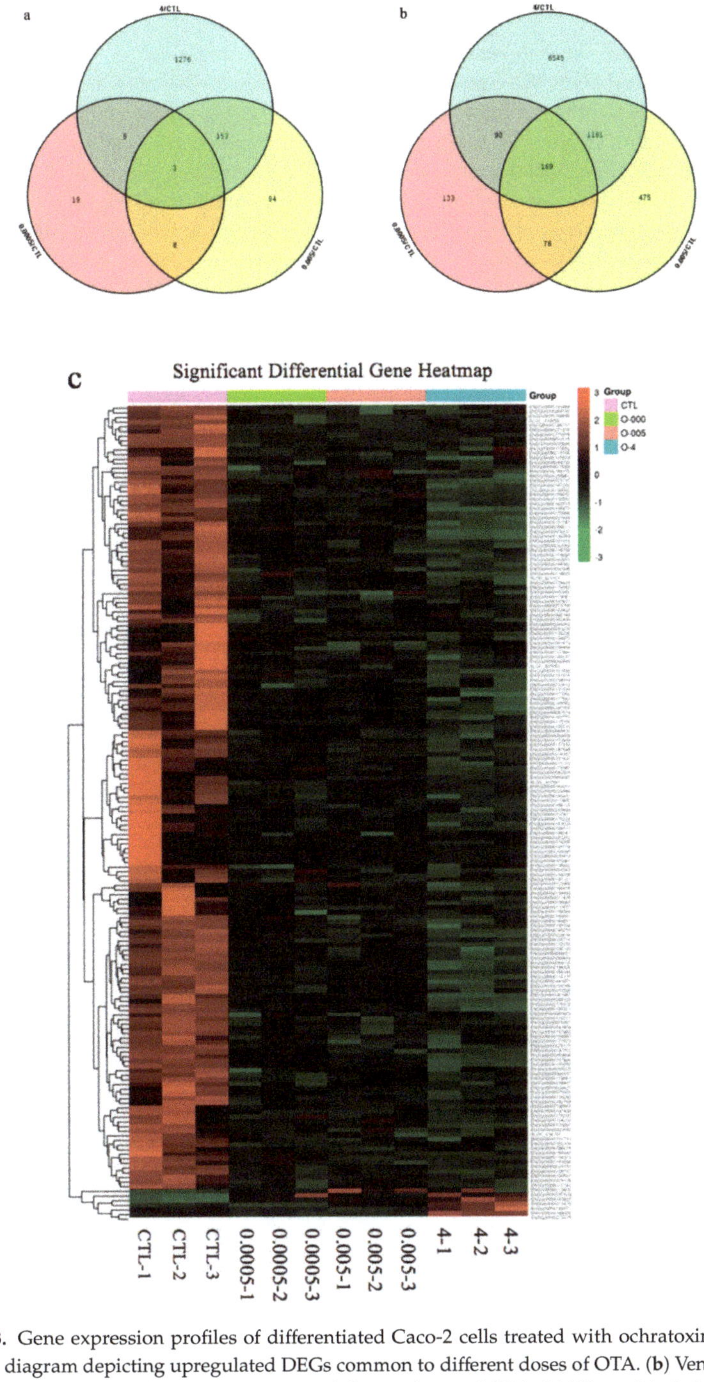


**Figure 3.** Gene expression profiles of differentiated Caco-2 cells treated with ochratoxin A (OTA). (**a**) Venn diagram depicting upregulated DEGs common to different doses of OTA. (**b**) Venn diagram depicting downregulated DEGs common to different doses of OTA. (**c**) Hierarchical clustering of common DEGs in differentiated Caco-2 cells based on log10-transformed expression values (fragments per kilobase of transcript per million fragments mapped, FPKM).

### 2.3. Gene Ontology (GO) Annotation and KEGG Enrichment Analysis of DEGs

Using the FC and $p$-value thresholds described in the Methods section above, we obtained 10,090 DEGs (compared with the control, the sum of DEGs of the OTA treatment at different concentrations), which could be clustered into eight profiles using the short time-series expression miner to obtain dynamic expression patterns of the DEGs. Among these eight profiles, two classic downregulated profiles (profiles 0 and 3) were significantly enriched (Supplementary Figure S2). A total of 7199 DEGs were mainly clustered into these two downregulated profiles, which contained 1883 and 5226 genes, respectively (Supplementary Figure S3). To discover the functions of the DEGs and the associated biological processes altered by OTA treatment of differentiated Caco-2 cells, we carried out a gene ontology (GO) (http://www.geneontology.org/) enrichment analysis, in which the DEGs were divided into three independent GO categories. Single DEGs could be annotated to more than two GO terms and the most enriched GO terms are displayed in Figure S3. The three main categories of the GO classification were assessed for enriched genes.

All the DEGs were mapped in the Kyoto Encyclopedia of Genes and Genomes (KEGG, https://www.kegg.jp) database to detect the response pathways altered by treatment with OTA. Of the DEGs that could be annotated to the KEGG pathway, most were associated with metabolism and signal transduction pathways. In profile 0, the enriched pathways were pyrimidine metabolism, the TNF signaling pathway, ribosome biogenesis in eukaryotes, and the Wnt signaling pathway. In profile 3, the enriched pathways were endocytosis, cell cycle, ubiquitin-mediated proteolysis, pyrimidine metabolism, and AMPK signaling (Figure 4).

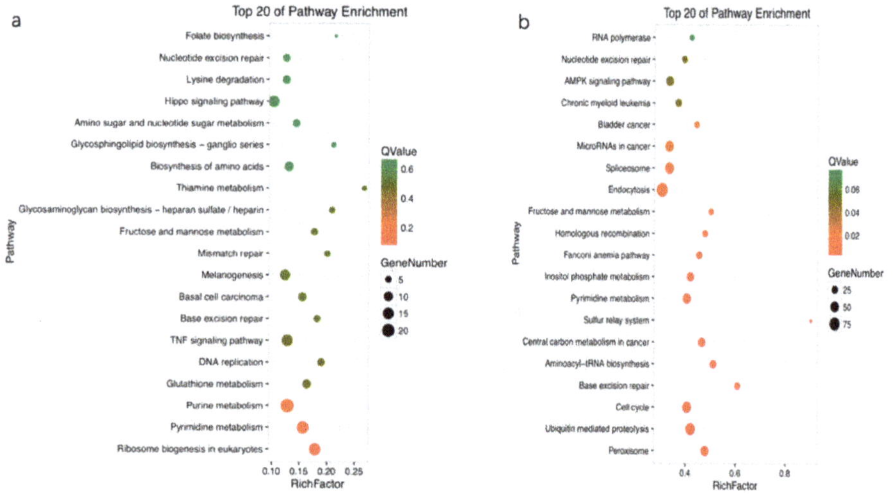


**Figure 4.** Scatter plots of the top 20 enriched Kyoto Encyclopedia of Genes and Genomes (KEGG) pathway terms (**a**), profile 0; (**b**), profile 3. Enriched items were measured by the rich factor, q value ($q < 0.05$), and number of genes. TNF, tumor necrosis factor.

### 2.4. Key Pathways and DEGs Related to Cell Apoptosis

Using the GO annotation and KEGG analysis, we can select the key pathways that are associated with the toxic effects of OTA in differentiated Caco-2 cells. DEGs from the key significantly enriched pathways, particularly those shared between the different concentrations of OTA, may be thought of as the key gene expression regulators that respond to treatment with OTA. These 10 key pathways, together with some key genes that participate in or regulate the cell cycle and cell apoptosis, are shown in Table 1.

**Table 1.** Key pathways and important related differentially expressed genes (DEGs) that are associated with the toxic effect of ochratoxin A (OTA) in differentiated Caco-2 cells. mTOR, mechanistic target of rapamycin kinase; MAPK, mitogen-activated protein kinase; TNF, tumor necrosis factor.

| Pathway | Pathway ID | Key DEGs from the Pathway |
|---|---|---|
| Cell cycle | ko04110 | MDM2, CDK1, TP53, EP300, ATM, CDKN1B, TGFB1, CHEK1, CDC25B, CCNB1, PDPK1 |
| P53 signaling pathway | ko04115 | MDM2, PMAIP1, CASP3, TP53AIP, CDK1, TP53, ATM, CYCS, TSC2, CHEK1, CASP9, CCNB1, BAX |
| HIF-1 signaling pathway | ko04066 | HIF1A, NFKB1, CDKN1B, MTOR, EP300, AKT1, PIK3R, EGFR, NOX1, INSR, PIK3CA |
| PI3k-Akt signaling pathway | ko04151 | CDKN1B, NFKB1, CCND1, BCL2L1, MYC, PIK3CA, EGFR, MDM2, TP53, IKBKB, AKT1, HRAS, TSC2, IL3RA, MAPK1, SOS1, CASP3, MTOR, INSR, BAD, CASP9, PDPK1 |
| mTOR signaling pathway | ko04150 | MTOR, TNF, IKBKB, PRKAA, PIK3CA, HRAS, TSC2, MAPK1, AKT1, SOS1, INSR, PDPK1 |
| Apoptosis | ko04210 | XIAP, BCL2L1, NFKB1, PIK3CA, CASP3, CYC, BAX, BAD, IL3RA, CASP9, CFLAR, TP53, ATM, HRAS, TRADD, MAPK1, RIPK1, CDKN1B, PMAIP1, TP53AIP, AKT1, TNF, IKBKB |
| Foxo signaling pathway | ko04068 | CDKN1B, PIK3CA, MDM2, PDPK1, EGFR1, FOXO1, AKT1, IRS1, INSR, MDM2, TGFB1, IKBKB, ATM, HRAS, MAPK1, SOS1, EGFR, EP300, CCNB1, TGFB1 |
| Insulin signaling pathway | ko04910 | MAPK1, SOS1, PIK3CA, AKT1, MTOR, IRS1, INSR, HRAS, TSC2, TRADD, MAPK1, CALM1, IKBKB, FOXO1 |
| MAPK signaling pathway | ko04010 | TNF, CASP3, NFKB1, TP53, MAPK14, TGFB1, PIK3CA, HRAS, SOS1, EGFR, MAPK1, TRAF2, CDC25B, AKT1, TNF, IKBKB |
| TNF signaling pathway | ko04668 | XIAP, TNF, NFKB1, CASP3, IKBKB, MAPK1, MAPK14, CASP8, TRADD, FADD, MAPK1, RIPK1, TRAF2, AKT1, PIK3CA |

As shown in Figure 5, the 50 DEGs that occurred frequently in these key pathways, or participated in individual key pathways, were combined and employed to construct a protein–protein interaction (PPI) network using STRING. Cytoscape 3.1 was then used for further filtering (Edge score > 0.8). The 10 key pathways and 24 key DEGs associated with cell apoptosis were identified mainly from those shared between the different concentrations of OTA in the GO and KEGG analysis, and these key pathways were largely associated with the regulation of cell apoptosis and the cell cycle. According to the degree of connectivity of each node, we selected the following 24 key enzymes: murine double minute 2 (MDM2), v-akt murine thymoma viral oncogene homolog 1 (AKT1), tumor protein p53 (TP53), caspase 3 (CASP3), caspase 9 (CASP9), hras proto-oncogene gtpase (HRAS), mechanistic target of rapamycin kinase (MTOR), epidermal growth factor receptor (EGFR), bcl-2-like protein 1 (BCL2L1), tumor necrosis factor (TNF), atm serine/threonine kinase (ATM), cytochrome C somatic (CYCs), mitogen-activated protein kinase 1 and 14 (MAPK1, MAPK14), ribosomal protein s6 kinase B1 (RPS6KB1), x-linked inhibitor of apoptosis (XIAP), nuclear factor kappa B subunit 1 (NFKB1), cyclin B1 (CCNB1), E1A binding protein p300 (EP300), inhibitor of nuclear factor kappa B kinase subunit beta (IKBKB), TSC complex subunit 2 (TSC2), phosphatidylinositol-4,5-bisphosphate 3-kinase catalytic subunit alpha (PIK3CA), cyclin dependent kinase 1 (CDK1), and forkhead box O1 (FOXO1).

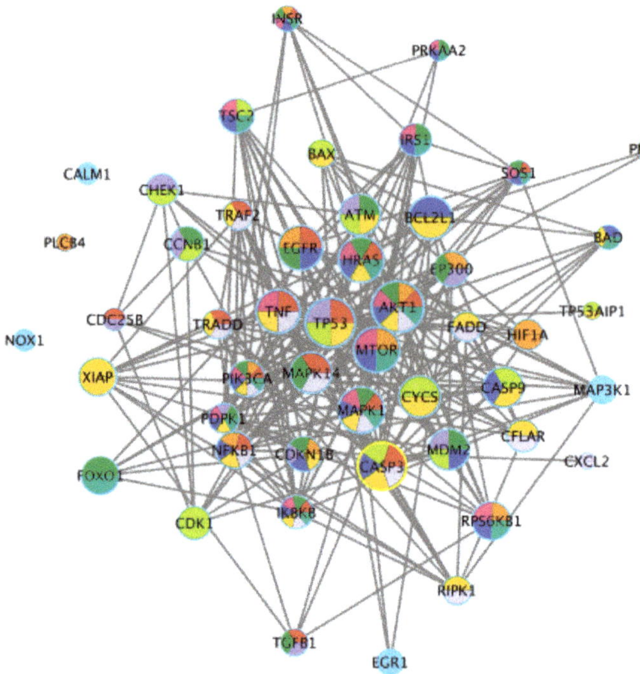


**Figure 5.** Protein–protein interaction (PPI) network for 50 important enzymes encoded by key differentially expressed genes (DEGs) of key pathways. Different nodes represent different enzymes. Interactions between these enzymes are represented by different size nodes; the larger the node, the stronger the connectivity.

### 2.5. *Validation of RNA-Seq Results by qRT-PCR*

Quantitative reverse transcription-polymerase chain reaction (qRT-PCR) analysis was performed to validate the high throughput data. We determined the expression of the following eight randomly selected genes: caspase 3 (CASP3), C–X–C motif chemokine ligand 2 (CXCL2), cell division cycle 25B (CDC25B), early growth response 1 (EGR1), FRY like transcription coactivator (FRYL), H2B histone family members (H2BFS), sedoheptulokinase (SHPK), and transcription factor EC (TFEC). Expression levels of CDC25B, SHPK, ERG1, FRYL, and TFEC significantly decreased after OTA treatment. In contrast, expression of CASP3, CXCL2, and H2BFS significantly increased (Figure 6a). These expression patterns were in good agreement with the data obtained by RNA-Seq, confirming the reliability of the two methods. There was a strong correlation ($r = 0.803$) between RNA-seq and qRT-PCR (Figure 6b). The protein levels of two randomly selected genes, MDM2 and CASP3, were measured by Western blotting. MDM2 levels significantly decreased and CASP3 levels increased after treatment with OTA (Figure 7).

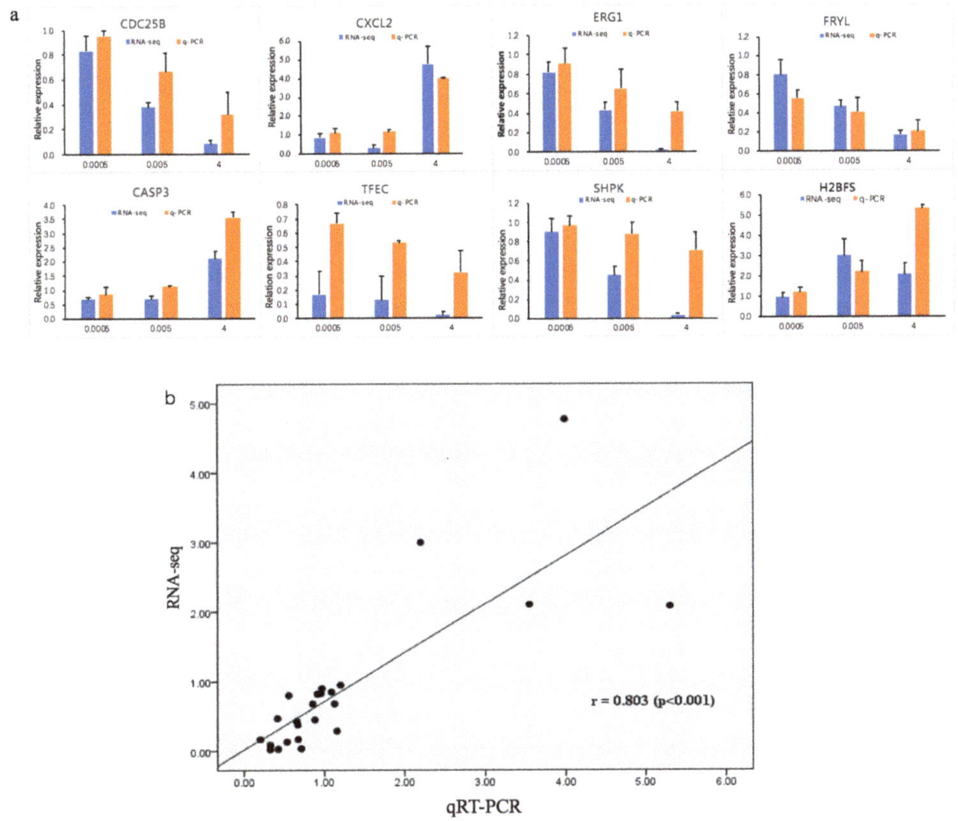


**Figure 6.** (**a**) Quantitative reverse transcription-polymerase chain reaction (qRT-PCR) results for eight DEGs compared with RNA-seq results. The blue bars represent RNA-seq data and the orange bars represent q-PCR data. (**b**) Correlation analysis between RNA-seq and qPCR.

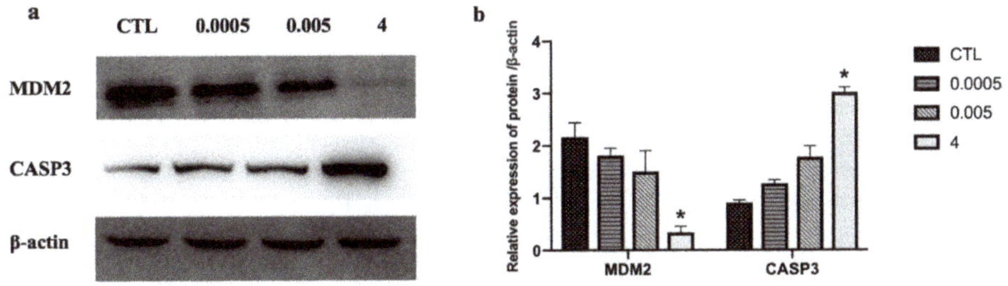


**Figure 7.** Effect of OTA (0.0005, 0.005, and 4 μg/mL) on cell apoptosis-related proteins in differentiated Caco-2 cells. Protein extracts were immunoblotted for candidate proteins (**a**) and band densities were quantified (**b**). Results are the mean of three separate experiments performed in triplicate ± SD. * $p < 0.05$, significantly different from control group.

## 3. Discussion

OTA has deleterious effects on humans and animals, resulting in worldwide illness and economic losses. Exposure to OTA occurs from ingestion of contaminated food and feed [42]. The small intestine is the main site of OTA absorption, with the largest absorption in the proximal jejunum [43]. Because of their location and function, intestinal epithelial cells are a potential target for the toxic effects of OTA. In the present study, flow cytometry showed that the number of apoptotic cells increased with increasing OTA concentration (Figure 1), which is consistent with previous studies demonstrating that OTA can induce apoptosis of intestinal cells [20,44,45]. Apoptosis, which is a form of programmed cell death, may disrupt the integrity of the intestinal barrier [46,47]. OTA induces apoptosis by modulating BcL-2 family members [30,48], and activation of MEK/ERK1-2 signaling has been shown to be crucial for OTA-induced apoptosis in HK-2 cells [49]. Although OTA-induced apoptosis has been studied previously, there has been a tendency to focus mainly on a particular pathway [20,49,50]. In this study, we chose instead to search for related pathways from a holistic perspective because transcriptome data can quickly and economically supply accurate genome information, particularly in identifying the effects of biological pathways and processes [51,52]. Elena et al. (2016) used transcriptomic analysis to reveal the different toxicity mechanisms of OTA and citrinin [53]. Hence, we used a transcriptomic study to provide a genome-wide biological view of changes that occurred after treatment of differentiated Caco-2 cells with different concentrations of OTA.

For the GO annotation, the main GO terms of the DEGs were cell processes and metabolic processes. Another microarray study demonstrated that OTA decreased mRNA levels of genes involved in liver cell metabolism [54]. KEGG enrichment analysis showed that there are key pathways, such as the cell cycle, the MAPK signaling pathway, the TNF signaling pathway, and the p53 signaling pathway, that are highly associated with cell apoptosis (Figure 4). These results indicate that OTA-induced cell apoptosis probably involves changes to the enriched pathways, such as the cell cycle, and other important signaling pathways. From the results obtained in this study, we speculate that cell apoptosis happens in an orderly manner and can be regulated by many mechanisms. Liang et al. [55] pointed out that OTA suppresses the cell cycle, particularly DNA replication, leading to cell cycle arrest and apoptosis. OTA has been shown to regulate apoptosis, the cell cycle, and cell fate following DNA damage by stimulating MAPK signaling pathways, such as p38 MAPK, ERK1/2, and JNK [56–58]. Apoptosis of liver and/or kidney cells has also been shown to be influenced by activation of certain signal transduction pathways, such as MAPK, ERK, p38, and JNK [56,59,60]. Another study obtained data that were of great importance in characterizing the modulatory effect of the TNF signaling pathway on apoptotic signaling [61]. Activation of the p53 pathway has also been shown to play a key role in OTA-induced apoptosis of human and monkey kidney cells [33]. These results are in agreement with reported research demonstrating that OTA triggers a p53-dependent apoptotic pathway in human hepatoma cells [62]. Using knockout mice, Hibi et al. showed that the p53 pathway plays a key role in OTA-induced genotoxicity [63]. Because previous research has highlighted the role of p53 signaling in OTA-induced apoptosis, in this study, we concentrated on the p53 pathway and analyzed its specific regulatory mechanism.

The p53 signaling pathway, which is amplified by different concentrations of OTA, plays a key role in regulating DNA repair mechanisms, oxidative stress, cell cycle arrest, and cell apoptosis [64,65]. In the renal outer medulla, OTA causes genotoxicity by deregulating molecular functions such as DNA double-strand break repair, cell cycle arrest in response to DNA damage, and p53-associated factors [66]. Alterations in oxidative stress and calcium homeostasis have also been associated with OTA-induced toxicity [67]. The proto-oncogene, MDM2, a nuclear protein that is the main cellular antagonist of p53, can regulate the potentially lethal activities of p53 by tightly combining with a p53 tumor suppressor protein and negatively regulating its stability and transcriptional activity [68]. Furthermore, MDM2 can not only inhibit the transactivation of p53 activity, but also stabilize p53 and reduce p53-mediated apoptosis [69]. The p53-MDM2 feedback loop may be important in regulating cell apoptosis. Previous studies have demonstrated that apoptotic pathways are regulated by proteins such as the tumor suppressor p53 and inhibitor of apoptosis (IAP) proteins, which are highly regulated by MDM2 through an autoregulatory feedback loop [70,71]. OTA may induce apoptosis in differentiated Caco-2 cells through the feedback loop interaction of MDM2 and the p53 signaling pathway. A study by Gu et al. [72] showed that gambogic acid induced apoptosis of wild-type p53-expressing cancer cells through downregulation of MDM2. Another study found that violacein decreased the expression of MDM2 and caused apoptosis of human breast cancer cells by activating PARP, CDKN1A, TNF-α, and p53 cleavage [73]. Our transcriptome analysis showed that OTA induced apoptosis in differentiated Caco-2 cells by activating key downstream genes in the p53 signaling pathway. In these key pathways, some DEGs, such as *CASP3*, *AKT1*, *MAPK1*, *HRAS*, *PIK3CA*, and *MDM2*, were highly involved (Figure 5), which appeared in the group 4 μg/mL specially instead of common DEGs (Figure 3). Several genes (*CASP3*, *CDC25B*, *CXCL*, and *EGR1*) were randomly selected from these key DEGs and common DEGs (*FRYL*, *TFEC*, *SHPK*, and *H2BFS*) were used for gene verification by qRT-PCR analysis. These key genes, and other DEGs, showed similar results in the RNA-seq analysis (Figure 6), and further study is needed to elucidate the relationships between the genes and regulation of cell apoptosis. In contrast to our own study, Kuroda et al. found that expression of the *CDK1* gene was increased by treatment with OTA [74]. We believe that the difference between the studies is because OTA increases DNA damage in *gpt* delta rats and CDK1 could accelerate the resection of DNA broken ends during the homologous recombination process [74–76]. Through analysis of the enrichment pathway, we found that p53 is a target signaling pathway and speculate that OTA probably induces cell apoptosis by downregulating MDM2 expression. Western blotting confirmed that OTA-induced cell apoptosis in differentiated Caco-2 cells is linked to perturbation of MDM2 (Figure 7).

In addition to the downregulation of MDM2, there are several important genes in the p53 signaling pathway that are upregulated in the apoptosis of differentiated Caco-2 cells. These are Noxa (phorbol-12-myristate-13-acetate-induced Protein1, PMAIP1), tumor protein p53 regulated apoptosis-inducing protein 1 (P53AIP1), and caspase 3 (cysteinyl aspartate proteases, CASP3). P53 transactivates noxa, bax, puma, and other apoptotic response genes, and their products trigger mitochondrial apoptosis pathways [50]. Noxa is a member of the pro-apoptotic B-cell lymphoma 2 (BCL-2) family and can not only promote activation of caspases and apoptosis, but also promote changes in the mitochondrial membrane and outflow of apoptogenic proteins from the mitochondria [77,78]. Functional studies have shown that P53AIP is a pro-apoptosis molecule, and it is believed to play a vital role in mediating p53-dependent apoptosis. P53AIP1 can lead to CASP3 activation and downstream activities by decreasing mitochondrial membrane potential and inducing release of cytochrome c. CASP3 plays a vital role in many events involved in cell apoptosis, including activation of the caspase cascade and the execution of apoptosis [79–81]. OTA-induced downregulation of MDM2 could regulate the downstream upregulation of Noxa and P53AIP1, and eventually activate CASP3 in the apoptosis of Caco-2 cells.

To conclude, we have shown that OTA-induced apoptosis in differentiated Caco-2 cells may involve downregulation of MDM2 and upregulation of CASP3, through activation of the p53-mediated cell apoptosis signaling pathway. A more exhaustive study is, however, needed to fully elucidate all of the underlying mechanisms. We have also demonstrated the intestinal toxicity of OTA and provided a genome-wide view of biological responses, which provides a theoretical basis for enterotoxicity and should be useful in establishing an MRL for OTA.

## 4. Materials and Methods

### 4.1. Chemicals and Reagents

OTA powder ($C_{20}H_{18}ClNO_6$; molecular weight, 403) was purchased from Pribolab (Qingdao, China). Human colon adenocarcinoma Caco-2 cells (passage number 18) were acquired from the American Type Culture Collection (Manassas, VA, USA). Fetal bovine serum (FBS) and Dulbecco's modified Eagle's medium (DMEM) were obtained from Gibco (Carlsbad, CA, USA). Nonessential amino acids (NEAA), trypsin (2.5%), antibiotics (100 units/mL penicillin, 100 μg/mL streptomycin), phosphate-buffered saline (PBS), Western and IP Cell Lysis Buffer, and an Annexin V-FITC apoptosis detection kit were supplied by Beyotime Biotechnology (Shanghai, China). A stock solution of OTA (1000 μg/mL) was obtained by dissolving OTA in methanol, and stored at −20 °C for later use. Rabbit anti-β-actin (58169S) and rabbit anti-MDM2 antibodies (86934S) were obtained from Cell Signaling Technology (Boston, MA, USA), and goat anti-rabbit IgG conjugated to horseradish peroxidase was obtained from Bioss (Beijing, China).

### 4.2. Cell Culture and Treatments

Differentiated Caco-2 cells were seeded into six-well Transwell chambers (Corning, NY, USA) at a density of $1 \times 10^5$ cells per well in DMEM containing 4.5 g/L glucose, 1% NEAA, 10% FBS, and antibiotics. The cells were incubated at 37 °C in a humidified atmosphere containing 5% $CO_2$. A polarized epithelial monolayer of differentiated Caco-2 cells was formed by replacing the medium every other day for 21 days. Because an MRL for OTA in milk has not yet been established and previous studies have indicated that OTA and aflatoxin M1 (AFM1) have the same cytotoxicity in human intestinal Caco-2 cells [82], we chose the concentration of 0.0005 μg/mL for OTA, based on the Chinese (0.5 μg/kg) limits for AFM1 in milk. We established a concentration gradient when measuring cell viability and transepithelial electrical resistance [83] and chose the 4 μg/mL concentration to investigate the effect of an upper concentration limit on intestinal injury, without affecting cell survival. After 48 h of treatment with OTA (0.0005, 0.005, and 4 μg/mL), serum-free medium containing the same concentration of methanol was added to the control group. Differentiated Caco-2 cells were collected after 48 h for subsequent cell apoptosis studies, transcriptomics analysis, and qRT-PCR.

### 4.3. Cell Apoptosis Assay by Annexin V-FITC/PI FACS

Following the instructions of the Annexin V-FITC apoptosis detection kit, the differentiated Caco-2 cells were washed twice with cold PBS after treatment with different concentrations of OTA for 48 h. Cell samples were trypsinized, transferred to centrifuge tubes, and centrifuged at 1000× *g* for 5 min. The supernatant was discarded and the cells were resuspended in PBS (1 mL). The cell suspension was transferred to a 1.5 mL centrifuge tube and centrifuged again at 1000× *g* for 5 min. The supernatant was discarded and the cells were gently resuspended by adding Annexin V-FITC (5 μL), propidium iodide (10 μL), and Annexin V-FITC binding solution (195 μL). The cells were gently vortexed and incubated for 10–20 min at room temperature. An FC 500 MCL flow cytometer (Becton Dickinson, Mountain View, CA, USA) was used to analyze the cell samples within 1 h.

### 4.4. RNA Extraction, Library Construction, and Transcriptome Sequencing

#### 4.4.1. RNA Extraction

After treatment with OTA (0.0005, 0.005, and 4 μg/mL) for 48 h, Trizol (Invitrogen, Camarillo, CA, USA) was used to extract total RNA from the differentiated Caco-2 cells in accordance with the manufacturer's instructions. Remaining DNA was then removed by treatment with RNase-free DNase I (Takara Bio, Kusatsu, Shiga, Japan) for 30 min at 37 °C. Triple replicates of each treatment of differentiated Caco-2 cells were combined into a sample to reduce sample variability. After purification using an RNeasy Mini Kit (Qiagen, Dusseldorf, Germany), a NanoDrop 2000 spectrophotometer (Thermo Scientific, Wilmington, DE, USA) was used to assess RNA quality and RNase-free agarose gel electrophoresis was used to assess quantity.

#### 4.4.2. Construction of cDNA Library and Illumina Sequencing

RNA-seq was performed on RNA samples from differentiated Caco-2 cells treated with each of the three concentrations of OTA described above. High-quality RNA from each sample was enriched using magnetic Oligo (dT) beads and used to construct and sequence a cDNA library. Suitable cDNA fragments were selected as templates for PCR amplification using index primers and NEB universal PCR primers. When constructed, the cDNA library was sequenced using a HiSeq™ 2500 RNA sequencing system (Illumina, San Diego, CA, USA).

4.4.3. De Novo Assembly and Quantification of Gene Abundance

Before data analysis, the quality of the original data was controlled and noise was reduced by data filtering. In order to obtain high-quality clean reads for subsequent information analysis, the clean reads were filtered more rigorously to remove reads containing adapters or more than 10% of unknown nucleotides (N), as well as all reads with more than 50% low-quality sequence ($q$-value ≤ 20). The transcriptome assembly program Trinity was used for de novo transcriptome reconstruction. The sequencing error rate was used to evaluate the quality of sequenced reads, the saturation of the library, and the randomness of sequencing. Cuffmerge was used to combine the transcripts from different replicates of one group into a comprehensive set of transcripts for subsequent differential analysis and to filter the unique annotation files for manually introduced assembly errors. Annotation of unigenes was obtained using Blast and compared with data obtained using GO, KEGG, KOG, NR, COG, and Swissprot databases. Gene expression levels were then calculated using both the "raw counts" mode and "FPKM" [84].

4.4.4. Differentially Expressed Genes and their Dynamic Expression Profile

The edge R package (http://www.rproject.org/) was used to determine the DEGs between different treatment groups [62]. Firstly, we used the general filtering standard (FDR (False Discovery Rate) < 0.05 and |log2FC|>1) to identify significant DEGs. All DEGs were analyzed using the short time-series expression miner [85]. GO annotation was analyzed using Blast2GO software [86]. Blast software was used against the KEGG database to determine the KEGG pathway annotation [75]. GO/KEGG functional enrichment analysis was carried out for the genes in each trend, and the $p$-value was calculated by the hypothesis test. After the $p$-value was corrected by FDR, the GO term and path satisfying this condition were assigned a $q$-value ≤ 0.05 threshold.

*4.5. Validation of RNA-Seq Results Using qRT-PCR*

A Prime Script™ II 1st Strand cDNA Synthesis Kit and TB Green™ Premix Ex Taq™ II (Takara, Kusatsu, Shiga, Japan) were used to reverse transcribe cDNAs. The qRT-PCR conditions were as follows: 95 °C for 30 s; 40 cycles at 95 °C for 5 s; 60 °C for 30 s; and, finally, 72 °C for 20 s. The sequences of the primers, which were synthesized by a commercial company (Sangon Biotech Co., Ltd., Shanghai, China), are shown in Table 2. The data were analyzed and 7500 Software v.2.0.1 (Applied Biosystems, Foster City, CA, USA) was then used to determine the cycle threshold (Ct). The GAPDH gene (house-keeping gene) was selected as an internal control to normalize the expression data. The $2^{-\Delta\Delta Ct}$ method was used to calculate the relative expression of genes, and the mean and standard deviation of three biologic replicates are shown as the results [87].

**Table 2.** Primer sequences for the quantification of genes by quantitative reverse transcription-polymerase chain reaction (qRT-PCR). CASP 3, caspase 3; CXCL2, C–X–C motif chemokine ligand 2; CDC25B, cell division cycle 25B; EGR1, early growth response 1 (EGR1), H2BFS, H2B histone family members; SHPK, sedoheptulokinase; TFEC, transcription factor EC.

| Genes | Product Length (bp) | Forward Primer Sequence (5′–3′) | Reverse Primer Sequence (5′–3′) |
|---|---|---|---|
| GAPDH | 235 | GGAGTCCACTGGCGTCTT | GAGTCCTTCCACGATACCAAA |
| CASP3 | 109 | TCCTGAGATGGGTTTATGT | TGTTTCCCTGAGGTTTGC |
| CXCL2 | 150 | CCAAACCGAAGTCATAGC | GAACAGCCACCAATAAGC |
| CDC25B | 296 | GTAGACGGAAAGCACCAAGA | TCCCTGATGAAACGGCAC |
| EGR1 | 229 | CACGAACGCCCTTACGCT | CATCGCTCCTGGCAAACT |
| H2BFS | 119 | TGCTCGTCTCAGGCTCGTAG | CTTCCTGCCGTCCTTCTTCT |
| SHPK | 58 | AGTAGATGCGGCAATGGT | TTGGTAGGGATGGCTGTG |
| TEFC | 94 | GCACTGGAGGGATAAATG | TAAAGACACCCGAAGGAT |

### 4.6. Western Blotting Assays

Western blotting was used to verify differentially expressed proteins. Caco-2 cells were cultured in transwell chambers, with or without OTA (0.0005, 0.005, and 4 μg/mL), for 48 h. First, the cell samples were lysed with Western and IP Cell Lysis Buffer, and then equal amounts of protein were subjected to sodium dodecyl sulfate polyacrylamide gel electrophoresis (SDS-PAGE). The samples were next transferred to polyvinylidene fluoride membranes by dry rotation and the membranes were blocked with 5% skim milk powder dissolved in Tris-buffered saline for 2 h at room temperature. The samples were then incubated for 2 h with specific primary antibodies (1:1000 in TBS), washed three times with TBST (TBS containing 0.1% Tween 20), and incubated for 2 h with secondary antibodies. The bands were imaged using a Tanon-5200 Chemiluminescent Imaging System (Tanon Science & Technology Co., Ltd.) and band densities were analyzed using Image J 2 × software (Version 2.1.0, National Institutes of Health, Bethesda, MD, USA, 2006). Intensity values were normalized to human β-actin.

### 4.7. Statistical Analysis

Analysis of data was performed using SPSS® Statistics version 19. Analysis of variance (ANOVA) followed by Tukey's multiple comparison was used to test statistical differences between the OTA treatment groups and the control group. An asterisk (*) indicates a $p$-value < 0.05, which was regarded as statistically significant.

**Supplementary Materials:** The following are available online at http://www.mdpi.com/2072-6651/12/1/23/s1, Figure S1: Venn diagram depicting the DEGs common to different dose of OTA exposure, Figure S2: DEGs expression profiles in ochratoxin A (OTA) treated differentiated Caco-2 cells, Figure S3: DEGs expression profile in the OTA treated differentiated Caco-2 cells.

**Author Contributions:** Conceptualization, X.Y., N.Z., Y.G., Q.Y. and J.W.; Formal analysis, X.Y., Y.G., S.Z. and X.B.; Project administration, N.Z. and J.W.; Supervision, N.Z. and Q.Y.; Writing—original draft, X.Y.; Writing—review & editing, X.Y., N.Z. and Y.G. All authors have read and agreed to the published version of the manuscript.

**Funding:** The study was supported by The National Key Research and Development Program (2017YFD0500502), The Scientific Research Project for Major Achievements of The Agricultural Science and Technology Innovation Program (ASTIP) (No.CAAS-ZDXT2019004), and Modern Agro-Industry Technology Research System of the PR China (CARS-36).

**Conflicts of Interest:** The authors declare no conflict of interest.

## References

1. Creppy, E.E. Update of survey, regulation and toxic effects of mycotoxins in Europe. *Toxicol. Lett.* **2002**, *127*, 19–28. [CrossRef]
2. Van der Merwe, K.J.; Steyn, P.S.; Fourie, L.; Scott, D.B.; Theron, J.J. Ochratoxin A, a toxic metabolite produced by Aspergillus ochraceus Wilh. *Nature* **1965**, *205*, 1112–1113. [CrossRef] [PubMed]
3. Duarte, S.C.; Pena, A.; Lino, C.M. A review on ochratoxin A occurrence and effects of processing of cereal and cereal derived food products. *Food Microbiol.* **2010**, *27*, 187–198. [CrossRef] [PubMed]
4. Clark, H.A.; Snedeker, S.M. Ochratoxin A: Its cancer risk and potential for exposure. *J. Toxicol. Environ. Health B Crit. Rev.* **2006**, *9*, 265–296. [CrossRef] [PubMed]
5. Kononenko, G.P.; Burkin, A.A.; Zotova, E.V.; Soboleva, N.A. Ochratoxin A: Study of grain contamination. *Prikl. Biokhim. Mikrobiol.* **2000**, *36*, 209–213. [PubMed]
6. Duarte, S.C.; Lino, C.M.; Pena, A. Food safety implications of ochratoxin A in animal-derived food products. *Vet. J.* **2012**, *192*, 286–292. [CrossRef]
7. Ringot, D.; Chango, A.; Schneider, Y.J.; Larondelle, Y. Toxicokinetics and toxicodynamics of ochratoxin A, an update. *Chem. Biol. Interact.* **2006**, *159*, 18–46. [CrossRef]
8. Capriotti, A.L.; Caruso, G.; Cavaliere, C.; Foglia, P.; Samperi, R.; Laganà, A. Multiclass mycotoxin analysis in food, environmental and biological matrices with chromatography/mass spectrometry. *Mass Spectrom. Rev.* **2012**, *31*, 466–503. [CrossRef]
9. Flores-Flores, M.E.; Lizarraga, E.; de Cerain, A.L.; Gonzalez-Penas, E. Presence of mycotoxins in animal milk: A review. *Food Control.* **2015**, *53*, 163–176. [CrossRef]

10. Joint FAO/WHO Expert Committee on Food Additives. *Safety Evaluation of Certain Mycotoxins in Food*; World Health Organization: Geneva, Switzerland, 2001.
11. Pattono, D.; Gallo, P.F.; Civera, T. Detection and quantification of Ochratoxin A in milk produced in organic farms. *Food Chem.* **2011**, *127*, 374–377. [CrossRef]
12. Huang, L.C.; Zheng, N.; Zheng, B.Q.; Wen, F.; Cheng, J.B.; Han, R.W.; Xu, X.M.; Li, S.L.; Wang, J.Q. Simultaneous determination of aflatoxin M1, ochratoxin A, zearalenone and alpha-zearalenol in milk by UHPLC-MS/MS. *Food Chem.* **2014**, *146*, 242–249. [CrossRef] [PubMed]
13. Elzupir, A.O.; Makawi, S.Z.A.; Elhussein, A.M. Determination of Aflatoxins and Ochratoxin a in Dairy Cattle Feed and Milk in Wad Medani, Sudan. *J. Anim. Vet. Adv.* **2009**, *8*, 2508–2511.
14. Cancer IAFO. *Some Naturally Occurring Substances: Food Items and Constituents, Heterocyclic Aromatic Amines and Mycotoxins*; International Agency for Research on Cancer: Geneva, Switzerland, 1993.
15. Gambacorta, L.; Pinton, P.; Avantaggiato, G.; Oswald, I.P.; Solfrizzo, M. Grape Pomace, an Agricultural Byproduct Reducing Mycotoxin Absorption: In Vivo Assessment in Pig Using Urinary Biomarkers. *J. Agric. Food Chem.* **2016**, *64*, 6762–6771. [CrossRef] [PubMed]
16. Bouhet, S.; Oswald, I.P. The effects of mycotoxins, fungal food contaminants, on the intestinal epithelial cell-derived innate immune response. *Vet. Immunol. Immunopathol.* **2005**, *108*, 199–209. [CrossRef] [PubMed]
17. Pfohl-Leszkowicz, A.; Manderville, R.A. Ochratoxin A: An overview on toxicity and carcinogenicity in animals and humans. *Mol. Nutr. Food Res.* **2007**, *51*, 61–99. [CrossRef]
18. Elling, F.; Hald, B.; Jacobsen, C.; Krogh, P. Spontaneous toxic nephropathy in poultry associated with ochratoxin A. *Acta Pathol. Microbiol. Scand. A* **1975**, *83*, 739–741. [CrossRef]
19. Gekle, M.; Silbernagl, S. Renal toxicodynamics of ochratoxin A: A pathophysiological approach. *Kidney Blood Press. Res.* **1996**, *19*, 225–235. [CrossRef]
20. Wang, H.; Chen, Y.; Zhai, N.; Chen, X.; Gan, F.; Li, H.; Huang, K. Ochratoxin A-Induced Apoptosis of IPEC-J2 Cells through ROS-Mediated Mitochondrial Permeability Transition Pore Opening Pathway. *J. Agric. Food Chem.* **2017**, *65*, 10630–10637. [CrossRef]
21. Gao, Y.; Li, S.; Wang, J.; Luo, C.; Zhao, S.; Zheng, N. Modulation of Intestinal Epithelial Permeability in Differentiated Caco-2 Cells Exposed to Aflatoxin M1 and Ochratoxin A Individually or Collectively. *Toxins* **2018**, *10*, 13. [CrossRef]
22. Maresca, M.; Fantini, J. Some food-associated mycotoxins as potential risk factors in humans predisposed to chronic intestinal inflammatory diseases. *Toxicon* **2010**, *56*, 282–294. [CrossRef]
23. Schrickx, J.; Lektarau, Y.; Fink-Gremmels, J. Ochratoxin A secretion by ATP-dependent membrane transporters in Caco-2 cells. *Arch. Toxicol.* **2006**, *80*, 243–249. [CrossRef] [PubMed]
24. Stoev, S.D.; Stefanov, M.; Denev, S.; Radic, B.; Domijan, A.M.; Peraica, M. Experimental mycotoxicosis in chickens induced by ochratoxin A and penicillic acid and intervention with natural plant extracts. *Vet. Res. Commun.* **2004**, *28*, 727–746. [CrossRef] [PubMed]
25. Dortant, P.M.; Peters-Volleberg, G.W.; Van Loveren, H.; Marquardt, R.R.; Speijers, G.J. Age-related differences in the toxicity of ochratoxin A in female rats. *Food Chem. Toxicol.* **2001**, *39*, 55–65. [CrossRef]
26. Solcan, C.; Pavel, G.; Floristean, V.C.; Chiriac, I.S.; Şlencu, B.G.; Solcan, G. Effect of ochratoxin A on the intestinal mucosa and mucosa-associated lymphoid tissues in broiler chickens. *Acta Vet. Hung.* **2015**, *63*, 30–48. [CrossRef]
27. Cano-Sancho, G.; González-Arias, C.A.; Ramos, A.J.; Sanchis, V.; Fernández-Cruz, M.L. Cytotoxicity of the mycotoxins deoxynivalenol and ochratoxin A on Caco-2 cell line in presence of resveratrol. *Toxicol. In Vitro* **2015**, *29*, 1639–1646. [CrossRef]
28. Revajová, V.; Levkut, M.; Levkutová, M.; Bořutová, R.; Grešaková, L.; Košiková, B.; Leng, L. Effect of lignin supplementation of a diet contaminated with Fusarium mycotoxins on blood and intestinal lymphocyte subpopulations in chickens. *Acta Vet. Hung.* **2013**, *61*, 354–365. [CrossRef]
29. Ranaldi, G.; Caprini, V.; Sambuy, Y.; Perozzi, G.; Murgia, C. Intracellular zinc stores protect the intestinal epithelium from Ochratoxin A toxicity. *Toxicol. In Vitro* **2009**, *23*, 1516–1521. [CrossRef]
30. Bouaziz, C.; Sharaf el dein, O.; Martel, C.; El Golli, E.; Abid-Essefi, S.; Brenner, C.; Lemaire, C.; Bacha, H. Molecular events involved in ochratoxin A induced mitochondrial pathway of apoptosis, modulation by Bcl-2 family members. *Environ. Toxicol.* **2011**, *26*, 579–590. [CrossRef]
31. Rached, E.; Pfeiffer, E.; Dekant, W.; Mally, A. Ochratoxin A: Apoptosis and aberrant exit from mitosis due to perturbation of microtubule dynamics? *Toxicol. Sci.* **2006**, *92*, 78–86. [CrossRef]

32. Gekle, M.; Sauvant, C.; Schwerdt, G. Ochratoxin A at nanomolar concentrations: A signal modulator in renal cells. *Mol. Nutr. Food Res.* **2005**, *49*, 118–130. [CrossRef]
33. Li, J.; Yin, S.; Dong, Y.; Fan, L.; Hu, H. P53 activation inhibits ochratoxin A-induced apoptosis in monkey and human kidney epithelial cells via suppression of JNK activation. *Biochem. Biophys. Res. Commun.* **2011**, *411*, 458–463. [CrossRef] [PubMed]
34. Cui, J.; Xing, L.; Li, Z.; Wu, S.; Wang, J.; Liu, J.; Wang, J.; Yan, X.; Zhang, X. Ochratoxin A induces G2 phase arrest in human gastric epithelium GES-1 cells in vitro. *Toxicol. Lett.* **2010**, *193*, 152–158. [CrossRef] [PubMed]
35. Chopra, M.; Link, P.; Michels, C.; Schrenk, D. Characterization of ochratoxin A-induced apoptosis in primary rat hepatocytes. *Cell Biol. Toxicol.* **2010**, *26*, 239–254. [CrossRef] [PubMed]
36. Artursson, P.; Palm, K.; Luthman, K. Caco-2 monolayers in experimental and theoretical predictions of drug transport. *Adv. Drug Deliv. Rev.* **2012**, *64*, 280–289. [CrossRef]
37. Akbari, P.; Braber, S.; Varasteh, S.; Alizadeh, A.; Garssen, J.; Fink-Gremmels, J. The intestinal barrier as an emerging target in the toxicological assessment of mycotoxins. *Arch. Toxicol.* **2017**, *91*, 1007–1029. [CrossRef]
38. Sambuy, Y.; De Angelis, I.; Ranaldi, G.; Scarino, M.L.; Stammati, A.; Zucco, F. The Caco-2 cell line as a model of the intestinal barrier: Influence of cell and culture-related factors on Caco-2 cell functional characteristics. *Cell Biol. Toxicol.* **2005**, *21*, 1–26. [CrossRef]
39. Derks, K.W.; Misovic, B.; van den Hout, M.C.; Kockx, C.E.; Gomez, C.P.; Brouwer, R.W.; Vrieling, H.; Hoeijmakers, J.H.; van IJcken, W.F.; Pothof, J. Deciphering the RNA landscape by RNAome sequencing. *RNA Biol.* **2015**, *12*, 30–42. [CrossRef]
40. Nagalakshmi, U.; Waern, K.; Snyder, M. RNA-Seq: A method for comprehensive transcriptome analysis. *Curr. Protoc. Mol. Biol.* **2010**, *11*, 1–13. [CrossRef]
41. Mutz, K.O.; Heilkenbrinker, A.; Lönne, M.; Walter, J.G.; Stahl, F. Transcriptome analysis using next-generation sequencing. *Curr. Opin. Biotechnol.* **2013**, *24*, 22–30. [CrossRef]
42. Peraica, M.; Flajs, D.; Domijan, A.M.; Ivić, D.; Cvjetković, B. Ochratoxin A Contamination of Food from Croatia. *Toxins* **2010**, *2*, 2098–2105. [CrossRef]
43. Sergent, T. Differential modulation of ochratoxin A absorption across Caco-2 cells by dietary polyphenols, used at realistic intestinal concentrations. *Toxicol. Lett.* **2005**, *159*, 60–70. [CrossRef] [PubMed]
44. Chen, R.; Deng, L.; Yu, X.; Wang, X.; Zhu, L.; Yu, T.; Zhang, Y.; Zhou, B.; Xu, W.; Chen, L.; et al. MiR-122 partly mediates the ochratoxin A-induced GC-2 cell apoptosis. *Toxicol. In Vitro* **2015**, *30*, 264–273. [CrossRef] [PubMed]
45. Giromini, C.; Rebucci, R.; Fusi, E.; Rossi, L.; Saccone, F.; Baldi, A. Cytotoxicity, apoptosis, DNA damage and methylation in mammary and kidney epithelial cell lines exposed to ochratoxin A. *Cell Biol. Toxicol.* **2016**, *32*, 249–258. [CrossRef] [PubMed]
46. Zhao, D.Y.; Zhang, W.X.; Qi, Q.Q.; Long, X.; Li, X.; Yu, Y.B.; Zuo, X.L. Brain-derived neurotrophic factor modulates intestinal barrier by inhibiting intestinal epithelial cells apoptosis in mice. *Physiol. Res.* **2018**, *67*, 475–485. [CrossRef] [PubMed]
47. Rai, M.F.; Tycksen, E.D.; Sandell, L.J.; Brophy, R.H. Advantages of RNA-seq compared to RNA microarrays for transcriptome profiling of anterior cruciate ligament tears. *J. Orthop. Res.* **2018**, *36*, 484–497. [CrossRef] [PubMed]
48. Assaf, H.; Azouri, H.; Pallardy, M. Ochratoxin A induces apoptosis in human lymphocytes through down regulation of Bcl-xL. *Toxicol. Sci.* **2004**, *79*, 335–344. [CrossRef]
49. Ozcan, Z.; Gul, G.; Yaman, I. Ochratoxin A activates opposing c-MET/PI3K/Akt and MAPK/ERK 1-2 pathways in human proximal tubule HK-2 cells. *Arch. Toxicol.* **2015**, *89*, 1313–1327. [CrossRef]
50. Bouaziz, C.; Sharaf El Dein, O.; El Golli, E.; Abid-Essefi, S.; Brenner, C.; Lemaire, C.; Bacha, H. Different apoptotic pathways induced by zearalenone, T-2 toxin and ochratoxin A in human hepatoma cells. *Toxicology* **2008**, *254*, 19–28. [CrossRef]
51. Vettorazzi, A.; van Delft, J.; de Cerain López, A. A review on ochratoxin A transcriptomic studies. *Food Chem. Toxicol.* **2013**, *59*, 766–783. [CrossRef]
52. Zhang, Y.; Qi, X.; Zheng, J.; Luo, Y.; Huang, K.; Xu, W. High-Throughput Tag-Sequencing Analysis of Early Events Induced by Ochratoxin A in HepG-2 Cells. *J. Biochem. Mol. Toxicol.* **2016**, *30*, 29–36. [CrossRef]
53. Vanacloig-Pedros, E.; Proft, M.; Pascual-Ahuir, A. Different Toxicity Mechanisms for Citrinin and Ochratoxin A Revealed by Transcriptomic Analysis in Yeast. *Toxins* **2016**, *8*, 273. [CrossRef] [PubMed]

54. Boesch-Saadatmandi, C.; Matzner, N.; Matzner, N.; Lang, F.; Blank, R.; Wolffram, S.; Blaschek, W.; Rimbach, G. Ochratoxin A lowers mRNA levels of genes encoding for key proteins of liver cell metabolism. *Cancer Genom. Proteom.* **2008**, *5*, 319–332.
55. Liang, R.; Shen, X.L.; Zhang, B.; Li, Y.; Xu, W.; Zhao, C.; Luo, Y.; Huang, K. Apoptosis Signal-regulating Kinase 1 promotes Ochratoxin A-induced renal cytotoxicity. *Sci. Rep.* **2015**, *5*, 8078–8089. [CrossRef] [PubMed]
56. Gekle, M.; Schwerdt, G.; Freudinger, R.; Mildenberger, S.; Wilflingseder, D.; Pollack, V.; Dander, M.; Schramek, H. Ochratoxin A induces JNK activation and apoptosis in MDCK-C7 cells at nanomolar concentrations. *J. Pharmacol. Exp. Ther.* **2000**, *293*, 837–844. [PubMed]
57. Darif, Y.; Mountassif, D.; Belkebir, A.; Zaid, Y.; Basu, K.; Mourad, W.; Oudghiri, M. Ochratoxin A mediates MAPK activation, modulates IL-2 and TNF-alpha mRNA expression and induces apoptosis by mitochondria-dependent and mitochondria-independent pathways in human H9 T cells. *J. Toxicol. Sci.* **2016**, *41*, 403–416. [CrossRef]
58. Kaminska, B. MAPK signalling pathways as molecular targets for anti-inflammatory therapy—From molecular mechanisms to therapeutic benefits. *Biochim. Biophys. Acta* **2005**, *1754*, 253–262. [CrossRef]
59. Horvath, A.; Upham, B.L.; Ganev, V.; Trosko, J.E. Determination of the epigenetic effects of ochratoxin in a human kidney and a rat liver epithelial cell line. *Toxicon* **2002**, *40*, 273–282. [CrossRef]
60. Sauvant, C.; Holzinger, H.; Gekle, M. The nephrotoxin ochratoxin A induces key parameters of chronic interstitial nephropathy in renal proximal tubular cells. *Cell Physiol. Biochem.* **2005**, *15*, 125–134. [CrossRef]
61. Sharma, R.P.; He, Q.; Johnson, V.J.; Voss, K.A. Increased expression of CD95-ligand and other apoptotic signaling factors by fumonisin B1, a hepatotoxic mycotoxin, in livers of mice lacking tumor necrosis factor $\alpha$. *Cytokine* **2003**, *24*, 226–236. [CrossRef]
62. Wang, L.; Feng, Z.; Wang, X.; Zhang, X. DEGseq: An R package for identifying differentially expressed genes from RNA-seq data. *Bioinformatics* **2010**, *26*, 136–138. [CrossRef]
63. Hibi, D.; Kijima, A.; Suzuki, Y.; Ishii, Y.; Jin, M.; Sugita-Konishi, Y.; Yanai, T.; Nishikawa, A.; Umemura, T. Effects of p53 knockout on ochratoxin A-induced genotoxicity in p53-deficient gpt delta mice. *Toxicology* **2013**, *304*, 92–99. [CrossRef] [PubMed]
64. Shangary, S.; Wang, S. Targeting the MDM2-p53 interaction for cancer therapy. *Clin. Cancer Res.* **2008**, *14*, 5318–5324. [CrossRef] [PubMed]
65. Fridman, J.S.; Lowe, S.W. Control of apoptosis by p53. *Oncogene* **2003**, *22*, 9030–9340. [CrossRef] [PubMed]
66. Hibi, D.; Kijima, A.; Kuroda, K.; Suzuki, Y.; Ishii, Y.; Jin, M.; Nakajima, M.; Sugita-Konishi, Y.; Yanai, T.; Nohmi, T.; et al. Molecular mechanisms underlying ochratoxin A-induced genotoxicity: Global gene expression analysis suggests induction of DNA double-strand breaks and cell cycle progression. *J. Toxicol. Sci.* **2013**, *38*, 57–69. [CrossRef] [PubMed]
67. Arbillaga, L.; Vettorazzi, A.; Gil, A.G.; van Delft, J.H.; García-Jalón, J.A.; de Cerain, A.L. Gene expression changes induced by ochratoxin A in renal and hepatic tissues of male F344 rat after oral repeated administration. *Toxicol. Appl. Pharmacol.* **2008**, *230*, 197–207. [CrossRef] [PubMed]
68. Vassilev, L.T.; Uesugi, M. In vivo activation of the p53 pathway by small-molecule antagonists of MDM2. *Science* **2004**, *303*, 844–848. [CrossRef]
69. De Rozieres, S.; Maya, R.; Oren, M.; Lozano, G. The loss of mdm2 induces p53-mediated apoptosis. *Oncogene* **2000**, *19*, 1691–1697. [CrossRef]
70. Silke, J.; Meier, P. Inhibitor of Apoptosis (IAP) Proteins-Modulators of Cell Death and Inflammation. *Cold Spring Harb. Perspect. Biol.* **2013**, *5*, 008730. [CrossRef]
71. Picksley, S.M.; Lane, D.P. The p53-mdm2 autoregulatory feedback loop: A paradigm for the regulation of growth control by p53? *Bioessays* **1993**, *15*, 689–690. [CrossRef]
72. Gu, H.; Wang, X.; Rao, S.; Wang, J.; Zhao, J.; Ren, F.L.; Mu, R.; Yang, Y.; Qi, Q.; Liu, W.; et al. Gambogic acid mediates apoptosis as a p53 inducer through down-regulation of mdm2 in wild-type p53-expressing cancer cells. *Mol. Cancer Ther.* **2008**, *7*, 3298–3305. [CrossRef]
73. Alshatwi, A.A.; Subash-Babu, P.; Antonisamy, P. Violacein induces apoptosis in human breast cancer cells through up regulation of BAX, p53 and down regulation of MDM2. *Exp. Toxicol. Pathol.* **2016**, *68*, 89–97. [CrossRef] [PubMed]
74. Kuroda, K.; Hibi, D.; Ishii, Y.; Takasu, S.; Kijima, A.; Matsushita, K.; Masumura, K.I.; Watanabe, M.; Sugita-Konishi, Y.; Sakai, H.; et al. Ochratoxin A induces DNA double-strand breaks and large deletion mutations in the carcinogenic target site of gpt delta rats. *Mutagenesis* **2014**, *29*, 27–36. [CrossRef] [PubMed]

75. Chapman, J.R.; Taylor, M.R.G.; Simon, J. Boulton, Playing the End Game: DNA Double-Strand Break Repair Pathway Choice. *Mol. Cell* **2012**, *47*, 497–510. [CrossRef] [PubMed]
76. Pfohl-Leszkowicz, A. MESNA protects rats against nephrotoxicity but not carcinogenity induced by Ochratoxin A, implicating two separate pathways. *Med. Biol.* **2002**, *9*, 6357–6361.
77. Guikema, J.E.; Amiot, M.; Eldering, E. Exploiting the pro-apoptotic function of NOXA as a therapeutic modality in cancer. *Expert Opin. Ther. Targets* **2017**, *21*, 767–779. [CrossRef]
78. Chen, H.C.; Kanai, M.; Inoue-Yamauchi, A.; Tu, H.C.; Huang, Y.; Ren, D.; Kim, H.; Takeda, S.; Reyna, D.E.; Chan, P.M.; et al. An interconnected hierarchical model of cell death regulation by the BCL-2 family. *Nat. Cell Biol.* **2015**, *17*, 1270–1281. [CrossRef]
79. Comim, C.M.; Tatiana, B.; Denis, G.; Felipe, D.P.; Joao, Q.; Stephen, L. Caspase-3 mediates in part hippocampal apoptosis in sepsis. *Mol. Neurobiol.* **2013**, *47*, 394–398. [CrossRef]
80. Larsen, B.D.; Sorensen, C.S. The caspase-activated DNase: Apoptosis and beyond. *FEBS J.* **2017**, *284*, 1160–1170. [CrossRef]
81. D'Amelio, M.; Sheng, M.; Cecconi, F. Caspase-3 in the central nervous system: Beyond apoptosis. *Trends Neurosci.* **2012**, *35*, 700–709. [CrossRef]
82. Gao, Y.N.; Wang, J.Q.; Li, S.L.; Zhang, Y.D.; Zheng, N. Aflatoxin M1 cytotoxicity against human intestinal Caco-2 cells is enhanced in the presence of other mycotoxins. *Food Chem. Toxicol.* **2016**, *96*, 79–89. [CrossRef]
83. Gao, Y.; Li, S.L.; Bao, X.Y.; Luo, C.C.; Yang, H.G.; Wang, J.Q.; Zhao, S.G.; Zheng, N. Transcriptional and Proteomic Analysis Revealed a Synergistic Effect of Aflatoxin M1 and Ochratoxin A Mycotoxins on the Intestinal Epithelial Integrity of Differentiated Human Caco-2 Cells. *J. Proteom. Res.* **2018**, *17*, 3128–3142. [CrossRef] [PubMed]
84. Trapnell, C.; Roberts, A.; Goff, L.; Pertea, G.; Kim, D.; Kelley, D.R.; Pimentel, H.; Salzberg, S.L.; Rinn, J.L.; Pachter, L. Differential gene and transcript expression analysis of RNA-seq experiments with TopHat and Cufflinks. *Nat. Protoc.* **2012**, *7*, 562–578. [CrossRef] [PubMed]
85. Ernst, J.; Bar-Joseph, Z. STEM: A tool for the analysis of short time series gene expression data. *BMC Bioinf.* **2006**, *7*, 191. [CrossRef] [PubMed]
86. Kanehisa, M.; Araki, M.; Goto, S.; Hattori, M.; Hirakawa, M.; Itoh, M.; Katayama, T.; Kawashima, S.; Okuda, S.; Tokimatsu, T.; et al. KEGG for linking genomes to life and the environment. *Nucleic Acids Res.* **2007**, *36*, 480–484. [CrossRef]
87. Livak, K.J.; Schmittgen, T.D. Analysis of relative gene expression data using real-time quantitative PCR and the 2(-Delta Delta, C.(T)) Method. *Methods* **2001**, *25*, 402–408. [CrossRef]

*toxins*

MDPI

*Article*

# Assessment of Toxic Effects of Ochratoxin A in Human Embryonic Stem Cells

**Slaven Erceg [1,*], Eva María Mateo [2], Iván Zipancic [3], Francisco Javier Rodríguez Jiménez [1], María Amparo Pérez Aragó [1], Misericordia Jiménez [2], José Miguel Soria [4] and Mª Ángeles Garcia-Esparza [5,*]**

1. Stem Cells Therapies in Neurodegenerative Diseases Lab, Research Center "Principe Felipe", Valencia 46012, Spain; frodriguez@cipf.es (F.J.R.J.); mparago@cipf.es (M.A.P.A.)
2. Department of Microbiology and Ecology, University of Valencia, Valencia 46100, Spain; eva.mateo@uv.es (E.M.M.); misericordia.jimenez@uv.es (M.J.)
3. Department of Biomedical Sciences, School of Health Sciences, Universidad Cardenal Herrera-CEU, CEU Universities, Valencia 46115, Spain; ivan.zipancic@uchceu.es
4. Department of Biomedical Sciences, School of Health Sciences, Universidad Cardenal Herrera-CEU, CEU Universities, Elche, Alicante 03204, Spain; Jose.soria@uchceu.es
5. Department of Pharmacy, School of Health Sciences, Universidad Cardenal Herrera-CEU, CEU Universities, Elche, Alicante 03204, Spain; Maria.garcia2@uchceu.es

* Correspondence: serceg@cipf.es (S.E.); maria.garcia2@uchceu.es (M.Á.G.-E.)

Received: 21 February 2019; Accepted: 4 April 2019; Published: 10 April 2019

**Abstract:** Ochratoxin A (OTA) is a mycotoxin produced by different *Aspergillus* and *Penicillium* species, and it is considered a common contaminant in food and animal feed worldwide. On the other hand, human embryonic stem cells (hESCs) have been suggested as a valuable model for evaluating drug embryotoxicity. In this study, we have evaluated potentially toxic effects of OTA in hESCs. By using in vitro culture techniques, specific cellular markers, and molecular biology procedures, we found that OTA produces mild cytotoxic effects in hESCs by inhibiting cell attachment, survival, and proliferation in a dose-dependent manner. Thus, we suggest that hESCs provide a valuable human and cellular model for toxicological studies regarding preimplantation stage of human fetal development.

**Keywords:** Ochratoxin A (OTA); human Stem Cells; mycotoxins; cells; cytotoxicity; cell culture

**Key Contribution:** OTA has a great impact in early stages of development. In vitro cell culture of hESCs in the presence of OTA at different concentrations reduced the viability, decreased cellular hESC proliferation, induced apoptosis, and increased the expression of oxygen stress markers. This work may contribute in elucidating the mechanisms underlying OTA embryotoxicity.

---

## 1. Introduction

Human pluripotent stem cells (hPSCs) represent heterogeneous populations, including induced pluripotent stem cells (iPSCs), endogenous plastic somatic cells, and embryonic stem cells (ESCs). Human ESCs (hESCs) are derived from the inner cell mass of the blastocyst, characterized by the ability to self-renew indefinitely and to give rise to all cell types of embryonic lineage (pluripotency) under the guidance of the appropriate chemical, mechanical, and environmental cues [1].

There are high expectations regarding the use of hESCs for treating injuries and degenerative diseases, for modelling complex illnesses and developments, for screening and testing of pharmacological products, and for examining toxicity, mutagenicity, teratogenicity, and potential carcinogenic effects of a variety of environmental factors, including mycotoxins [2,3].

Ochratoxin A (OTA) is the most abundant and toxic member of the ochratoxins, a group of secondary metabolites produced by fungi belonging to the genera *Aspergillus* and *Penicillium* [4–7].

OTA can contaminate a wide variety of foods because of fungal infection in crops, in fields during growth, at harvest, or during storage and shipment. Besides cereals and cereal products, OTA is also found in a range of other food commodities, including coffee, cocoa, wine, beer, pulses, spices, dried fruits, grape juice, pig kidney, and other meat and meat products from non-ruminant animals exposed to foodstuffs contaminated with this mycotoxin [8].

Research into the toxicity of this mycotoxin is mostly centered on its teratogenic [9], nephrotoxic [10], immunotoxic [10], neurotoxic [11–13], and carcinogenic [14] effects that result from exposure to a range of different food types, particularly of plant origin, that may be contaminated by OTA [15,16]. The kidney has been considered as the key target organ of OTA toxicity in most of the mammalian species [17]. Additionally, in humans OTA has been found in blood plasma [5,18], and frequent exposure to OTA is attributed to its nephrotoxic effects, especially in children [19]. Several studies have highlighted OTA as a possible causative agent of Balkan endemic nephropathy, an endemic, severe, progressive, and fatal kidney disease found in the Balkan countries [14,19,20].

Furthermore, investigations in animal models showed OTA as a neurotoxic agent [21,22]. In addition, different studies in vitro have demonstrated a direct relationship between some environmental products and prenatal development [23]. Thus, although OTA appears to exert multiple biological actions, and is cytotoxic, few studies conducted to date have explored whether OTA negatively affects embryonic development [24,25].

During normal embryogenesis, the process of apoptosis removes abnormal or redundant cells from pre-implantation embryos [26]. Induction of apoptosis during early stages of embryogenesis (i.e., following exposure to a teratogen) compromises embryonic development [27,28]. The main methods to study teratogens are either through epidemiological studies in human populations or by controlled exposure in animal models. Previous studies found that OTA induced apoptosis in mammalian cells, including monkey and human kidney epithelial cells, porcine kidney PK15 cells, and human OK cells [29–31]. Although these methods are still essential, more reliable and indicative human-based toxicity tests are needed to represent toxicity effects in humans. Due to the ethical issues regarding teratogenic effect assessment of OTA in human embryos, in this study we have used hESCs as an in vitro model for teratogen screening in a human developmental setting using physiologically relevant doses. There is clear evidence that hESCs represent faithful in vitro toxicity models, as a wide range of chemicals were tested and showed adverse effects in these cells [32–35] with no toxicity in animal models, such as in the case of thalidomide [36]. As hESCs are cells derived from the blastocyst stage, toxicity assays with hESCs can provide toxicity information at a very early stage after fertilization. Having unique proliferation and differentiation capacities toward a wide range of cells in the human body, hESCs closely mimic human embryogenesis [37], thus they offer a unique cellular, developmental, functional, and reproductive human in vitro model for toxicological testing.

The purpose of this study was to assess and determine toxicity of OTA using hESCs as a model for preimplantation embryos. Our data show that (1) hESCs can be used to measure toxicity of food contaminants such as OTA, and (2) OTA exerts its effect through possible mechanisms of apoptosis and oxidative stress.

## 2. Results

### 2.1. *Ochratoxin A Reduces the Viability and Decreases the Cellular Proliferation of Human Embryonic Stem Cells (hESCs)*

OTA treatment (1–100 ppm) reduced the viability of hESCs in a dose-dependent manner. Evident toxic effects of OTA were observed after 8 h when approximately 60% of cells survived at a concentration of 10 ppm. Similar effects were observed with a concentration of 50 ppm of OTA, and this was considered the 50% effective concentration ($EC_{50}$) (Figure 1A,B). In all treatments, the percentage of colonies that underwent shrinkage during exposure exponentially increased (data not shown).

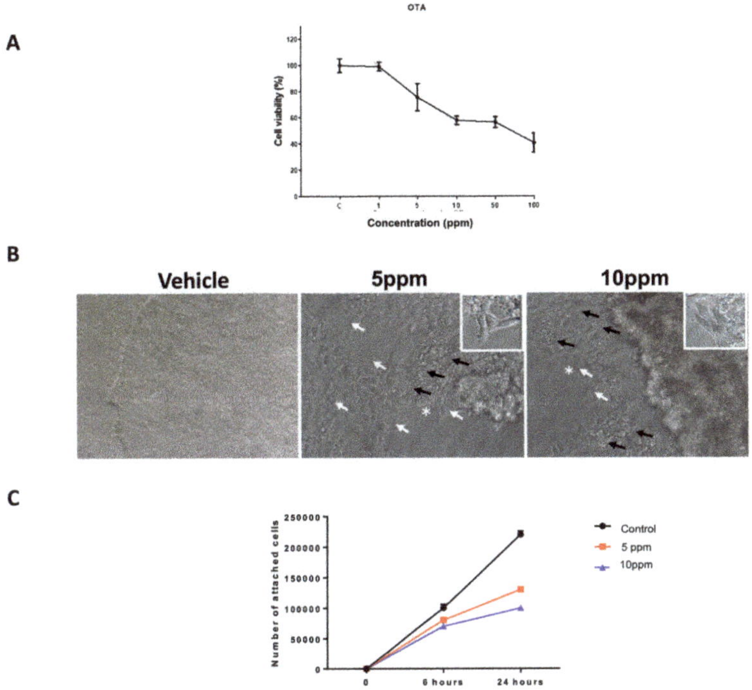


**Figure 1.** (**A**) Dose-dependent survival rate (MTS assay) of human embryonic stem cells (hESC) at 8 h shows decrease of cell survival to 60% at doses of 10 ppm ($n$ = 6). (**B**) Representative bright field micrographs of hESC colonies treated with vehicle (ethanol) or OTA (5 and 10 ppm). White arrows indicate surviving cells and black arrows indicate dead cells. Micrographs show the suitable aspect and shape of surviving cells. White asterisks indicate the area from which the photographs were taken. (**C**) Number of attached cells after 6 and 24 h in two experimental groups compared to control. Magnification times: 20×.

Since the major OTA effects on cell death were observed with concentrations of 5 and 10 ppm, further experiments were performed using these concentrations. Thus, to determine how OTA solutions affected proliferation of hESCs, the surviving cells after 5 and 10 ppm treatments were detached, seeded, and used in subsequent experiments to assess cell attachment and growth during the following 24 h (Figure 1C). Throughout this process, video data of colonies in each group were collected using the IncuCyte System. All videos were first analyzed to determine whether colonies grew, shrunk, or died during incubation. During the 24 h, an evident decrease of cell growth and attachment was observed in comparison with non-treated cells (Figure 1C).

In order to investigate the role of OTA on cell death and apoptotic processes, the cells were stained with nucleic acid IncuCyte®Cytotox Red Reagent for counting necrotic cells, which was able to penetrate and dye compromised cell membranes associated with dead or dying cells, followed by imaging with the IncuCyte ZOOM every 4 h over a 24 h period. A dose-dependent increase in cell death when treated with OTA was observed across all hESCs (Figure 2A, (A1, A3 and A5) and Figure 2B. The same results regarding cell death were observed over 24 h.

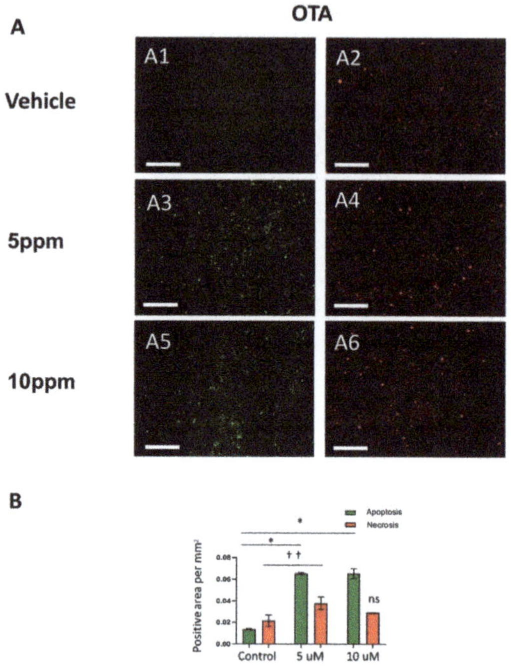


**Figure 2.** Ochratoxin A (OTA) increases necrotic cells and apoptosis in hESCs at 5 and 10 ppm. (**A**) Representative fluorescent micrographs of hESC colonies treated with vehicle (ethanol in A1, A2), OTA (5 ppm in A3, A4), and (10 ppm in A5, A6) captured after 8 h with the IncuCyte ZOOM. IncuCyte®Cytotox Red Reagent was used for counting necrotic cells (red) and caspase-mediated apoptosis using a kinetic caspase 3/7 reagent (Essen Bioscience) (green). (**B**) The number of "objects" per well was calculated using IncuCyte software and graphed, showing a significant increase in the number of cells undergoing necrosis (red) or caspase-mediated apoptosis when treated with OTA (green) compared to ethanol. ($n = 3$; *, † = $p \leq 0.05$). Scale bar: 300 μm. Magnification times: 20×.

### 2.2. Ochratoxin A (OTA) Induces Caspase-Mediated Apoptosis in hESCs

In addition to cytotoxicity quantification, hESCs were also stained and imaged for caspase-mediated apoptosis using a kinetic caspase 3/7 reagent (Essen BioScience, 300 West Morgan Road, Ann Arbor, MI, USA). The number of "caspase-3 objects" per well was calculated using IncuCyte integrated analysis software and graphed, showing a significant increase in the number of cells undergoing caspase-mediated apoptosis when treated with OTA compared to vehicle treated cells (Figure 2A, (A2, A4 and A6) and Figure 2B). The trend in caspase 3/7 activation in hESCs correlated with their $EC_{50}$ value.

### 2.3. OTA Increases the Expression of Oxygen Stress Markers in hESCs

After apoptosis and cytotoxicity assays, the cells were collected, and RT-PCR for main oxidative markers was performed to determine the role of oxidative stress in OTA cytotoxicity. In cells treated with OTA, analysis of reactive oxygen stress markers showed a significant but not dose-dependent increase of the expression of glutathione synthetase (gss), superoxide dismutases 1 (sod1), superoxide dismutases 2 (sod2) and activating transcription factor 3 (atf3) in reactive oxygen species (ROS) for both doses: 5 and 10 ppm (Figure 3). A greater fold-change compared to vehicle control was observed in hESCs, strongly suggesting OTA-induced cell death.

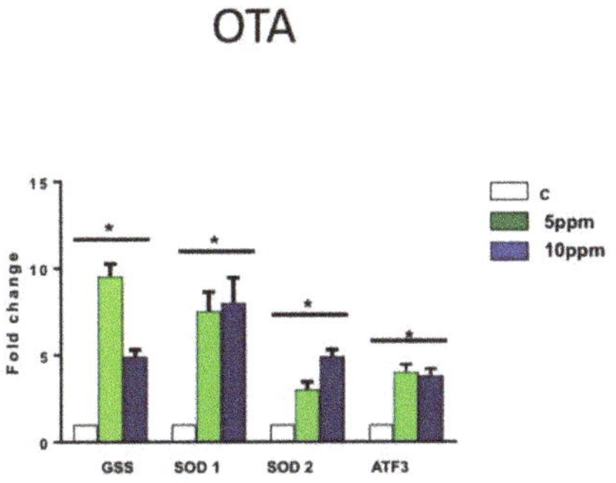


**Figure 3.** OTA significantly increases the expression of oxygen stress markers in hESCs. Analysis of reactive oxygen stress markers showed a dose-dependent increase of the expression of glutathione synthetase (GSS), superoxide dismutases 1 (SOD1), superoxide dismutases 1 (SOD2), and activating transcription factor 3 (ATF3) as main markers involved in oxidative stress. ($n = 3$; * = $p \leq 0.05$).

## 3. Discussion

OTA exposure studies have been developed on different cell lines of human and animal models, especially describing the mechanisms associated with increased levels of oxidative stress, DNA, and lipid and protein damage [38]. Embryos are generally more sensitive to chemicals than adults are, and for this reason it is essential to develop faithful human cell assays for preimplantation stages of human development when possible [39]. OTA is a mycotoxin commonly found in food, which can produce serious toxic effects in the organism and, specifically, in the developing brain [40,41]. In this study, we evaluated the impact of OTA exposure in hESCs as a model for pre- and post-implantation of human embryos. OTA showed toxic, dose-dependent effects only after 4 h of treatment. The mechanism through which OTA induces toxicity in vitro is mainly attributed to multiple effects on various subcellular structures, such as loss of membrane integrity, confirmed by LDH leakage assay in other cells [42,43]. In the present study, OTA exhibited cell toxicity via cell mortality, confirmed by MTS, and through mechanisms of apoptosis and oxidative stress. Our results are in line with earlier studies, which have demonstrated that OTA-induced oxidative stress leads to cytotoxicity and apoptosis in Neuro-2a cells [43], highlighting that elevated ROS is a principle event in oxidative stress in cells treated with OTA. Our results corroborate other findings where OTA was confirmed as a potent ROS inducer [44–46]. Results of our study suggest that OTA cytotoxicity is mediated by oxidative stress in a dose-dependent manner. Although the oxidative species were not measured, the significant increase of expression of main oxidative stress markers, such as GSS, SOD 1, SOD2, and ATF3, strongly indicate that oxidative stress is one of the underlying mechanisms for OTA-induced loss of cell viability and DNA damage. Since mitochondria events are the major generator of ROS, mitochondria could play a crucial role in toxicity of OTA [47]. Generation of free radicals and other oxidative species triggers lipid peroxidation and permeability of the mitochondrial membrane, which produces apoptotic cell death [47,48]. Indeed, it was previously shown that OTA treatment leads to loss of mitochondrial membrane potential and DNA damage in a dose-dependent manner [43]. Our study confirms results obtained by Sava et al. [11,22], in which the authors tested neural stem/progenitor cells (NSCs) prepared from the hippocampus of an adult mouse brain for their vulnerability to OTA in vitro. In that study the authors observed that OTA caused a dose- and time-dependent decrease in viability of both proliferating and differentiating NSCs. Along with decreased viability, OTA elicited pronounced oxidative stress, evidenced by a robust increase in total and mitochondrial SOD activity. This study concluded that greater vulnerability to the toxin exhibited proliferating number of NSCs compared to differentiated, more mature neurons, despite robust DNA repair and antioxidant responses. Further studies need to be performed in order to clarify whether the same mechanisms of oxidative stress are triggered in hESC by OTA. Our results are in line with previous studies, which have reported OTA as a trigger for the caspase-9 and caspase-3 activation with potential mitochondrial membrane loss in different human primary cells [49–51]. To our knowledge, the present study is the first one describing the effects of OTA in a prenatal human cellular model, demonstrating the importance of assessing toxicity in early stages of development. In this context, it is crucial to develop new simple and faithful in vitro assays that are able to screen the effects of environmental and food chemicals in various stages of the developing fetus. To this purpose, many assays, such as explants of rodent embryos [52,53] or embryonic bodies derived from mESC to model post-implantation development, have been developed [54]. The approach used in this study represents a quick and simple human in vitro method for assessing environmental toxicants in hESCs, a model for the inner cell mass of preimplantation embryos already used for other environmental pollutants [55] such as tobacco smoke [35] or thalidomide [56]. This study may contribute to elucidating the mechanisms underlying OTA teratogenicity in the early days of human fetal development.

## 4. Materials and Methods

### 4.1. Undifferentiated hESC Line Maintenance

WA09 hESCs were obtained from the WiCell Research Institute (Madison, WI, USA) and were maintained in feeder-free conditions using mTeSR1 media (StemCell Technologies, Vancouver, BC, Canada) on hESC-qualified Matrigel (BD Biosciences, San Jose, CA, USA) coated plates. To maintain the undifferentiated stem cell population, differentiated colonies were removed daily through aspiration and medium was replaced. Additionally, the hESCs were only used in experiments up to passage 40 and were karyotyped approximately every 10 passages to minimize and monitor the potential for genetic instability. hESCs were passaged at 90%–95% confluence (approximately every 7 days) using Accutase. Cell cultures were maintained at 37 °C under 5% $CO_2$.

### 4.2. In vitro Culture of hESCs

All experimental treatments were carried out in 96-well plates coated with Matrigel. To minimize plating variability and increase reproducibility, hESCs were removed from a 6-well plate using TrypLE (Life Technologies). The cells were washed with DMEM/F12 (Dulbecco´s Modified Eagle Medium F-12 Nutrient Mixture (Ham), GIBCO, Paisley, Scotland, UK) and re-suspended in mTeSR1 that contained 10 uM/L Y27632 Rho-associated kinase inhibitor (Merck KGaA/Calbiochem, Darmstadt, Germany). The rho-associated kinase inhibitor was added to the plating media to increase plating efficiency by decreasing dissociation-induced apoptosis. Five thousand hESCs were plated as a single cell suspension and maintained in an undifferentiated state until 80% confluence was reached.

### 4.3. Analysis of Cellular Viability

Analysis of cellular viability in the presence of respiratory inhibitors was performed using MTS assay (Promega, G1111, Promega Corporation, Madison, WI, USA) according to the manufacturer's instructions. Briefly, hESCs were seeded at a density of 5000 cells per well in Matrigel-treated 96-well culture microplates in 100 µL of culture media, and they were incubated for 4 h at 37 °C. The cells were used when 80% confluence was reached. After 24 h of compound (ethanol) treatment, 20 µL of MTS reagent was applied to each well of a 96-well plate. Absorbance at 490 nm was recorded after 2 h incubation. Sextuplets were prepared for each condition.

### 4.4. hESC Compound Exposures

hESCs were treated with OTA at different concentrations equivalent to previous and published in vitro studies [21]. To test OTA exposure, all compound stock solutions were made with ethanol.

### 4.5. Toxin Preparation

A standard of OTA was supplied by Sigma-Aldrich (Alcobendas, Spain). The OTA standard was dissolved in ethanol (Ethanol HPLC 99.5%-gradient grade, Burker, Deventer, Netherlands) to give a stock solution of 1000 μg/mL (ppm). OTA solutions of 100, 50, 10, 5, and 1 ppm were prepared by dilution of suitable aliquots of the stock solution with ethanol. An aliquot of these mycotoxin solutions was added to the wells containing the cell cultures to obtain the final concentration of the toxin. Blank controls having no mycotoxin, but the same volume of solvent, were performed in parallel.

### 4.6. RNA Extraction and Reverse Transcriptase Polymerase Chain Reaction (RT-PCR and qRT-PCR)

Cells were collected by centrifugation, and total RNA was isolated with the RNeasy Mini Kit (Qiagen, Hilden, Germany) following the manufacturer´s instructions. They were treated with DNase1 to remove any genomic DNA contamination. QuantiTect Reverse Transcription Kit (Qiagen) was used to carry out cDNA synthesis from 1 μg of total RNA according to the manufacturer's instructions. For quantitative real-time PCR (qRT-PCR), the relative quantification analysis was performed using a CFX96 RealTime PCR Detection system and C1000 Thermal Cycler (Bio-Rad, Hercules, CA, USA). The PCR cycling program consisted of denaturing at 95 °C for 10 min followed by 40 cycles of 95 °C for 15 s and anncaling/clongation at 60 °C for 1 min. The reactions were done in triplicate using TaqMan Gene Expression Master Mix and the following TaqMan probes (Applied Biosystems, Foster City, CA, USA): SOD1 (Hs00533490_mL), SOD2 (Hs00167309_mL), GSS (Hs00609286_mL), and ATF3 (Hs00231069_mL). PCR was done in triplicate, and the expression of polymerase 2A (POL2A; Hs00172187_mL) was used as three endogenous controls to normalize the variations in cDNA quantities from different samples. The results were analyzed using Bio-Rad CFX software (CFX Maestro Software for Bio-Rad CFX Real-Time PCR Systems) and Microsoft Excel (software version 16.16.8 (190312), 2018, Microsoft, Redmond, WA, USA).

### 4.7. Cytotoxicity and Apoptosis Assays

IncuCyte ZOOM Live-Cell Imaging system (Essen Bioscience, Ann Arbor, MI, USA) was used for kinetic monitoring of cytotoxicity and apoptotic activity of OTA in hESCs. These two assays were performed at the same time. Five thousand hESC cells were seeded at day 3 in mTESR medium in each of the 96-well plates, in such manner that by day 1 the cell confluence was approximately 30%. Cells were treated with increasing two concentrations (5 and 10 ppm) of OTA in the presence of 5 μM of Caspase 3/7 Apoptosis Assay Reagent (Essen Bioscience). The Caspase 3/7 reagent labeled apoptotic cells yielding green fluorescence. At the same time, IncuCyte®Cytotox Red Reagent for counting dead cells was applied. This reagent labeled dead cells yielding red fluorescence. The plate was scanned, and fluorescent and phase-contrast images were acquired in real time every 4 h from 0 to 48 hours post treatment. Normalized green object count per well at each time point and quantified time-lapse curves were generated by IncuCyte ZOOM software (IncuCyte®ZOOM Live-Cell Analysis Systems, 2018. Essen BioScience, 300 West Morgan Road, Ann Arbor, MI, USA). Ratios of caspase 3/7 level in OTA-treated cells compared to vehicle were plotted in Microsoft Excel. The cells were monitored for confluence. At a confluence of 50% we performed the experiment, monitoring cell growth using the IncuCyte System to capture phase contrast images every 2 h, and analyzed results using the integrated confluence algorithm. Caspase 3/7 diluted reagent at 1:1000 (5 μM final concentration) and Cytotox Red Reagent (final volume of 50 μL/well) or vehicle (ethanol) were added to the wells. Then, the medium was aspirated. The images were captured every 2–3 h (10× or 20×) in the IncuCyte® System.

### 4.8. Statistical Analysis

Statistical analyses of qRT-PCR data from at least three biological replicates were calculated using Student's t-test using GraphPad Prism 5.02 (GraphPad Software 2365 Northside 560 San Diego, CA, USA).

**Author Contributions:** Conceptualization, M.A.G.-E., J.M.S., S.E. and M.J.; Data curation, F.J.R.J. and E.M.M.; Formal analysis, I.Z. and M.A.P.A.; Investigation, M.A.G.-E., J.M.S., S.E., M.A.P.A. and E.M.M.; Supervision, M.A.G.-E., J.M.S. and S.E.; Validation, M.A.G.E., J.M.S. and S.E.; Writing original draft, M.A.G.-E., J.M.S., S.E., I.Z. and M.J.; Writing review and editing, M.A.G.-E., J.M.S., S.E.I.Z., M.J. and I.Z. All the authors approved the final version of the manuscript.

**Funding:** This research was funded by: (1) Ayudas a la Consolidación de Indicadores en Investigación Programa Banco Santander Universidad CEU Cardenal Herrera (grant number: INDI 18/43). Principal investigator: José Miguel Soria. (2) Ministry of Economy and Competitiveness, Spanish Government and European Regional Development Fund (grant number AGL2014-53928-C2-1-R). Principal investigator: Misericordia Jiménez. (3) Ayudas a la Consolidación de Indicadores en Investigación Programa Banco Santander Universidad CEU Cardenal Herrera (grant number: INDI 18/17). Principal investigator Mª Ángeles Garcia-Esparza.

**Acknowledgments:** We acknowledge the University CEU Cardenal Herrera, University of Valencia and Research Center Principe Felipe for the help, support and facilities.

**Conflicts of Interest:** The authors declare no conflict of interest.

## References

1. Thomson, J.A.; Itskovitz-Eldor, J.; Shapiro, S.S.; Waknitz, M.A.; Swiergiel, J.J.; Marshall, V.S.; Jones, J.M. Embryonic stem cell lines derived from human blastocysts. *Science* **1998**, *282*, 1145–1147. [CrossRef] [PubMed]
2. Shinde, V.; Klima, S.; Sureshkumar, P.S.; Meganathan, K.; Jagtap, S.; Rempel, E.; Rahnenfuhrer, J.; Hengstler, J.G.; Waldmann, T.; Hescheler, J.; et al. Human Pluripotent Stem Cell Based Developmental Toxicity Assays for Chemical Safety Screening and Systems Biology Data Generation. *J. Vis. Exp.* **2015**, *100*, e52333. [CrossRef]
3. Sokolov, M.V.; Neumann, R.D. Changes in human pluripotent stem cell gene expression after genotoxic stress exposures. *World J. Stem Cells* **2014**, *6*, 598–605. [CrossRef] [PubMed]
4. Larsen, T.O.; Svendsen, A.; Smedsgaard, J. Biochemical characterization of ochratoxin A-producing strains of the genus Penicillium. *Appl. Environ. Microbiol.* **2001**, *67*, 3630–3635. [CrossRef] [PubMed]
5. Medina, A.; Mateo, E.M.; Roig, R.J.; Blanquer, A.; Jimenez, M. Ochratoxin A levels in the plasma of healthy blood donors from Valencia and estimation of exposure degree: comparison with previous national Spanish data. *Food Addit. Contam. Part A Chem. Anal. Control Expo. Risk Assess.* **2010**, *27*, 1273–1284. [CrossRef] [PubMed]
6. Van der Merwe, K.J.; Steyn, P.S.; Fourie, L.; Scott, D.B.; Theron, J.J. Ochratoxin A, a toxic metabolite produced by Aspergillus ochraceus Wilh. *Nature* **1965**, *205*, 1112–1113. [CrossRef] [PubMed]
7. Abarca, M.L.; Bragulat, M.R.; Castella, G.; Cabanes, F.J. Ochratoxin A production by strains of Aspergillus niger var. niger. *Appl. Environ. Microbiol.* **1994**, *60*, 2650–2652. [PubMed]
8. Todescato, F.; Antognoli, A.; Meneghello, A.; Cretaio, E.; Signorini, R.; Bozio, R. Sensitive detection of Ochratoxin A in food and drinks using metal-enhanced fluorescence. *Biosens. Bioelectron.* **2014**, *57*, 125–132. [CrossRef]
9. Arora, R.G.; Frolen, H.; Fellner-Feldegg, H. Inhibition of ochratoxin A teratogenesis by zearalenone and diethylstilboestrol. *Food Chem. Toxicol.* **1983**, *21*, 779–783. [CrossRef]
10. Haubeck, H.D.; Lorkowski, G.; Kolsch, E.; Roschenthaler, R. Immunosuppression by ochratoxin A and its prevention by phenylalanine. *Appl. Environ. Microbiol.* **1981**, *41*, 1040–1042.
11. Sava, V.; Reunova, O.; Velasquez, A.; Sanchez-Ramos, J. Can low level exposure to ochratoxin-A cause parkinsonism? *J. Neurol. Sci.* **2006**, *249*, 68–75. [CrossRef]
12. Wilk-Zasadna, I.; Minta, M. Developmental toxicity of Ochratoxin A in rat embryo midbrain micromass cultures. *Int. J. Mol. Sci.* **2009**, *10*, 37–49. [CrossRef]
13. Razafimanjato, H.; Garmy, N.; Guo, X.J.; Varini, K.; Di Scala, C.; Di Pasquale, E.; Taieb, N.; Maresca, M. The food-associated fungal neurotoxin ochratoxin A inhibits the absorption of glutamate by astrocytes through a decrease in cell surface expression of the excitatory amino-acid transporters GLAST and GLT-1. *Neurotoxicology* **2010**, *31*, 475–484. [CrossRef] [PubMed]
14. Pfohl-Leszkowicz, A.; Manderville, R.A. Ochratoxin A: An overview on toxicity and carcinogenicity in animals and humans. *Mol. Nutr. Food Res.* **2007**, *51*, 61–99. [CrossRef]

15. Torovic, L. Aflatoxins and ochratoxin A in flour: A survey of the Serbian retail market. *Food Addit. Contam. Part B* **2018**, *11*, 26–32. [CrossRef]
16. Clarke, R.; Connolly, L.; Frizzell, C.; Elliott, C.T. Challenging conventional risk assessment with respect to human exposure to multiple food contaminants in food: A case study using maize. *Toxicol. Lett.* **2015**, *238*, 54–64. [CrossRef] [PubMed]
17. Jilani, K.; Lupescu, A.; Zbidah, M.; Abed, M.; Shaik, N.; Lang, F. Enhanced apoptotic death of erythrocytes induced by the mycotoxin ochratoxin A. *Kidney Blood Press Res.* **2012**, *36*, 107–118. [CrossRef]
18. Coronel, M.B.; Sanchis, V.; Ramos, A.J.; Marin, S. Review. Ochratoxin A: presence in human plasma and intake estimation. *Food Sci. Technol. Int.* **2010**, *16*, 5–18. [CrossRef]
19. Hope, J.H.; Hope, B.E. A review of the diagnosis and treatment of Ochratoxin A inhalational exposure associated with human illness and kidney disease including focal segmental glomerulosclerosis. *J. Environ. Public Health* **2012**, *2012*, 835059. [CrossRef]
20. Petkova-Bocharova, T.; Castegnaro, M.; Michelon, J.; Maru, V. Ochratoxin A and other mycotoxins in cereals from an area of Balkan endemic nephropathy and urinary tract tumours in Bulgaria. *IARC Sci. Publ.* **1991**, *115*, 83–87.
21. Belmadani, A.; Tramu, G.; Betbeder, A.M.; Creppy, E.E. Subchronic effects of ochratoxin A on young adult rat brain and partial prevention by aspartame, a sweetener. *Hum. Exp. Toxicol.* **1998**, *17*, 380–386. [CrossRef]
22. Paradells, S.; Rocamonde, B.; Llinares, C.; Herranz-Perez, V.; Jimenez, M.; Garcia-Verdugo, J.M.; Zipancic, I.; Soria, J.M.; Garcia-Esparza, M.A. Neurotoxic effects of ochratoxin A on the subventricular zone of adult mouse brain. *J. Appl. Toxicol.* **2015**, *35*, 737–751. [CrossRef]
23. Talbot, P. In vitro assessment of reproductive toxicity of tobacco smoke and its constituents. *Birth Defects Res. C Embryo Today* **2008**, *84*, 61–72. [CrossRef]
24. Hayes, A.W.; Hood, R.D.; Lee, H.L. Teratogenic effects of ochratoxin A in mice. *Teratology* **1974**, *9*, 93–97. [CrossRef]
25. Wangikar, P.B.; Dwivedi, P.; Sharma, A.K.; Sinha, N. Effect in rats of simultaneous prenatal exposure to ochratoxin A and aflatoxin B1. II. Histopathological features of teratological anomalies induced in fetuses. *Birth Defects Res. B Dev. Reprod. Toxicol.* **2004**, *71*, 352–358. [CrossRef]
26. Hardy, K. Cell death in the mammalian blastocyst. *Mol. Hum. Reprod.* **1997**, *3*, 919–925. [CrossRef]
27. Chan, W.H. Impact of genistein on maturation of mouse oocytes, fertilization, and fetal development. *Reprod. Toxicol.* **2009**, *28*, 52–58. [CrossRef]
28. Chan, W.H. Effects of citrinin on maturation of mouse oocytes, fertilization, and fetal development in vitro and in vivo. *Toxicol. Lett.* **2008**, *180*, 28–32. [CrossRef]
29. Klaric, M.S.; Zeljezic, D.; Rumora, L.; Peraica, M.; Pepeljnjak, S.; Domijan, A.M. A potential role of calcium in apoptosis and aberrant chromatin forms in porcine kidney PK15 cells induced by individual and combined ochratoxin A and citrinin. *Arch. Toxicol.* **2012**, *86*, 97–107. [CrossRef]
30. Li, J.; Yin, S.; Dong, Y.; Fan, L.; Hu, H. p53 activation inhibits ochratoxin A-induced apoptosis in monkey and human kidney epithelial cells via suppression of JNK activation. *Biochem. Biophys. Res. Commun.* **2011**, *411*, 458–463. [CrossRef]
31. Sauvant, C.; Holzinger, H.; Gekle, M. Proximal tubular toxicity of ochratoxin A is amplified by simultaneous inhibition of the extracellular signal-regulated kinases 1/2. *J. Pharmacol. Exp. Ther.* **2005**, *313*, 234–241. [CrossRef]
32. Flora, S.J.; Mehta, A. Monoisoamyl dimercaptosuccinic acid abrogates arsenic-induced developmental toxicity in human embryonic stem cell-derived embryoid bodies: Comparison with in vivo studies. *Biochem. Pharmacol.* **2009**, *78*, 1340–1349. [CrossRef]
33. He, X.; Imanishi, S.; Sone, H.; Nagano, R.; Qin, X.Y.; Yoshinaga, J.; Akanuma, H.; Yamane, J.; Fujibuchi, W.; Ohsako, S. Effects of methylmercury exposure on neuronal differentiation of mouse and human embryonic stem cells. *Toxicol. Lett.* **2012**, *212*, 1–10. [CrossRef]
34. Lin, S.; Tran, V.; Talbot, P. Comparison of toxicity of smoke from traditional and harm-reduction cigarettes using mouse embryonic stem cells as a novel model for preimplantation development. *Hum. Reprod.* **2009**, *24*, 386–397. [CrossRef]
35. Lin, S.; Fonteno, S.; Weng, J.H.; Talbot, P. Comparison of the toxicity of smoke from conventional and harm reduction cigarettes using human embryonic stem cells. *Toxicol. Sci.* **2010**, *118*, 202–212. [CrossRef]

36. Meganathan, K.; Jagtap, S.; Wagh, V.; Winkler, J.; Gaspar, J.A.; Hildebrand, D.; Trusch, M.; Lehmann, K.; Hescheler, J.; Schluter, H.; et al. Identification of thalidomide-specific transcriptomics and proteomics signatures during differentiation of human embryonic stem cells. *PLoS ONE* **2012**, *7*, e44228. [CrossRef]
37. Schuldiner, M.; Yanuka, O.; Itskovitz-Eldor, J.; Melton, D.A.; Benvenisty, N. Effects of eight growth factors on the differentiation of cells derived from human embryonic stem cells. *Proc. Natl. Acad. Sci. USA* **2000**, *97*, 11307–11312. [CrossRef]
38. Muller, G.; Rosner, H.; Rohrmann, B.; Erler, W.; Geschwend, G.; Grafe, U.; Burkert, B.; Moller, U.; Diller, R.; Sachse, K.; et al. Effects of the mycotoxin ochratoxin A and some of its metabolites on the human cell line THP-1. *Toxicology* **2003**, *184*, 69–82. [CrossRef]
39. Grandjean, P.; Bellinger, D.; Bergman, A.; Cordier, S.; Davey-Smith, G.; Eskenazi, B.; Gee, D.; Gray, K.; Hanson, M.; van den Hazel, P.; et al. The faroes statement: human health effects of developmental exposure to chemicals in our environment. *Basic Clin. Pharmacol. Toxicol.* **2008**, *102*, 73–75. [CrossRef]
40. Fukui, Y.; Hayasaka, S.; Itoh, M.; Takeuchi, Y. Development of neurons and synapses in ochratoxin A-induced microcephalic mice: A quantitative assessment of somatosensory cortex. *Neurotoxicol. Teratol.* **1992**, *14*, 191–196. [CrossRef]
41. Miki, T.; Fukui, Y.; Uemura, N.; Takeuchi, Y. Regional difference in the neurotoxicity of ochratoxin A on the developing cerebral cortex in mice. *Brain Res. Dev. Brain Res.* **1994**, *82*, 259–264. [CrossRef]
42. Bennett, J.W.; Klich, M. Mycotoxins. *Clin. Microbiol. Rev.* **2003**, *16*, 497–516. [CrossRef] [PubMed]
43. Bhat, P.V.; Pandareesh, M.; Khanum, F.; Tamatam, A. Cytotoxic Effects of Ochratoxin A in Neuro-2a Cells: Role of Oxidative Stress Evidenced by N-acetylcysteine. *Front. Microbiol.* **2016**, *7*, 1142. [CrossRef]
44. Renzulli, C.; Galvano, F.; Pierdomenico, L.; Speroni, E.; Guerra, M.C. Effects of rosmarinic acid against aflatoxin B1 and ochratoxin-A-induced cell damage in a human hepatoma cell line (Hep G2). *J. Appl. Toxicol.* **2004**, *24*, 289–296. [CrossRef] [PubMed]
45. Hibi, D.; Suzuki, Y.; Ishii, Y.; Jin, M.; Watanabe, M.; Sugita-Konishi, Y.; Yanai, T.; Nohmi, T.; Nishikawa, A.; Umemura, T. Site-specific in vivo mutagenicity in the kidney of gpt delta rats given a carcinogenic dose of ochratoxin A. *Toxicol. Sci.* **2011**, *122*, 406–414. [CrossRef]
46. Palabiyik, S.S.; Erkekoglu, P.; Zeybek, N.D.; Kizilgun, M.; Baydar, D.E.; Sahin, G.; Giray, B.K. Protective effect of lycopene against ochratoxin A induced renal oxidative stress and apoptosis in rats. *Exp. Toxicol. Pathol.* **2013**, *65*, 853–861. [CrossRef]
47. Doi, K.; Uetsuka, K. Mechanisms of mycotoxin-induced neurotoxicity through oxidative stress-associated pathways. *Int. J. Mol. Sci.* **2011**, *12*, 5213–5237. [CrossRef]
48. Van Gurp, M.; Festjens, N.; van Loo, G.; Saelens, X.; Vandenabeele, P. Mitochondrial intermembrane proteins in cell death. *Biochem. Biophys. Res. Commun.* **2003**, *304*, 487–497. [CrossRef]
49. Assaf, H.; Azouri, H.; Pallardy, M. Ochratoxin A induces apoptosis in human lymphocytes through down regulation of Bcl-xL. *Toxicol. Sci.* **2004**, *79*, 335–344. [CrossRef] [PubMed]
50. Darif, Y.; Mountassif, D.; Belkebir, A.; Zaid, Y.; Basu, K.; Mourad, W.; Oudghiri, M. Ochratoxin A mediates MAPK activation, modulates IL-2 and TNF-alpha mRNA expression and induces apoptosis by mitochondria-dependent and mitochondria-independent pathways in human H9 T cells. *J. Toxicol. Sci.* **2016**, *41*, 403–416. [CrossRef] [PubMed]
51. Raghubeer, S.; Nagiah, S.; Chuturgoon, A.A. Acute Ochratoxin A exposure induces inflammation and apoptosis in human embryonic kidney (HEK293) cells. *Toxicon* **2017**, *137*, 48–53. [CrossRef]
52. Joschko, M.A.; Dreosti, I.E.; Tulsi, R.S. The teratogenic effects of nicotine in vitro in rats: a light and electron microscope study. *Neurotoxicol. Teratol.* **1991**, *13*, 307–316. [CrossRef]
53. Zhao, Z.; Reece, E.A. Nicotine-induced embryonic malformations mediated by apoptosis from increasing intracellular calcium and oxidative stress. *Birth Defects Res. B Dev. Reprod. Toxicol.* **2005**, *74*, 383–391. [CrossRef]
54. Seiler, A.E.; Buesen, R.; Visan, A.; Spielmann, H. Use of murine embryonic stem cells in embryotoxicity assays: The embryonic stem cell test. *Methods Mol. Biol.* **2006**, *329*, 371–395. [CrossRef]

55. Yamane, J.; Aburatani, S.; Imanishi, S.; Akanuma, H.; Nagano, R.; Kato, T.; Sone, H.; Ohsako, S.; Fujibuchi, W. Prediction of developmental chemical toxicity based on gene networks of human embryonic stem cells. *Nucleic Acids Res.* **2016**, *44*, 5515–5528. [CrossRef]
56. Aikawa, N.; Kunisato, A.; Nagao, K.; Kusaka, H.; Takaba, K.; Ohgami, K. Detection of thalidomide embryotoxicity by in vitro embryotoxicity testing based on human iPS cells. *J. Pharmacol. Sci.* **2014**, *124*, 201–207. [CrossRef]

toxins

MDPI

Article

# Deoxynivalenol Induces Inflammation in IPEC-J2 Cells by Activating P38 Mapk And Erk1/2

**Hua Zhang [1], Xiwen Deng [1], Chuang Zhou [2], Wenda Wu [1,3,*] and Haibin Zhang [1,*]**

1 College of Veterinary Medicine, Nanjing Agricultural University, Nanjing 210095, China; 2016207033@njau.edu.cn (H.Z.); 9171310404@njau.edu.cn (X.D.)
2 Jiangsu Vocational College of Agriculture and Forestry, Jurong 212400, China; zhouchuang@jsafc.edu.cn
3 Department of Chemistry, Faculty of Science, University of Hradec Kralove, 500 03 Hradec Kralove, Czech Republic
* Correspondence: wuwenda@njau.edu.cn (W.W.); haibinzh@njau.edu.cn (H.Z.); Tel.: +86-152-5185-0173 (W.W.); +86-139-0515-1215 (H.Z.)

Received: 11 February 2020; Accepted: 4 March 2020; Published: 13 March 2020

**Abstract:** Fusarium-derived mycotoxin deoxynivalenol (DON) usually induces diarrhea, vomiting and gastrointestinal inflammation. We studied the cytotoxic effect of DON on porcine small intestinal epithelium using the intestinal porcine epithelial cell line IPEC-J2. We screened out differentially expressed genes (DEGs) using RNA-seq and identified 320 upregulated genes and 160 downregulated genes. The enrichment pathways of these DEGs focused on immune-related pathways. DON induced proinflammatory gene expression, including cytokines, chemokines and other inflammation-related genes. DON increased IL1A, IL6 and TNF-α release and DON activated the phosphorylation of extracellular signal-regulated kinase-1 and-2 (ERK1/2), JUN N-terminal kinase (JNK) and p38 MAPK. A p38 inhibitor attenuated DON-induced IL6, TNF-α, CXCL2, CXCL8, IL12A, IL1A, CCL20, CCL4 and IL15 production, while an ERK1/2 inhibitor had only a small inhibitory effect on IL15 and IL6. An inhibitor of p38 MAPK decreased the release of IL1A, IL6 and TNF-α and an inhibitor of ERK1/2 partly attenuated protein levels of IL6. These data demonstrate that DON induces proinflammatory factor production in IPEC-J2 cells by activating p38 and ERK1/2.

**Keywords:** deoxynivalenol; IPEC-J2 cells; RNA-seq; inflammation; MAPKs

**Key Contribution:** DON induces proinflammatory gene expression, including cytokines, chemokines and other inflammation-related genes. DON enhances inflammation in IPEC-J2 via p38 and ERK1/2.

## 1. Introduction

Deoxynivalenol (DON; vomitoxin) is a type B trichothecene mycotoxin produced by strains of *Fusarium graminearum* and *F. culmorum* [1]. DON mainly contaminates cereal, especially barley, oats, wheat, corn and their subsequent products. In addition, DON accumulation is a potential sign for the occurrence of other mycotoxins [2]. Due to its adverse effects on animals, DON is known as one of the most significant mycotoxins in animal production.

Consumption of DON-contaminated foods and feeds has been associated with a spectrum of adverse effects and the immunotoxic effects of DON are of increasing concern for farm animals, as well as for humans [2,3]. According to the dose, timing of exposure, time and functional immune assay being used, DON may exert immunosuppressive or immunostimulatory effects [4]. Our preliminary experiments indicate that exposure to DON induces the overexpression of cytokines and chemokines, leading to immune stress, which caused immune function damage [5,6].

The intestinal epithelium forms an important physical barrier against external matter and it is highly sensitive to mycotoxins and important for maintaining health [7]. Consuming DON-contaminated food is related to gastroenteritis flare-ups and DON exposure leads to intestinal lesions in vivo (animals studies), ex vivo (intestinal explants) and in vitro (cell line) [8–10]. Numerous studies have concluded that DON upregulates the expression of cytokines, chemokines and inflammatory genes [11–13]. However, the mechanism underlying DON-induced inflammation in intestinal epithelial cells (IECs) remains unclear.

MAPKs, including p38 MAPK, extracellular signal-regulated kinase-1 and-2 (ERK1/2) and JUN N-terminal kinase (JNK), modulate many cellular processes associated with cell proliferation, differentiation, survival and death [14]. MAPK signaling has basic functions in immunoregulation and immunopathology, including inflammatory responses and enteritis. Recent research has suggested that DON and other trichothecenes induce the activation of MAPKs in IPEC-J2 cells [15–17], which contributes to autophagy, oxidative stress, epithelial tight junction disruption and intestinal barrier dysfunction. However, few correlative studies have investigated the interaction of MAPK signaling with DON-induced inflammation in the intestinal epithelium.

Therefore, the aims of the present study were to use the IPEC-J2 cell line, an in vitro model of porcine small IECs, to investigate the capacity of DON to induce inflammation and relate the immunomodulatory effects of DON to MAPK activation.

## 2. Results

### *2.1. DON Decreases the Viability and Induces Inflammation in IPEC-J2 Cells*

IPEC-J2 cells were treated for different time periods (2, 6, 12 and 24 h) and with different concentrations of DON (0.25, 0.5, 1, 2 and 4 μg/mL). As presented in Figure 1a, DON (≥0.5 μg/mL) significantly reduced IPEC-J2 cell viability in a time- and concentration-dependent manner.

DON at concentrations of 1.0 and 2.0 μg/mL markedly enhanced the gene expression levels of IL6, IL1A and TNF-α at 2 h compared to the control group (Figure 1b,d,f). After treatment with DON at concentrations of 1.0 and 2.0 μg/mL, the expression of IL1A and IL6 was significantly increased at 6 h (Figure 1b,f) and the expression of IL6 was significantly increased at 12 h (Figure 1b). Moreover, IL6, IL1A and TNF-α protein release into the incubation medium was elevated after treatment with DON at concentrations of 1.0 and 2.0 μg/mL (Figure 1c,e,g). To investigate the immunomodulatory effects of DON, IPEC-J2 cells were exposed to 2 μg/mL DON for 2 h in subsequent experiments.

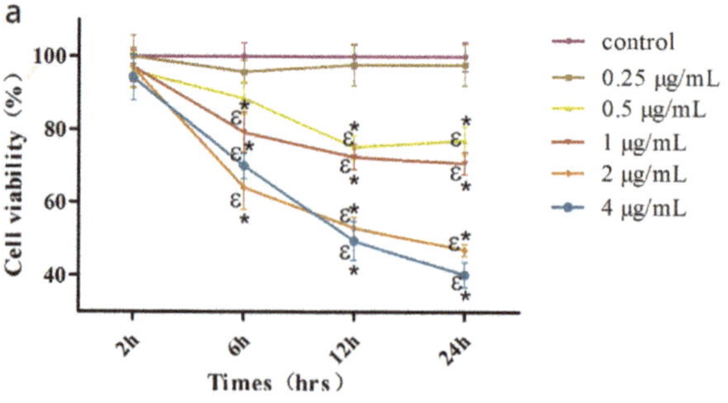


**Figure 1.** *Cont.*

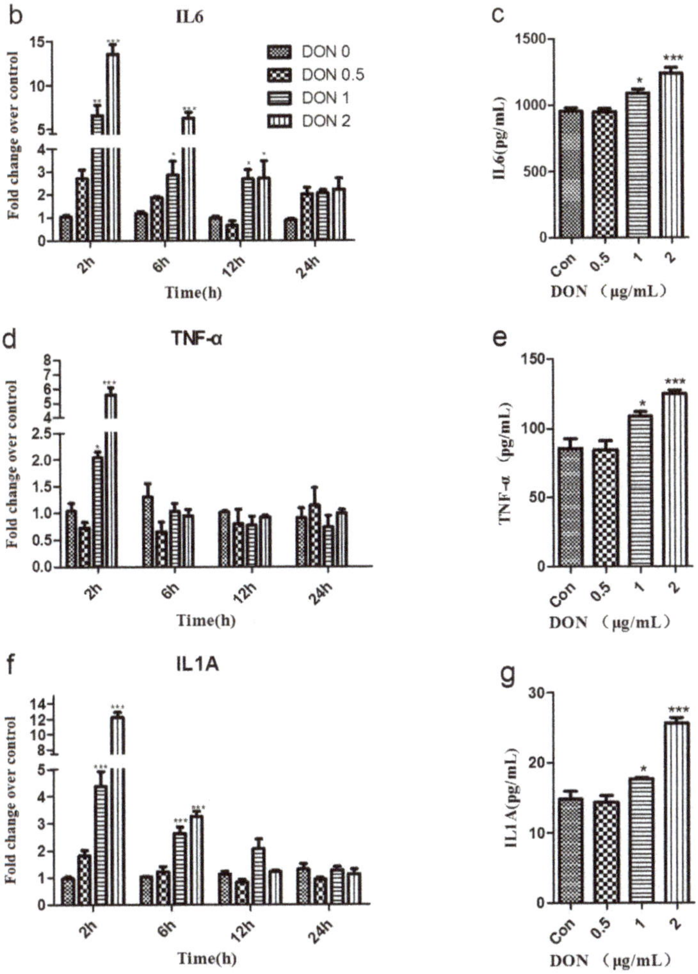


**Figure 1.** Deoxynivalenol (DON) decreases the viability and induces inflammation in IPEC-J2 cells (**a**) Cell viability in IPEC-J2 cells with or without DON. Two-way ANOVA using Holm-Sidak method was used to assess significant differences in cell viability compared with of the control. Symbols: * indicates difference in cell viability relative to the control at specific time point ($p < 0.05$) and ε indicates difference in cell viability relative to the 2h exposure time at specific dose ($p < 0.05$). Effects of DON on IL6 (**b**), TNF-α (**d**) and IL1A (**f**) gene expression. and IL6 (**c**), TNF-α (**e**) and IL1A (**g**) cytokine release in IPEC-J2 cells. Samples were collected after 2, 6, 12 and 24 h (mRNA) or 12 h (protein release). One-way ANOVA with a Holm-Sidak test was used to assess significant differences in the mRNA and protein release of IL6, TNF-α and IL1A compared with of the control. The data are expressed as the mean ± SEM. * $p < 0.05$, ** $p < 0.01$ and *** $p < 0.001$ versus control.

### 2.2. Identification and Functional Enrichment Analysis of Differentially Expressed Genes (DEGs)

Based on the RNA-seq data, we obtained 480 differentially expressed genes (DEGs) with 320 upregulated genes and 160 downregulated genes (Supplementary Materials: Table S1). In Figure 2, the heatmap and volcano plot show that these genes were clearly separated (Figure 2a,b). According to the Gene Ontology (GO) terms (Figure 2c), 71 genes were enriched in the immune system process. Kyoto Encyclopedia of Genes and Genomes (KEGG) pathway analysis revealed that the upregulated DEGs were mainly enriched in the following immune-related pathways: TNF signaling pathway, cytokine-cytokine receptor interaction, MAPK signaling pathway, NF-kappa B signaling pathway, Jak-STAT signaling pathway, Toll-like receptor signaling pathway and NOD-like receptor signaling pathway (Figure 2d). Table 1 shows several enriched pathway terms and 15 DEGs were enriched in the MAPK signaling pathway. These results suggest that DON-induced inflammation may associate with the MAPK signaling pathway.

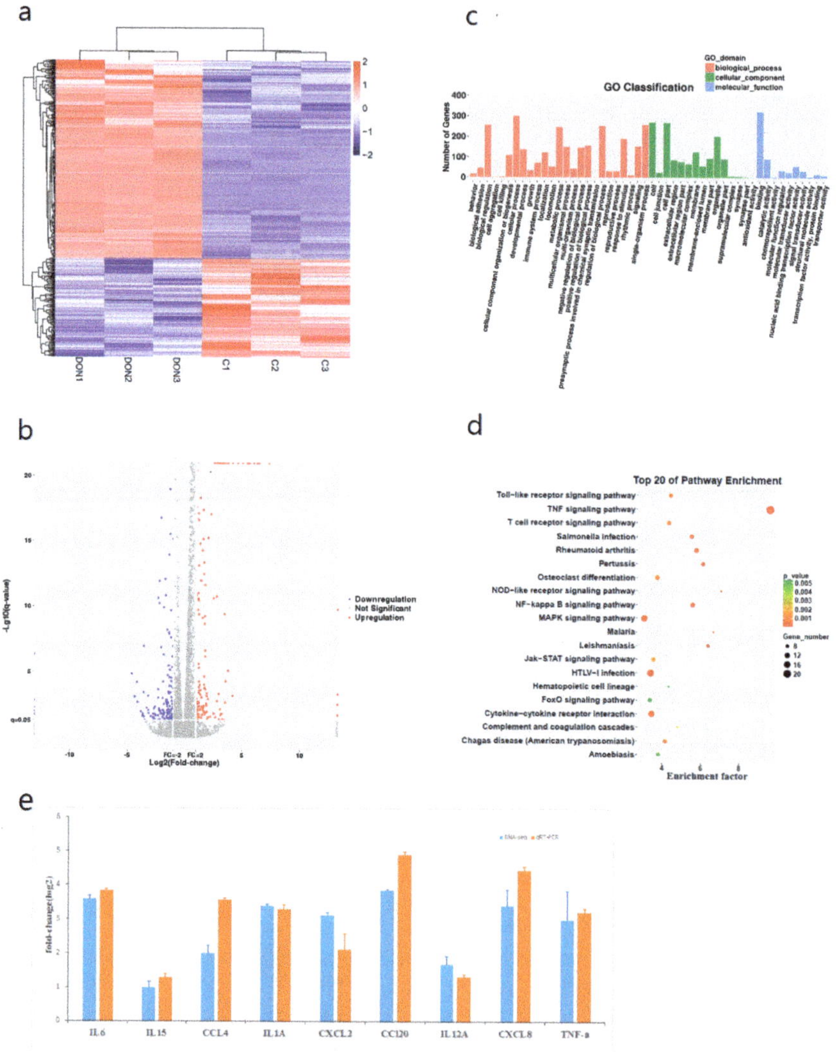


**Figure 2.** (**a**) Cluster heatmap. A change in color from blue to red indicates that the expression level of the gene was relatively high. (**b**) Volcano plot of the DEGs. Blue indicates downregulated genes and red indicates upregulated genes. (**c**) Gene ontology (GO) analysis classified the DEGs into 3 groups: molecular function, biological process and cellular component. (**d**) Bubbles of Kyoto Encyclopedia of Genes and Genomes (KEGG) pathways of the DEGs. The coloring indicates higher enrichment in red and lower enrichment in green. The point size indicates the number of DEGs enriched in a certain pathway. Lower q-values indicate more significant enrichment. (**e**) Validation of DEG data by real-time quantitative PCR (RT-qPCR). The x-axis represents the mRNAs and the y-axis is the fold change between the RT-qPCR and sequencing values.

**Table 1.** Pathway enrichment analysis of the differentially expressed genes (DEGs).

| Pathways | Number | Gene upregulation | Gene downregulation | Q-value |
|---|---|---|---|---|
| TNF signaling pathway | 21 | TNFAIP3, MAP3K8, CCL20, CSF2, LIF, EDN1, CXCL2, IL15, NFKBIA, FOS, MAP3K14, CSF1, TNF, IL6, VCAM1, JUN, MAP3K5, PTGS2, SOCS3, BIRC3, JUNB | - | $2.03 \times 10^{-14}$ |
| HTLV-I infection | 17 | FZD5, EGR1, CSF2, ATF3, MYC, IL15 NFKBIA, FOS, MAP3K14, TNF, IL6, VCAM1, FOSL1, JUN, EGR2, ETS1, ETS2 | - | $3.47 \times 10^{-05}$ |
| MAPK signaling pathway | 15 | RASA1, GADD45G, DUSP1, MAP3K8, DUSP5, IL1A, GADD45B, MYC, FOS, MAP3K14, TNF, JUN, DUSP10, MAP3K5, DUSP6 | - | 0.000375 |
| Cytokine-cytokine receptor interaction | 13 | CCL4, IL6, IL1A, CCL20, CSF2, KDR, TSLP, IL12A, LIF, IL15, CSF1, TNF, CXCL8 | - | 0.000191 |
| NF-kappa B signaling pathway | 10 | VCAM1, TNF, PTGS2, CXCL8, NFKBIA, BIRC3, PLAU, CCL4, TNFAIP3, MAPK3K14 | - | $6.84 \times 10^{-05}$ |
| Jak-STAT signaling pathway | 10 | CSF2, TSLP, IL12A, LIF, MYC, MCL1, IL15, PIM1, IL6, SOCS3 | - | 0.001979 |
| Rheumatoid arthritis | 10 | IL1A, CCL20, CSF2, IL15, FOS, CSF1, TNF, IL6, CXCL8, JUN | - | $5.21 \times 10^{-05}$ |
| Toll-like receptor signaling pathway | 9 | CCL4, IL12A, NFKBIA, FOS, TNF, IL6, CXCL8, JUN, SPP1 | - | 0.000926 |

### *2.3. Integration of Protein-Protein Interaction (PPI) Network Analysis*

To further investigate regulatory pathways of DON, a protein-protein interaction (PPI) network was formulated based on the data in the Search Tool for the Retrieval of Interacting Genes/Proteins (STRING) database with a total of 371 nodes and 729 relationship pairs (Figure 3a). The top 10 hub genes were TNF, IL6, JUN, MYC, CXCL8, FOS, EGR1, CSF2, EDN1 and ATF3 and they were key node proteins in the PPI network. To better analyze the interaction of the proteins, we detected two modules using the Cytoscape plugin Molecular Complex Detection (MCODE) with a score >5 and the top module is shown in Figure 3b. Pathway enrichment analysis of the top module showed that it was mainly related to the MAPK signaling pathway, cytokine-cytokine receptor interaction and TNF signaling pathway.

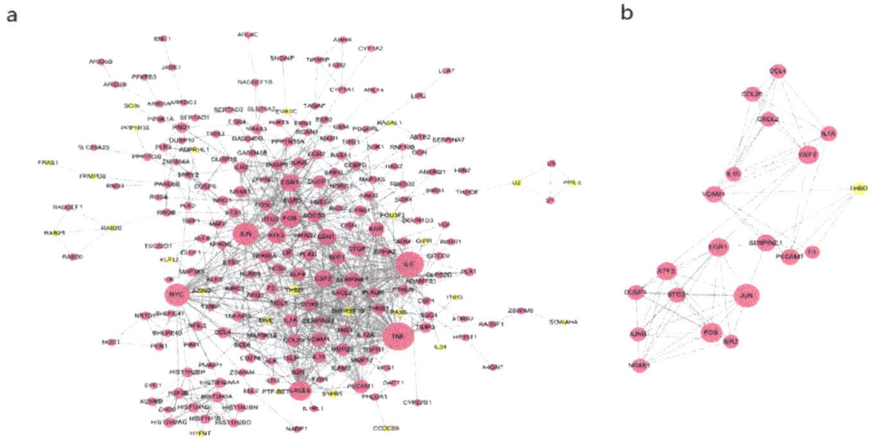


**Figure 3.** Protein-protein interaction (PPI) network of the DEGs (**a**) and the most significant modules (**b**). Purple nodes represent upregulated genes and yellow nodes represent downregulated genes.

## 2.4. *Validation of the Expression Profile Analysis by RT-qPCR*

Ten genes were selected from the significant DEGs for RT-qPCR analysis to validate their expression levels. The transcriptional levels according to the sequencing and RT-qPCR data were consistent (Figure 2e), thus confirming that the sequencing information was reliable.

## 2.5. *DON Promotes the Expression of Inflammatory Factors and Induces Inflammation in IPEC-J2 Cells Through p38 and ERK1/2*

We hypothesized that there may be a link between the activation of the MAPK pathway and DON-induced inflammation. We measured the phosphorylated protein levels of p38, ERK1/2 and JNK. DON effectively increased the phosphorylation of p38, ERK1/2 and JNK (Figure 4).

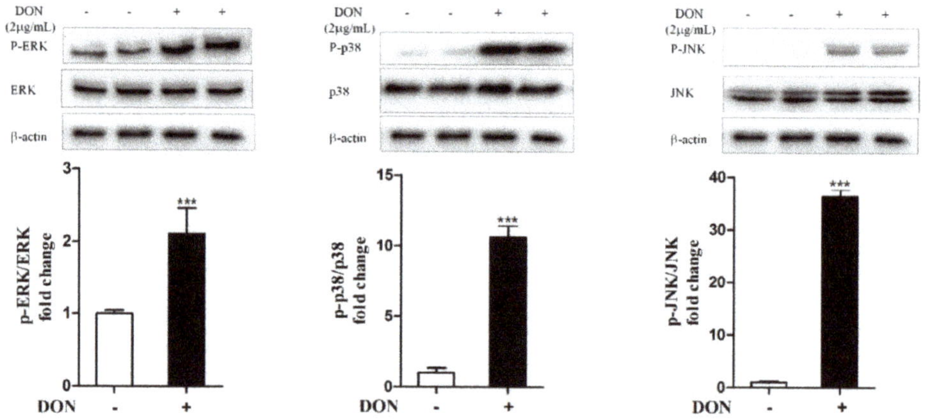


**Figure 4.** DON induces MAPK activation in IPEC-J2 cells. The levels of p-ERK, p-p38 and p-JNK were detected by western blotting. Data analyzed as described in Figure 1b legend. The quantitative data are presented as the mean ± SEM. * $p < 0.05$, ** $p < 0.01$ and *** $p < 0.001$ versus control.

To gain insight into the mechanism of MAPKs in DON-induced inflammatory factor upregulation, IPEC-J2 cells were pretreated with inhibitors, including U0126 (ERK 1/2 inhibitor, 10 mM), SP600125 (JNK inhibitor, 20 mM) and SB203580 (p38 inhibitor, 10 mM), before DON treatment. As shown in Figure 5, the inhibition of p38 significantly attenuated DON-induced IL6, TNF-α, CXCL2, CXCL8, IL12A, IL1A, CCL20, CCL4 and IL15 production, whereas the inhibition of JNK had no effect. In addition, the inhibition of ERK 1/2 attenuated DON-induced IL15 and IL6 production. In contrast, CCL4, CCL20 and CXCL2 production increased after treatment with the ERK 1/2 and JNK inhibitors. DON treatment did not significantly affect CCL2 production. In addition, the inhibition of p38 significantly attenuated IL6, IL1A and TNF-α protein release and the inhibition of ERK 1/2 partly attenuated DON-induced IL6 protein release (Figure 6). These results suggest that both p38 and ERK 1/2 contribute to DON-induced inflammation.

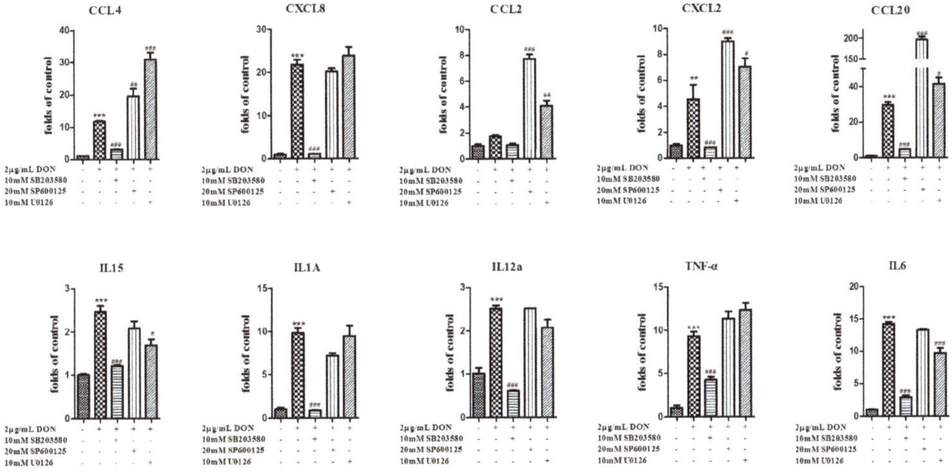


**Figure 5.** DON promotes the expression of inflammatory factors through p38 and ERK1/2. Data analyzed as described in Figure 1b legend. The data are expressed as the mean ± SEM. * $p < 0.05$, ** $p < 0.01$ and *** $p < 0.001$ versus control. # $p < 0.05$, ## $p < 0.01$ and ### $p < 0.001$ versus control-DON.

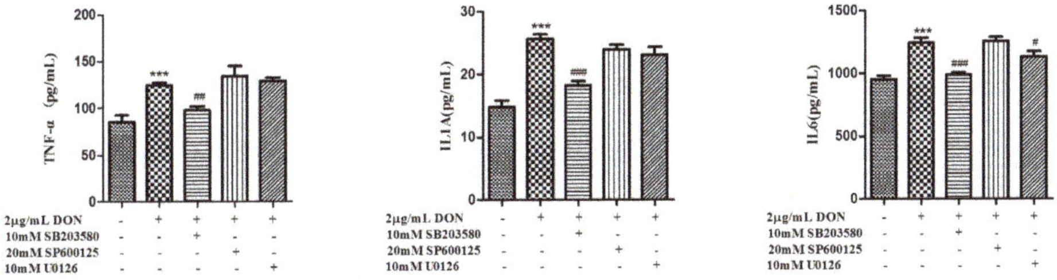


**Figure 6.** DON induces inflammation in IPEC-J2 cells through p38 and ERK1/2. Data analyzed as described in Figure 1b legend. The data are expressed as the mean ± SEM. * $p < 0.05$, ** $p < 0.01$ and *** $p < 0.001$ versus control. # $p < 0.05$, ## $p < 0.01$ and ### $p < 0.001$ versus control-DON.

## 3. Discussion

The mycotoxin DON is a frequent contaminant of cereals and co-products. The intestine, which serves as the first barrier against food contaminants, shows high sensitivity to DON and related mycotoxins [7,13,18]. After pigs are exposed to DON, most absorption occurs in jejunal epithelial cells. DON mainly causes oxidative stress, disrupts epithelial tight junctions and induces intestinal barrier dysfunction [15,17]. However, the mechanism underlying DON-induced inflammation in IECs is not completely clear. To gain insight into the genes and pathways related to DON in IPEC-J2 cells, we conducted RNA-seq analysis to identify the top inflammatory factors and molecular pathways following DON treatment.

DON robustly upregulates proinflammatory gene expression [4]. DON increased the expression of genes and proteins associated with inflammation, such as TNF-α and IL6 in IPEC-J2 cells, which was consistent with a previous study [19]. TNF-α and interleukins are classic proinflammatory factors that are quickly secreted and cause inflammation when the body is exposed to exogenous stimulation [20]. Overabundant production of TNF-α causes excess secretion of other inflammatory factors, such as IL1β, IL2 and IL8, thereby inducing intestinal mucosal injury [20–22]. Accordingly, inflammatory factors play roles in intestinal immunity. Our data showed that DON significantly upregulated the levels of proinflammatory factors in a concentration-dependent manner in IPEC-J2 cells, indicating that DON enhances the production of inflammatory mediators.

Apart from proinflammatory cytokine upregulation, DON upregulates the transcription levels of several chemokines, including CXCL2, CCL2 and CCL20 [6,23,24]. In our study, DON upregulated the chemokines CXCL2, CXCL8, CCL4 and CCL20. The chemokine CXCL2 is a cytokine secreted by IPEC-J2 cells and a chemotactic for polymorphonuclear leukocytes [25]. CXCL8 is a proinflammatory chemokine that acts as a strong chemoattractant but can create tissue injury with long-term exposure [26]. CCL4 serves as a chemoattractant for monocytes, natural killer cells and a variety of other immune cells [27] and CCL20 is strongly chemotactic for lymphocytes [28]. DON induces the release of CXCL8 in several intestinal epithelial cell lines [29,30]. These previous results are in agreement with our study. Thereby, the inflammation effects of DON may, in part, be influenced by the leukocyte chemotaxis induced by chemokine dysfunction.

The KEGG pathway enrichment analysis showed that the significant DEGs were enriched in immunological pathways and that the MAPK signaling pathway was one of the main signaling pathway enriched in 15 DEGs. Pathway enrichment analysis of the top module showed that it was mainly associated with MAPKs. MAPKs are a type of protein kinase that is pivotal for the development of inflammation [31]. MAPK pathways are activated by kinases, cytoskeletal proteins, transcription factors and other enzymes [32]. The first step to their activation consists of relieving their autoinhibition by a smaller ligand (such as Ras for c-Ra and GADD45 for MEKK4) [33]. DUSPs negatively regulate some MAPKs. DUSP5 and DUSP6 inactivate ERK1/2 and DUSP1 interacts with p38-$\alpha$, ERK2 and JNK1 [34,35]. MAP3K8, MAP3K5 and MAP3K14 are important MAP3 kinases. The transcription factors JUN, MYC and FOS regulate the expression of inflammation- and immune-related genes [4]. In our study, the upregulation of GADD45B, GADD45G, RASA1, MAP3K8, MAP3K14, MAP3K5, IL1A, MYC, FOS, TNF and JUN, which are related to the MAPK pathway, contributed to MAPK activation and the expression of inflammatory factors. According to the RNA-seq analysis, DON may induce inflammation via the MAPK pathway.

MAPK contributes to DON-induced transactivation and the mRNA stabilization of inflammatory factors [36,37]. To determine whether DON induces porcine intestinal epithelium cell inflammation via the MAPK pathway, MAPK inhibition assays were performed. It has been reported that the MAPK pathway is one of the main pathways for DON to induce inflammation [11,22]. The results in the present study showed that DON induced activation of MAPKs. The p38 inhibitor attenuated DON-induced gene expression levels of IL6, TNF-$\alpha$, CXCL2, CXCL8, IL12A, IL1A, CCL20, CCL4 and IL15 as well as protein expression levels of IL1A, IL6 and TNF-$\alpha$. The ERK1/2 inhibitor had only a small inhibitory effect on IL1A and IL6 gene expression levels as well as IL6 protein levels, while the JNK inhibitor had no effect. We demonstrated that DON induced the expression of proinflammatory cytokines and chemokines via the p38 MAPK and ERK1/2 signaling pathways. CXCL8 secretion were upregulated in various human intestinal epithelial cell lines exposed to DON [29,30,38]. In response to DON, dose-dependent increases in IL-8 secretion were observed in Caco-2 cells and this was linked to the ribotoxic-associated activation of PKR, NF-kB and p38 [29,38]. DON elevates CXCL8 generation via ERK1/2 but not p38 in human embryonic epithelial intestine 407 (Int407) cells [30]. This discrepancy may be due to the maturation status of the cells: differentiated mature Caco-2 cells and IPEC-J2 vs. undifferentiated Int407 cells.

In conclusion, the results of the present study indicate that DON induces inflammation in IPEC-J2 cells. This discovery provides a theoretical basis for further exploring the molecular mechanisms of IEC inflammation induced by DON.

## 4. Materials and Methods

### 4.1. Reagents

DON was obtained from Sigma-Aldrich (St. Louis, MO, USA). Cell culture medium and supplements were purchased from Life Technologies (Grand Island, NY, USA). Anti-phospho-p38 (4511), anti-p38 (8690), anti-phospho-JNK (4668), anti-JNK (9252), anti-phospho-ERK (4370), anti-ERK

(4695) and anti-β-actin (4970) antibodies were purchased from Cell Signaling Technology (Beverly, MA, USA). SB203580 was obtained from Promega (Madison, WI, USA). U0126 and SP600125 were acquired from Cayman Chemicals (Ann Arbor, MI, USA).

### 4.2. Cell Culture and Treatment

The IPEC-J2 cell line was a gift from Professor Qian Yang, Nanjing Agricultural University, Nanjing, China. Cells were grown in DMEM/F12 medium supplemented with antibiotics and 10% fetal bovine serum. Cells were maintained in the exponential growth phase by passages at intervals of 2–3 days. Compounds were prepared as stock solutions and diluted with the cell culture medium before use. The working concentrations were as follows: DON (0.25, 0.5, 1, 2 and 4 μg/mL), U0126 (10 μM), SP600125 (20 μM) and SB203580 (10 μM). The final concentration of dimethyl sulfoxide (DMSO) was less than 0.1%, which exerted no effect on cell viability. Cells were treated with or without DON and the indicated test compounds for various times according to the experimental protocol.

### 4.3. Cell Viability Assay

Cell viability was measured using the MTT (Sigma, M5655) method according to the manufacturer's instructions after DON treatments for 2, 6, 12 and 24 h. The optical density of the control group was considered to be 100% viable.

### 4.4. Quantitative Real-Time PCR (qRT-PCR) Assay

Total RNA was isolated using TRIzol reagent (Takara, Dalian, China). cDNA was obtained by reverse transcription using a cDNA transcription kit (Takara, Dalian, China). Real-time PCR was performed in 96-well optical plates on an ABI StepOne Plus Real-time PCR system using SYBR Premix Ex Taq™ (Takara, Dalian, China). The primers used for RT-PCR are shown in Table 2. Analysis of the relative gene expression level was achieved using the $2^{-\Delta\Delta CT}$ method and gene expression levels were normalized to GAPDH.

**Table 2.** Primer sequences of RT-PCR target genes.

| Gene | Primer sequence (5′-3′) | |
|---|---|---|
| | Sense | Antisense |
| GAPDH | CGTCAAGCTCATTTCCTGGT | TGGGATGGAAACTGGAAGTC |
| IL6 | AGCAAGGAGGTACTGGCAGA | CAGGGTCTGGATCAGTGCTT |
| TNF-α | AACCTCCTCTCTGCCATCAA | TAGACCTGCCCAGATTCAGC |
| CXCL2 | CACAGACCCTCCGAGCTAAG | TGACTTCCGTTTGGTCACAG |
| CXCL8 | GCCTCATTCCTGTGCTGGTCAG | AACAACGTGCATGGGACACTGG |
| IL12A | AAGCCCTCCCTGGAAGAACTGG | TCACCGCACGAATTCTGAAGGC |
| IL1A | CGAACCCGTGTTGCTGAAGGAG | TGGATGGGCGGCTGATTTGAAG |
| CCL20 | GATGTCGGTGCTGCTGCTCTAC | ATTGGCGAGCTGCTGTGTGAAG |
| CCL2 | CACCAGCAGCAAGTGTCCTA | GGGCAAGTTAGAAGGAAATGAA |
| CCL4 | TGGTCCTGGTCGCTGCCTTC | TTCCGCACGGTGTATGTGAAGC |
| IL15 | TGCATCCAGTGCTACTTGTGTT | GACCTGCACTGATACAGCCC |

### 4.5. Cytokine Detection by ELISA

IPEC-J2 cell supernatants were collected after treatment with 2.0 mg/mL DON for 12 h. Porcine IL6, IL1A and TNF-α ELISAs (MEIMIAN, Jiangsu, China) were performed according to the manufacturer's instructions. Samples were analyzed in duplicate.

### 4.6. RNA-seq Analysis

After 2 h of exposure to DON, IPEC-J2 cells were collected. Total RNA was extracted using the miRNeasy Mini Kit (Qiagen, Hilden, Germany) following the manufacturer's instructions. cDNA library construction and sequencing with an Illumina HiSeq 2000 sequencer were performed at Shanghai Biotechnology Corporation (Shanghai, China). The resulting RNA-seq reads were mapped onto the reference genome of Sscrofa11.1. The generated RNA-seq data were deposited in the National Center for Biotechnology Information (NCBI) Sequence Read Archive (SRA) repository with accession number PRJNA578240. The expression of transcripts was quantified as fragments per kilobase of exon model per million mapped reads (FPKM). Genes with differential expression levels were identified using edgeR [39]. Differential expression P-values were false discovery rate (FDR)-adjusted using the q-value Bioconductor package. Genes with a q-value ≤0.05 and |fold change| ≥2 were defined as differentially expressed. We analyzed the enrichment of the DEGs using GO functional enrichment analysis and KEGG pathway analysis. ClusterProfiler is a R package applied to perform GO function and KEGG pathway enrichment analyses on DEGs. The terms were considered to be significantly enriched if q-value ≤ 0.05.

### 4.7. PPI Network Analysis

The STRING online tool (https://string-db.org/cgi/input.pl) was used to construct a PPI network of the DEGs with a confidence score >0.4 defined as significant [40]. We then imported the interaction data into Cytoscape (version 3.6.0, http://chianti.ucsd.edu/cytoscape-3.6.0/) to map the PPI network [41]. The MCODE plugin for Cytoscape was used to analyze the interaction relationships of the DEGs with their encoded proteins and to screen the hub genes.

### 4.8. Western Blot Analyses

After 2 h of exposure to DON, IPEC-J2 cells were collected and lysed in cell lysis buffer (Beyotime, Haimen, China). Protein concentrations were determined using a BCA protein assay kit (Beyotime, China). Proteins were separated by electrophoresis and transferred to PVDF membranes. Anti-phospho-p38 (1:1000), anti-p38 (1:1000), anti-phospho-JNK (1:1000), anti-JNK (1:1000), anti-phospho-ERK (1:2000), anti-ERK (1:1000) and anti-β-actin antibodies were used as primary antibodies. Proteins bound by the primary antibodies were visualized with an appropriate secondary antibody (1:5000) and then detected by an ECL Chemiluminescence kit (Vazyme, E411-05). Protein bands were quantified using NIH ImageJ software (available in the public domain) and detected using a Bio-Rad imaging system (Bio-Rad, Hercules, CA, USA).

### 4.9. Statistical Analysis

All data were statistically analyzed using SigmaPlot 11 for Windows (Jandel Scientific; San Rafael, CA, USA). Data of cell viability were analyzed by a two-way ANOVA using the Holm–Sidak method. Other test were assessed by one-way ANOVA with Holm-Sidak tests. Data were considered to be statistically significant difference if $p < 0.05$.

**Supplementary Materials:** The following are available online at http://www.mdpi.com/2072-6651/12/3/180/s1, Table S1: All the identified DEGs.

**Author Contributions:** Conceptualization, H.Z. (Hua Zhang), H.Z. (Haibin Zhang) and W.W.; Methodology, H.Z. (Hua Zhang), X.D., C.Z.; Software, H.Z. (Hua Zhang); Validation, H.Z. (Hua Zhang), C.Z.; Formal Analysis, H.Z. (Hua Zhang), X.D.; Investigation, H.Z. (Hua Zhang), X.D. and C.Z.; Resources, H.Z. (Haibin Zhang); Data Curation, H.Z. (Hua Zhang); Writing – Original Draft Preparation, H.Z. (Hua Zhang); Writing – Review & Editing, W.W.; Visualization, X.D., C.Z.; Supervision, H.Z. (Haibin Zhang), W.W.; Project Administration, H.Z. (Haibin Zhang), W.W.; Funding Acquisition, H.Z. (Haibin Zhang). All authors have read and agreed to the published version of the manuscript.

**Funding:** This work was supported by the National Natural Science Foundation of China (31572576), National Key R & D Program (2016YFD0501207, 2016YFD0501009), China Postdoctoral Science Foundation (2016T90477), PAPD, Excelence project PrF UHK 2212/2019.

**Conflicts of Interest:** The authors declare that there are no conflict of interest.

## References


1. Wu, Q.; Wang, X.; Nepovimova, E.; Miron, A.; Liu, Q.; Wang, Y.; Su, D.; Yang, H.; Li, L.; Kuca, K. Trichothecenes: Immunomodulatory effects, mechanisms and anti-cancer potential. *Arch. Toxicol.* **2017**, *91*, 3737–3785. [CrossRef]
2. Sobrova, P.; Adam, V.; Vasatkova, A.; Beklova, M.; Zeman, L.; Kizek, R. Deoxynivalenol and its toxicity. *Interdiscip. Toxicol.* **2010**, *3*, 94–99. [CrossRef]
3. Pestka, J.J. Deoxynivalenol: Mechanisms of action, human exposure and toxicological relevance. *Arch. Toxicol.* **2010**, *84*, 663–679. [CrossRef]
4. Pestka, J.J. Deoxynivalenol-induced proinflammatory gene expression: Mechanisms and pathological sequelae. *Toxins* **2010**, *2*, 1300–1317. [CrossRef] [PubMed]
5. Wu, W.; Zhang, H. Role of tumor necrosis factor-alpha and interleukin-1beta in anorexia induction following oral exposure to the trichothecene deoxynivalenol (vomitoxin) in the mouse. *J. Toxicol. Sci.* **2014**, *39*, 875–886. [CrossRef] [PubMed]
6. Wu, W.; He, K.; Zhou, H.R.; Berthiller, F.; Adam, G.; Sugita-Konishi, Y.; Watanabe, M.; Krantis, A.; Durst, T.; Zhang, H.; et al. Effects of oral exposure to naturally-occurring and synthetic deoxynivalenol congeners on proinflammatory cytokine and chemokine mRNA expression in the mouse. *Toxicol. Appl. Pharmacol.* **2014**, *278*, 107–115. [CrossRef] [PubMed]
7. Pinton, P.; Oswald, I.P. Effect of deoxynivalenol and other Type B trichothecenes on the intestine: A review. *Toxins* **2014**, *6*, 1615–1643. [CrossRef] [PubMed]
8. Lucioli, J.; Pinton, P.; Callu, P.; Laffitte, J.; Grosjean, F.; Kolf-Clauw, M.; Oswald, I.P.; Bracarense, A.P. The food contaminant deoxynivalenol activates the mitogen activated protein kinases in the intestine: Interest of ex vivo models as an alternative to in vivo experiments. *Toxicon Off. J. Int. Soc. Toxinol.* **2013**, *66*, 31–36. [CrossRef]
9. Pinton, P.; Tsybulskyy, D.; Lucioli, J.; Laffitte, J.; Callu, P.; Lyazhri, F.; Grosjean, F.; Bracarense, A.P.; Kolf-Clauw, M.; Oswald, I.P. Toxicity of deoxynivalenol and its acetylated derivatives on the intestine: Differential effects on morphology, barrier function, tight junction proteins and mitogen-activated protein kinases. *Toxicol. Sci. Off. J. Soc. Toxicol.* **2012**, *130*, 180–190. [CrossRef]
10. Garcia, G.R.; Payros, D.; Pinton, P.; Dogi, C.A.; Laffitte, J.; Neves, M.; Gonzalez Pereyra, M.L.; Cavaglieri, L.R.; Oswald, I.P. Intestinal toxicity of deoxynivalenol is limited by Lactobacillus rhamnosus RC007 in pig jejunum explants. *Arch. Toxicol.* **2018**, *92*, 983–993. [CrossRef]
11. Ying, C.; Hong, W.; Nianhui, Z.; Chunlei, W.; Kehe, H.; Cuiling, P. Nontoxic concentrations of OTA aggravate DON-induced intestinal barrier dysfunction in IPEC-J2 cells via activation of NF-kappaB signaling pathway. *Toxicol. Lett.* **2019**, *311*, 114–124. [CrossRef] [PubMed]
12. Yang, W.; Huang, L.; Wang, P.; Wu, Z.; Li, F.; Wang, C. The Effect of Low and High Dose Deoxynivalenol on Intestinal Morphology, Distribution and Expression of Inflammatory Cytokines of Weaning Rabbits. *Toxins* **2019**, *11*, 473. [CrossRef] [PubMed]
13. Alassane-Kpembi, I.; Puel, O.; Pinton, P.; Cossalter, A.M.; Chou, T.C.; Oswald, I.P. Co-exposure to low doses of the food contaminants deoxynivalenol and nivalenol has a synergistic inflammatory effect on intestinal explants. *Arch. Toxicol.* **2017**, *91*, 2677–2687. [CrossRef] [PubMed]
14. Pearson, G.; Robinson, F.; Beers Gibson, T.; Xu, B.E.; Karandikar, M.; Berman, K.; Cobb, M.H. Mitogen-activated protein (MAP) kinase pathways: Regulation and physiological functions. *Endocr. Rev.* **2001**, *22*, 153–183. [CrossRef] [PubMed]
15. Zhang, Z.Q.; Wang, S.B.; Wang, R.G.; Zhang, W.; Wang, P.L.; Su, X.O. Phosphoproteome Analysis Reveals the Molecular Mechanisms Underlying Deoxynivalenol-Induced Intestinal Toxicity in IPEC-J2 Cells. *Toxins* **2016**, *8*, 270. [CrossRef]
16. Wang, H.; Li, H.; Chen, X.; Huang, K. ERK1/2-mediated autophagy is essential for cell survival under Ochratoxin A exposure in IPEC-J2 cells. *Toxicol. Appl. Pharmacol.* **2018**, *360*, 38–44. [CrossRef] [PubMed]
17. Springler, A.; Hessenberger, S.; Schatzmayr, G.; Mayer, E. Early Activation of MAPK p44/42 Is Partially Involved in DON-Induced Disruption of the Intestinal Barrier Function and Tight Junction Network. *Toxins* **2016**, *8*, 264. [CrossRef]
18. Maresca, M. From the gut to the brain: Journey and pathophysiological effects of the food-associated trichothecene mycotoxin deoxynivalenol. *Toxins* **2013**, *5*, 784–820. [CrossRef]

19. Kang, R.; Li, R.; Dai, P.; Li, Z.; Li, Y.; Li, C. Deoxynivalenol induced apoptosis and inflammation of IPEC-J2 cells by promoting ROS production. *Environ. Pollut.* **2019**, *251*, 689–698. [CrossRef]
20. Dong, N.; Xu, X.; Xue, C.; Wang, C.; Li, X.; Bi, C.; Shan, A. Ethyl pyruvate inhibits LPS induced IPEC-J2 inflammation and apoptosis through p38 and ERK1/2 pathways. *Cell Cycle* **2019**, *18*, 2614–2628. [CrossRef]
21. Sugimoto, M.; Yamaoka, Y.; Furuta, T. Influence of interleukin polymorphisms on development of gastric cancer and peptic ulcer. *World J. Gastroenterol.* **2010**, *16*, 1188–1200. [CrossRef] [PubMed]
22. Ishiguro, Y. Mucosal proinflammatory cytokine production correlates with endoscopic activity of ulcerative colitis. *J. Gastroenterol.* **1999**, *34*, 66–74. [CrossRef] [PubMed]
23. He, K.; Pan, X.; Zhou, H.R.; Pestka, J.J. Modulation of inflammatory gene expression by the ribotoxin deoxynivalenol involves coordinate regulation of the transcriptome and translatome. *Toxicol. Sci. Off. J. Soc. Toxicol.* **2013**, *131*, 153–163. [CrossRef] [PubMed]
24. Nagashima, H.; Nakagawa, H. Differences in the Toxicities of Trichothecene Mycotoxins, Deoxynivalenol and Nivalenol, in Cultured Cells. *Jpn. Agric. Res. Q.* **2014**, *48*, 393–397. [CrossRef]
25. Al-Alwan, L.A.; Chang, Y.; Mogas, A.; Halayko, A.J.; Baglole, C.J.; Martin, J.G.; Rousseau, S.; Eidelman, D.H.; Hamid, Q. Differential roles of CXCL2 and CXCL3 and their receptors in regulating normal and asthmatic airway smooth muscle cell migration. *J. Immunol.* **2013**, *191*, 2731–2741. [CrossRef]
26. Pestka, J.J.; Uzarski, R.L.; Islam, Z. Induction of apoptosis and cytokine production in the Jurkat human T cells by deoxynivalenol: Role of mitogen-activated protein kinases and comparison to other 8-ketotrichothecenes. *Toxicology* **2005**, *206*, 207–219. [CrossRef]
27. Bystry, R.S.; Aluvihare, V.; Welch, K.A.; Kallikourdis, M.; Betz, A.G. B cells and professional APCs recruit regulatory T cells via CCL4. *Nat. Immunol.* **2001**, *2*, 1126–1132. [CrossRef]
28. Hieshima, K.; Imai, T.; Opdenakker, G.; Van Damme, J.; Kusuda, J.; Tei, H.; Sakaki, Y.; Takatsuki, K.; Miura, R.; Yoshie, O.; et al. Molecular cloning of a novel human CC chemokine liver and activation-regulated chemokine (LARC) expressed in liver. Chemotactic activity for lymphocytes and gene localization on chromosome 2. *J. Biol. Chem.* **1997**, *272*, 5846–5853. [CrossRef]
29. Van De Walle, J.; Romier, B.; Larondelle, Y.; Schneider, Y.J. Influence of deoxynivalenol on NF-kappaB activation and IL-8 secretion in human intestinal Caco-2 cells. *Toxicol. Lett.* **2008**, *177*, 205–214. [CrossRef]
30. Moon, Y.; Yang, H.; Lee, S.H. Modulation of early growth response gene 1 and interleukin-8 expression by ribotoxin deoxynivalenol (vomitoxin) via ERK1/2 in human epithelial intestine 407 cells. *Biochem. Biophys. Res. Commun.* **2007**, *362*, 256–262. [CrossRef]
31. Fecher, L.A.; Amaravadi, R.K.; Flaherty, K.T. The MAPK pathway in melanoma. *Curr. Opin. Oncol.* **2008**, *20*, 183–189. [CrossRef] [PubMed]
32. Qi, M.; Elion, E.A. MAP kinase pathways. *J. Cell Sci.* **2005**, *118*, 3569–3572. [CrossRef] [PubMed]
33. Miyake, Z.; Takekawa, M.; Ge, Q.; Saito, H. Activation of MTK1/MEKK4 by GADD45 through induced N-C dissociation and dimerization-mediated trans autophosphorylation of the MTK1 kinase domain. *Mol. Cell. Biol.* **2007**, *27*, 2765–2776. [CrossRef] [PubMed]
34. Slack, D.N.; Seternes, O.M.; Gabrielsen, M.; Keyse, S.M. Distinct binding determinants for ERK2/p38alpha and JNK map kinases mediate catalytic activation and substrate selectivity of map kinase phosphatase-1. *J. Biol. Chem.* **2001**, *276*, 16491–16500. [CrossRef] [PubMed]
35. Patterson, K.I.; Brummer, T.; O'Brien, P.M.; Daly, R.J. Dual-specificity phosphatases: Critical regulators with diverse cellular targets. *Biochem. J.* **2009**, *418*, 475–489. [CrossRef]
36. Moon, Y.; Pestka, J.J. Vomitoxin-induced cyclooxygenase-2 gene expression in macrophages mediated by activation of ERK and p38 but not JNK mitogen-activated protein kinases. *Toxicol. Sci.* **2002**, *69*, 373–382. [CrossRef]
37. Zhou, H.R.; Islam, Z.; Pestka, J.J. Rapid, sequential activation of mitogen-activated protein kinases and transcription factors precedes proinflammatory cytokine mRNA expression in spleens of mice exposed to the trichothecene vomitoxin. *Toxicol. Sci.* **2003**, *72*, 130–142. [CrossRef] [PubMed]
38. Van De Walle, J.; During, A.; Piront, N.; Toussaint, O.; Schneider, Y.J.; Larondelle, Y. Physio-pathological parameters affect the activation of inflammatory pathways by deoxynivalenol in Caco-2 cells. *Toxicol. In Vitro* **2010**, *24*, 1890–1898. [CrossRef]
39. Robinson, M.D.; McCarthy, D.J.; Smyth, G.K. edgeR: A Bioconductor package for differential expression analysis of digital gene expression data. *Bioinformatics* **2010**, *26*, 139–140. [CrossRef]

40. Szklarczyk, D.; Franceschini, A.; Wyder, S.; Forslund, K.; Heller, D.; Huerta-Cepas, J.; Simonovic, M.; Roth, A.; Santos, A.; Tsafou, K.P.; et al. STRING v10: Protein-protein interaction networks, integrated over the tree of life. *Nucleic Acids Res.* **2015**, *43*, D447–D452. [CrossRef]
41. Shannon, P.; Markiel, A.; Ozier, O.; Baliga, N.S.; Wang, J.T.; Ramage, D.; Amin, N.; Schwikowski, B.; Ideker, T. Cytoscape: A software environment for integrated models of biomolecular interaction networks. *Genome Res.* **2003**, *13*, 2498–2504. [CrossRef] [PubMed]

*toxins*

MDPI

*Article*

# T-2 Toxin Induces Oxidative Stress, Apoptosis and Cytoprotective Autophagy in Chicken Hepatocytes

**Huadong Yin †, Shunshun Han †, Yuqi Chen †, Yan Wang, Diyan Li and Qing Zhu ***

Farm Animal Genetic Resources Exploration and Innovation Key Laboratory of Sichuan Province, Sichuan Agricultural University, Chengdu 611130, Sichuan, China; yinhuadong@sicau.edu.cn (H.Y.); hanshunshun@stu.sicau.edu.cn (S.H.); chenyuqi@stu.sicau.edu.cn (Y.C.); as519723614@163.com (Y.W.); diyanli@sicau.edu.cn (D.L.)

* Correspondence: zhuqing@sicau.edu.cn; Tel.: +86-028-8629-0991

† These authors contributed equally to this work.

Received: 13 December 2019; Accepted: 27 January 2020; Published: 29 January 2020

**Abstract:** T-2 toxin is type A trichothecenes mycotoxin, which produced by fusarium species in cereal grains. T-2 toxin has been shown to induce a series of toxic effects on the health of human and animal, such as immunosuppression and carcinogenesis. Previous study has proven that T-2 toxin caused hepatotoxicity in chicken, but the regulatory mechanism is unclear. In the present study, we assessed the toxicological effect of T-2 toxin on apoptosis and autophagy in hepatocytes. The total of 120 1-day-old healthy broilers were allocated randomly into four groups and reared for 21 day with complete feed containing 0 mg/kg, 0.5 mg/kg, 1 mg/kg or 2 mg/kg T-2 toxin, respectively. The results showed that the apoptosis rate and pathological changes degree hepatocytes were aggravated with the increase of T-2 toxin. At the molecular mechanism level, T-2 toxin induced mitochondria-mediated apoptosis by producing reactive oxygen species, promoting cytochrome c translocation between the mitochondria and cytoplasm, and thus promoting apoptosomes formation. Meanwhile, the expression of the autophagy-related protein, ATG5, ATG7 and Beclin-1, and the LC3-II/LC3-I ratio were increased, while p62 was downregulated, suggesting T-2 toxin caused autophagy in hepatocytes. Further experiments demonstrated that the PI3K/AKT/mTOR signal may be participated in autophagy induced by T-2 toxin in chicken hepatocytes. These data suggest a possible underlying molecular mechanism for T-2 toxin that induces apoptosis and autophagy in chicken hepatocytes

**Keywords:** T-2 toxin; hepatocyte; apoptosis; autophagy; chicken

**Key Contribution:** T-2 toxin-induced hepatotoxicity was characterized by the induction of mitochondrial-mediated apoptosis and PI3K/AKT/mTOR-mediated autophagy in chicken.

## 1. Introduction

Mycotoxins are the main secondary metabolites of molds and lead to widespread contamination on crop plants and fruits. Among the most important mycotoxins, T-2 toxin is a mycotoxin that can cause multiple effects in organisms [1]. T-2 toxin is a type A trichothecene produced by several *Fusarium* species [2], which shows the most potent cytotoxicity [3]. Furthermore, T-2 toxin leads to the effects of cytotoxin radiomimetic, which is due to impaired protein synthesis. T-2 toxin hampers synthesis of DNA and RNA in eukaryotic cells, which ultimately triggers cell apoptosis in vitro and in vivo [4]. Many studies have shown that T-2 toxin induces apoptotic cell death in hematopoietic tissue [5], spleen, liver [6], skin and intestinal crypt in mice [7]. In chickens, apoptosis induced by T-2 toxin was detected in the thymus, bursa of Fabricius and primary hepatocytes [8,9]. Previous studies have demonstrated a crosstalk between autophagy and apoptosis, as apoptosis increases when the autophagic pathway is completely inhibited [10].

T-2 toxin contamination is usually found on cereals, such as maize, wheat and oats, which are the main food and feed resources for human and livestock [11]. The presence of T-2 toxin can be reduced but not completely eliminated. T-2 toxin can cause chronic toxicity in organisms after oral exposure, dermal exposure and inhalation. In livestock, this results in anorexia, reduced body weight and nutritional efficiency, altered neuro-endocrine system, and immune modulation [12]. In addition, residues of the T-2 toxin and its metabolites in animal products are an important human health problem. Poultry is extremely sensitive to the toxic effects of T-2 toxins, leading to yellow cheese-like necrosis at the edge of the septum, hard mucosal mucosa and typical angular cheilitis of the mouth and tongue [13]. In addition, chickens exposed to T-2 toxin show enhanced mortality from *Salmonella* infection and low-resistance titers for Newcastle disease and infectious bursal disease [14,15].

Multiple studies have examined the effects of T-2 toxin in inducing of hepatotoxicity in chickens. However, the relationship between T-2-induced autophagy and apoptosis has not been examined. Here, we investigated the effects of T-2 toxin on hepatocyte apoptosis and autophagy and provide experimental evidence for the potential molecular mechanism of T-2 toxin-induced hepatotoxicity in broiler chickens.

## 2. Results

### 2.1. Pathological Lesions

To determine the effect of T-2 toxin on chicken livers, we examined the pathomorphological changes in the liver. In the control group, the liver tissue structure was normal, the cell structure was intact, and the cells were arranged neatly (Figure 1A). In the 0.5 mg/kg T-2 toxin treatment group, the liver pathological changes were mild; the hepatocyte volume was increased and mild swelling manifested as blisters, with occasional inflammatory cell infiltration (Figure 1B). In the 1 mg/kg and 2 mg/kg treatment groups, the hepatocytes were swollen and showed balloon-like deformation; the cytoplasm was vacuolated, and the nucleus was located in the center of the vacuole or squeezed on one side. Additionally, hepatic sinus stenosis, a small amount of red blood cell deposits, focal inflammatory cell infiltration and massive proliferation of interlobular bile duct epithelial cells were observed in the 1 mg/kg and 2 mg/kg treatment groups (Figure 1C,D).

### 2.2. T-2 Triggers Apoptosis in Hepatocytes

We next performed flow cytometry to determine if T-2 toxin induced apoptosis in hepatocytes from T-2 treated chickens. The amounts of apoptotic cells in the treatment groups were significantly higher ($p < 0.01$) than that in the control, and this difference was dose-dependent (Figure 2A,B). Western blot results showed cleavage of rapamycin (PARP) in the T-2 treatment groups; furthermore, pro-caspase-3 and pro-caspase-9 expressions were reduced in a dose-dependent manner, whereas the cleaved form of caspase-3 and caspase-9 increased (Figure 2C,D). These data further indicate that T-2 toxin induced apoptosis in hepatocytes.

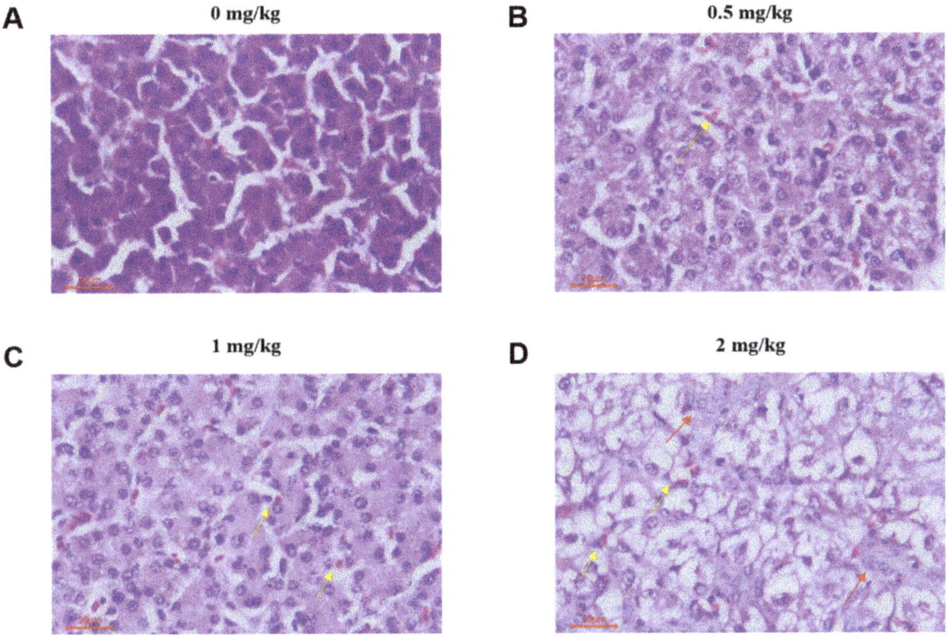


**Figure 1.** Photomicrographs of hematoxylin and eosin stained chicken liver sections of 21 day chicken after treatment of T-2 toxin with different concentration of 0, 0.5, 1 and 2 mg/kg. (**A**) No obvious pathological changes were observed in hepatocytes. (**B**) Hepatocytes with mild steatosis and slight congestion. (**C**) Hepatocytes were slightly swollen, with vacuolar degeneration and lymphocyte neutrophil infiltration. (**D**) The liver showed slight congestion, local vacuolar degeneration was obvious, and the bile duct epithelium and cells demonstrated slight hyperplasia. Red arrow: red blood cell; yellow arrow: bile duct epithelial cell; hematoxylin and eosin (H&E); bar, 20 μm.

### *2.3. The Mitochondrial Pathway is Activated by T-2 Toxin*

To evaluate whether the mitochondrial pathway participates in the T-2 toxin-induced apoptosis, we first examined the mitochondrial reactive oxygen species (ROS) levels in hepatocytes from T-2 treated chickens by flow cytometry. Low intracellular ROS levels were found in the untreated group, whereas they increased dramatically in the 1 mg/kg and 2 mg/kg T-2 toxin treatment groups (Figure 3A,B). In addition, T-2 toxin significantly suppressed the activity of the antioxidant enzymes GSH-Px, CAT and SOD, but the MDA level was significantly higher in treatment groups than in the control group (Figure 3C). We next evaluated the protein expression of Bax and Bcl-2 and found that Bax protein abundance was upregulated, whereas Bcl-2 abundance was downregulated in a dose-dependent manner, with an increase in Bax/Bcl-2 ratio (Figure 3D). We also examined the mitochondrial release of cytochrome (cyt c) during T-2 toxin-induced apoptosis. The level of mitochondrial cyt c decreased with the increase of T-2 toxin concentration, whereas the level of cytosolic cyt c increased (Figure 3E).

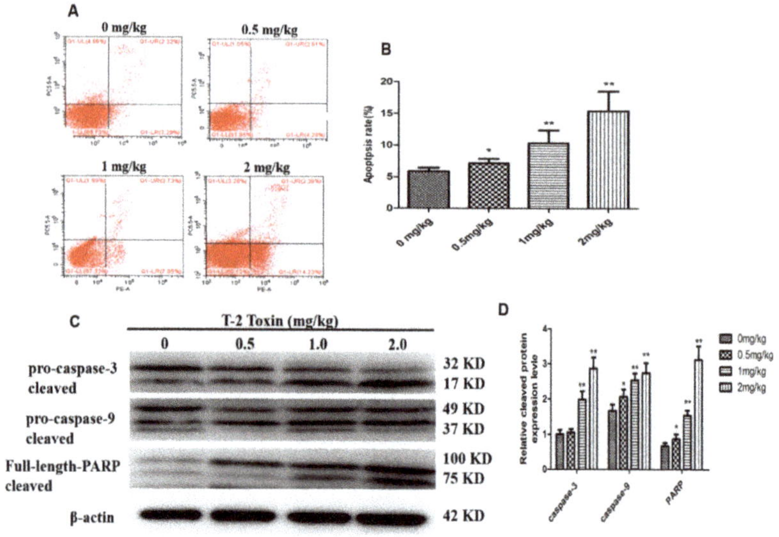


**Figure 2.** Effect of different concentration (0, 0.5, 1 and 2 mg/kg, respectively) of T-2 toxin on hepatocyte apoptosis. (**A**) Scattergram and (**B**) apoptosis rate of apoptotic hepatocytes. (**C**) The protein levels of PARP, caspase-3 and caspase-9, and their cleaved forms in hepatocytes. (**D**) The bar showed the relative protein cleaved level of caspase-3, caspase-9 and PARP. The data are presented as the means ± standard error of the mean (SEM) of three independent experiments. * $p < 0.05$ and ** $p < 0.01$, compared with the control group.

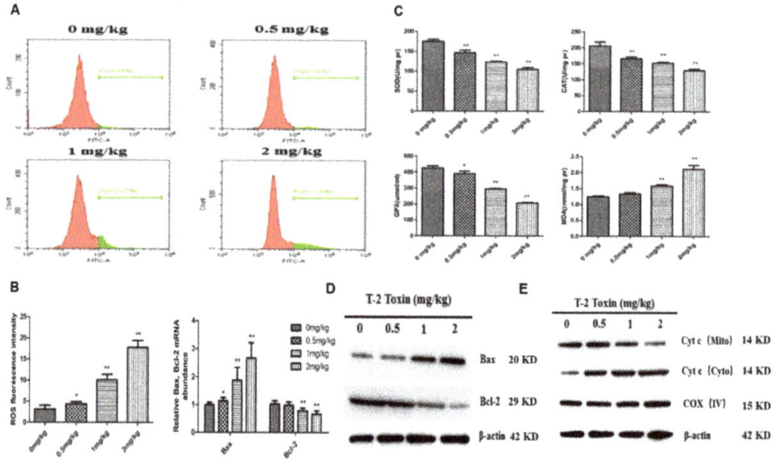


**Figure 3.** T-2 toxin induced hepatocyte apoptosis via activation of the mitochondria-dependent pathway. (**A**,**B**) Intracellular reactive oxygen species (ROS) levels in hepatocytes from chickens treated with T-2 toxin of different concentration at 0, 0.5, 1 and 2 mg/kg. (**C**) The activity of antioxidant enzymes SOD, CAT, GPX-Sh and MDA content in hepatocytes from chickens treated with T-2 toxin of different concentration at 0, 0.5, 1 and 2 mg/kg. (**D**) The Bax and Bcl-2 mRNA and protein levels in hepatocytes from chickens treated with T-2 toxin of different concentration at 0, 0.5, 1 and 2 mg/kg. (**E**) The cytosolic and mitochondrial cyt c level in hepatocytes from chickens treated with T-2 toxin of different concentration at 0, 0.5, 1 and 2 mg/kg. All the data are presented as means ± SEM of three independent experiments. * $p < 0.05$ and ** $p < 0.01$, compared with the control group.

### 2.4. *T-2 Toxin Triggers Autophagy in Hepatocytes*

To determine if T-2 toxin induces autophagy in hepatocytes from T-2 treated chickens, we measured the transcript levels of autophagy genes including ATG5, ATG7 and Beclin-1 genes (Figure 4A). T-2 toxin treatments induced greater expression levels of ATG5, ATG7 and Beclin-1 genes compared with controls. Furthermore, the ratio of LC3-II/LC3-I increased with the T-2 toxin dosage, while the protein abundance of p62 decreased (Figure 4B). In addition, the cell ultrastructure changed; typical autophagy features were observed and the number of autophagosomes increased in the treatment groups compared with controls (Figure 4C).

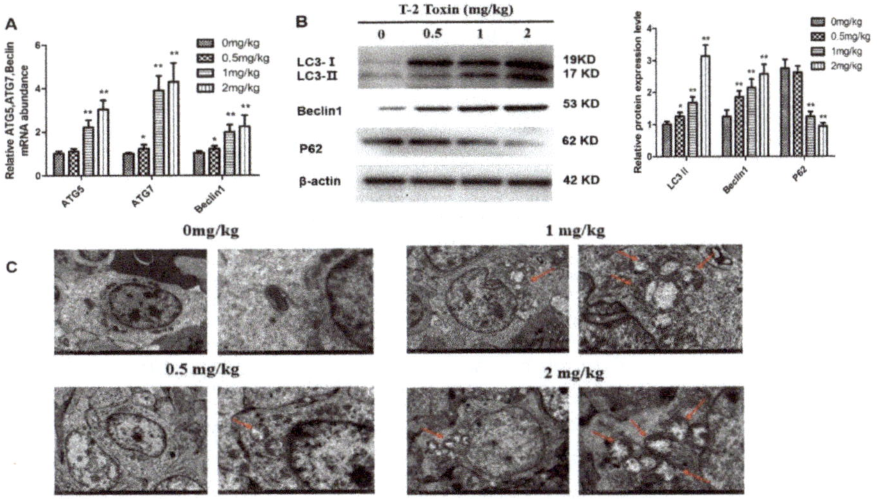


**Figure 4.** Effect of T-2 toxin on autophagy in chicken hepatocytes. (**A**) The mRNA levels of Beclin-1, Atg5 and Atg7 in hepatocytes from chickens treated with T-2 toxin of different concentration at 0, 0.5, 1 and 2 mg/kg. (**B**) The protein expression levels of LC3, p62 and Beclin-1 in hepatocytes from chickens treated with T-2 toxin of different concentration at 0, 0.5, 1 and 2 mg/kg. (**C**) Morphological observation of autophagy in hepatocytes from chickens treated with T-2 toxin of different concentration at 0, 0.5, 1 and 2 mg/kg, autophagic vacuoles (red arrows, magnification from left to right: ×1200, ×5000). All the data are presented as means ± SEM of three independent experiments. * $p < 0.05$ and ** $p < 0.01$, compared with the control group.

### 2.5. *Autophagy Protects Apoptosis in T-2 Treated Hepatocytes*

Increased autophagy is considered a protective mechanism against apoptosis as both autophagy and apoptosis share common proteins. To explore the relationship between autophagy and apoptosis, the specific autophagy inhibitor 3-methyladenine (3MA) and autophagy inducer rapamycin (RAP) were used on T-2 toxin-treated hepatocytes. Immunofluorescence showed that T-2 toxin treatment significantly increased the numbers of LC3B puncta, and autophagy flux was further enhanced after the addition of RAP, but autophagy intensity was significantly decreased after the addition of 3MA (Figure 5A,B). When autophagy was inhibited by 3MA, the levels of caspase-3 and caspase-9 cleavage were significantly enhanced after T-2 treatment. Conversely, when autophagy was induced by RAP, the levels of caspase-3 and caspase-9 cleavage were significantly decreased (Figure 5C,D). These results may suggest that autophagy hinders apoptosis in T-2 toxin-treated hepatocytes.

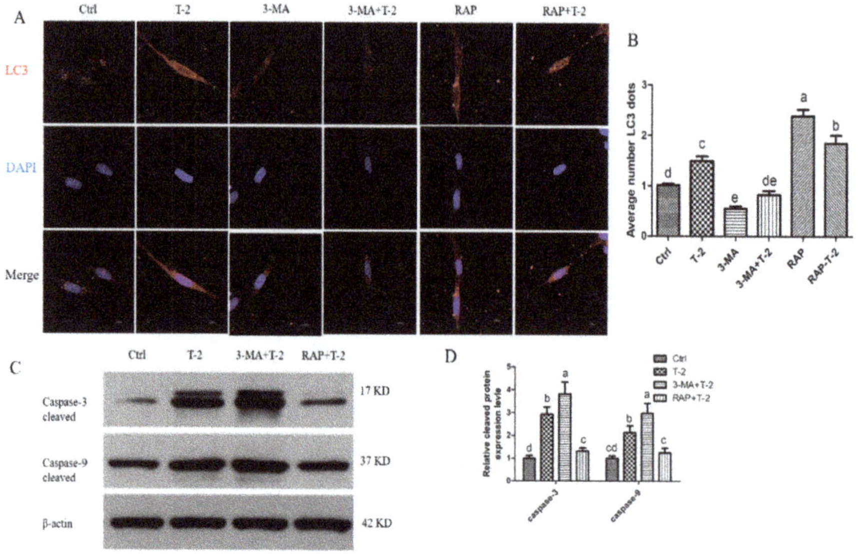


**Figure 5.** Autophagy delays apoptosis in T-2 treated hepatocytes. (**A**) Hepatocytes stained with LC3 (red) antibody using a confocal microscope (600x), Nuclei were stained with 4,6-diamino-2-phenyl indole (DAPI) (blue; bar = 10 μm). (**B**) The bar showed the number of LC3 dots. (**C**) Western blots showed the expression levels of caspase-3 and caspse-9 cleaved in hepatocytes. (**D**) The bar showed the protein level of cleaved caspase-3 and caspase-9. All the data are presented as means ± SEM of three independent experiments. * $p < 0.05$ and ** $p < 0.01$, compared with the control group.

### 2.6. T-2 Toxin Inhibits the PI3K/Akt/mTOR Signal Pathway

To determine if T-2 toxin regulates the PI3K/Akt/mTOR signal pathway in hepatocytes from T-2 treated chickens, we next examined the protein abundance of the tumor suppressor factor, phosphatase and tensin homolog (PTEN), which has a dual-specificity phosphatase activity. PTEN expression level increased in hepatocytes with the increase in T-2 toxin concentration (Figure 6A). In addition, we examined the protein abundance and phosphorylation levels of PI3K, Akt, mTOR and p70S6K, which are key proteins in the PI3K/Akt/mTOR pathway. We found that the protein abundances of PI3K, Akt, mTOR and p70S6K did not differ among the treatment groups, but their phosphorylation levels gradually decreased with the increase in T-2 toxin concentration (Figure 6B,C). These results may suggest that T-2 toxin inhibits the PI3K/Akt/mTOR signal pathway in hepatocytes.

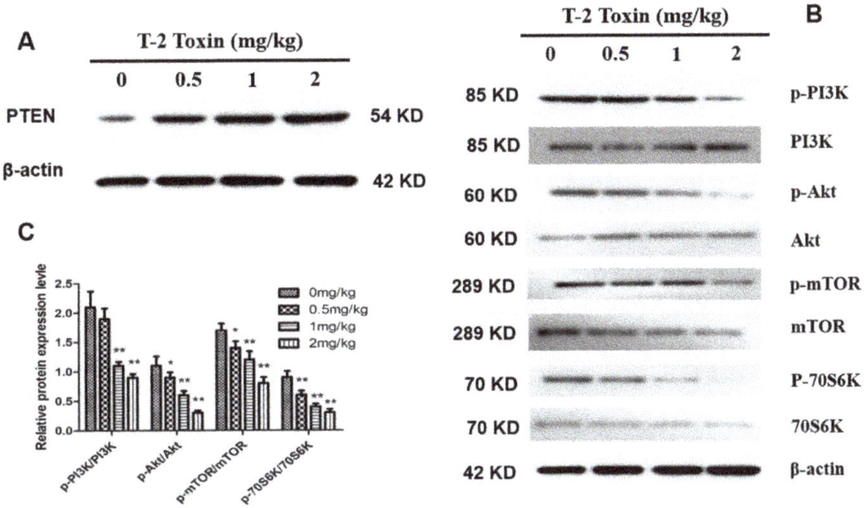


**Figure 6.** Effect of T-2 toxin on PI3K/Akt/mTOR in hepatocytes. (**A**) Protein abundance of phosphatase and tensin homolog (PTEN) in hepatocytes from chickens treated with T-2 toxin of different concentration at 0, 0.5, 1 and 2 mg/kg. (**B**) Representative blots showed the expression abundance of p-PI3K, PI3K, p-Akt, Akt, p-mTOR, mTOR, p-70S6K and 70S6K in hepatocytes from chickens treated with T-2 toxin of different concentration at 0, 0.5, 1 and 2 mg/kg. (**C**) The bar graphs showed the ratio of p-PI3K/PI3K, p-Akt/Akt, p-mTOR/mTOR, and p-p70S6K/p70S6K. All the data are presented as means ± SEM of three independent experiments. * $p < 0.05$ and ** $p < 0.01$, compared with the control group.

## 3. Discussion

The T-2 toxin has harmful mutagenic, carcinogenic and teratogenic effects on humans and animals [16–18]. Although various studies have examined hepatocyte apoptosis in broilers treated with T-2 toxin [19,20], no reports have focused on the relationship between autophagy and T-2 toxin-induced apoptosis. Herein, we reported that T-2 toxin-induced hepatotoxicity was characterized by the induction of mitochondrial-mediated apoptosis and PI3K/AKT/mTOR-mediated autophagy in chicken.

The liver is the main organ of metabolism in which foreign substances accumulate and are detoxified. The T-2 toxin suppresses hepatocyte protein synthesis and inhibits metabolic enzyme activity and liver fat peroxidation, which ultimately leads to hepatocyte apoptosis [21–23]. In the current study, histopathological analysis showed that T-2 toxin caused pathological changes in liver tissue, including hepatocyte swelling, volume increase and more granules in the cytoplasm, suggesting that T-2 toxin leads to hepatocyte apoptosis. Our results were consistent with the report by Meissonnier et al. who showed that exposure of pigs to T-2 toxin via diet for 28 days caused liver histopathological changes, excessive hepatic glycogen accumulation and mild interstitial inflammatory cell infiltration [24].

Apoptosis is a crucial physiological cell death process that can be induced by toxic stimuli [25]. Previous studies have shown that T-2 toxin injection can strongly induce cell apoptosis in different tissues, such as thymus, spleen and liver, particularly in the liver [6]. Yang et al. incubated primary chicken hepatocytes with T-2 toxin for 24 h and found that the cell activity was significantly reduced and apoptosis gradually increased in a dose-dependent manner [9], which was similar to our finding that hepatocyte apoptosis gradually increased with the increasing dosage of T-2 toxin.

The mitochondrial pathway has a vital role in the intrinsic apoptosis pathway [26], which depends on the translocation of the apoptogenic protein, cyt c, into the cytoplasm. This occurs via the Bax/Bcl-2 pathway, as their relative levels determine cell destiny by activating death-driving proteolytic proteins known as caspases [27]. In the current study, several findings suggested that T-2 toxin induced the mitochondrial apoptotic pathway in hepatocytes: (1) Bcl-2 was downregulated and Bax was upregulated, thus increasing the Bax/Bcl-2 ratio; and (2) cyt c was released from the mitochondria into the cytosol, followed by apoptosome formation with the apoptotic proteases Apaf-1 and caspase-9. In addition, T-2 toxin treatment lead to an increase in ROS and MDA levels and a decrease in the activities of SOD, CAT, and GSH-Px, resulting in oxidative stress and a concentration-dependent increase in apoptotic cells. Mu et al found that T-2 toxin can induce the ROS accumulation and an increase in mitochondrial mass, which indicated that oxidative stress and mitochondrial enhancement occurred in T-2 toxin-treated primary hepatocytes, which is similar to our result [28]. In addition to our results, other studies have shown apoptosis induced by T-2 toxin via the ROS-mediated mitochondrial pathway in other cells, such as ovarian granulosa cells [29], embryonic stem cells and fibroblast 3T3 cells [30] in mouse.

Autophagy is a crucial homeostasis mechanism that is involved in multiple physiological and pathological processes [31]. Autophagy also shows a complex relationship with apoptosis, as autophagy not only increases caspase-dependent cell death, but also promotes cell survival [32]. In the present study, the increase in gene expression of Atg5, Atg7 and Beclin-1, which are autophagy marker genes, suggested that T-2 toxin induced autophagy in hepatocytes. Moreover, we found an increase in the LC3-II/LC3-I ratio and Beclin-1 protein abundance and a decrease in expression of p62 protein, further suggesting that T-2 toxin induced autophagy in hepatocytes. Bcl-2 and Beclin-1 participate in the regulation of both apoptosis and autophagy [33], and Bcl-2 interacts with Beclin-1 to suppress Beclin-1-dependent autophagy [34]. In our study, we found that Beclin-1 was activated by T-2 toxin, but Bcl-2 was suppressed, and T-2 toxin-induced apoptosis can be delayed by autophagy. Wang et al showed that autophagy may reduce zearalenone-induced cytotoxicity and prevent rat Leydig cell apoptosis [35]. Wu et al found that autophagy plays a role in protecting human cells from T-2 toxin-induced apoptosis, because autophagy may decrease toxic responses induced by T-2 toxin [36]. Our results were consistent with these reports.

The PI3K/AKT/mTOR/p70S6K signaling pathway plays a vital role in autophagy regulation in eukaryotic cells [37]. PI3K induces a signaling cascade and phosphorylates the serine/threonine kinase, mTOR, by activating the serine/threonine kinase, Akt [38]. PTEN has also been proven to suppress the Akt/mTOR signal [39]. As the major upstream modulator, the PI3K pathway regulates autophagy by phosphorylating AKT, which affects the downstream factors p70S6K and 4E-BP1 [40]. Several mycotoxins induce autophagy by inhibiting the PI3K/Akt/mTOR axis, such as zearalenone in donkey granulosa cells [41], aflatoxin B2 in chicken hepatocytes [16] and sterigmatocystin in human gastric epithelium cells [42]. In this study, T-2 toxin inhibited the phosphorylation of PI3K, Akt, mTOR and p70S6K, whereas it activated PTEN, suggesting that the PI3K/AKT/mTOR/p70S6K pathway may be participated in the autophagic process induced by toxicity effect of T-2 toxin. These findings are similar to a previous study that showed that deoxypodophyllotoxin induced cytoprotective autophagy against apoptosis through inhibition of the PI3K/AKT/mTOR pathway in osteosarcoma U2OS cells [42].

In summary, T-2 toxin treatment activates the mitochondrial apoptotic pathway by triggering ROS production and Bcl-2 family protein expression, resulting in hepatocyte apoptosis. In addition, T-2 toxin may involve in the PI3K/AKT/mTOR signal to regulate hepatocellular autophagy. This study provides new insights into the mechanisms underlying the toxicological effect of T-2 toxin in chicken hepatocytes.

## 4. Materials and Methods

### 4.1. Ethics Approval

All experimental operations were approved by the Animal Ethics Committee of Sichuan Agricultural University, and the approved number was 2018-2121 (21 May 2018). Relevant guidelines and regulations were followed while performing all the methods.

### 4.2. Animals

A total of 120 ROSS 308 male chickens at one-day of age were used in this study. After being weighted, chickens were randomly divided into four groups (n = 30 per group); each treatment had six replicates with five chickens. Experimental replicates were raised in separate cages. The four groups were maintained under the same condition and received general nutrient composition and levels that met the requirement of ROSS 308, with T-2 toxin in feed as follows: 0 mg/kg (control), 0.5 mg/kg, 1 mg/kg, and 2 mg/kg. Feed and water were freely available during the whole trial period.

### 4.3. Exposure of Chickens

All the feed was made up by the processing-workshop of feedstuff in the Animal Nutrition Institute of Sichuan Agricultural University, which meet the nutritional requirement of ROSS 308. There were no common mycotoxins, such as aflatoxins, deoxynivalenol, ochratoxin A, zearalenone and T-2 toxin, were found in this feed by the ELISA kit (Huaan Mangech Biotech, Beijing, China). Firstly, the T-2 toxin (purity ≥ 98%; Sigma Aldrich, St. Louis, MO, USA) powder was dissolved by 95% ethanol, and mixed in 1 kg feed and dry it. Then, the mixture was added into feed to get the get the target concentration (0 mg/kg, 0.5 mg/kg, 1 mg/kg, and 2 mg/kg, respectively) of T-2 toxin. At last, we used the ELISA kit (Huaan Mangech Biotech) to confirm the final concentration of toxins in the feed.

### 4.4. Sample Collection and Preparation

After 21 days of feeding, six chickens (one chicken for every replicate) were randomly selected from the same treatment and euthanized. Livers were collected to determine the pathological histology and hepatocyte apoptosis rate. Fresh livers were dissected, minced, and stored at − 80 °C for extracting RNA and protein.

### 4.5. Pathological Observation

Liver tissues were fixed overnight in 4% phosphate-buffered paraformaldehyde (Jianke Biotech, Chengdu, Sichuan, China) and then paraffin-embedded blocks were archived. We sliced 5 μm thick tissue sections from paraffin-embedded tumor blocks and mounted the sections onto glass slides. Hematoxylin and eosin (H&E) staining was performed on tissue sections, and pathological examination was performed using an optical microscope (Olympus, Tokyo, Japan).

### 4.6. Apoptosis Detection

Livers were minced in pre-cold phosphate-buffered saline (PBS; Beyotime, Shanghai, China), and the suspension was passed through a 300 mesh nylon filter. After filtration, the hepatocyte suspensions were washed in PBS twice. Hepatocytes were re-suspended in 1× binding buffer (BD Pharmingen, Santiago, CA, USA) to obtain a concentration of $1 \times 10^6$ cells/mL. Next, 100 μL were transferred into a culture tube and 5 μL of propidium iodide (PI; BD Pharmingen, Shanghai China) and 5 μL of Annexin V-FITC (BD Pharmingen, Shanghai, China) were added. After mixing, the cells were incubated at 25 °C for 15 min in the dark and then 400 μL of 1× binding buffer (BD Pharmingen, Shanghai, China) was added. Cells were then analyzed by FACSCanto II flow cytometry (BD Bioscience, San Diego, CA, USA).

### 4.7. Real-Time PCR

Total RNA of the livers were isolated by Trizol reagent (TaKaRa, Dalian, China). First-strand complementary cDNA was synthesized by PrimeScirptTM RT reagent kit with gDNA eraser (TaKaRa, Dalian, China) following the manufacturer's protocol, and then was stored at − 20 °C for RT-PCR. PCR amplifications were performed as follows: 95 °C for 5 min and 36 cycles each with 95 °C for 10 s, 60 °C for 30 s and 72 °C for 20 s, then 65 °C for 5 s and 95 °C for 5 s using the BIO-RAD CFX Connect™ real time system (Bio-Rad, Hercules, CA, USA). All PCR reactions were performed in triplicate. β-actin was used as the endogenous reference gene. Specific primers are referenced to Chen et al [16] or designed by the software of Primer Premier 5.0 (Ottawa, Ontario, Canada, 2007), and the primer sequences are listed in Table 1.

**Table 1.** Table: Gene-special primers for RT-PCR.

| Gene | Forward Primer | Reverse Primer | NCBI Accession no | Tm/°C | Product/bp |
|---|---|---|---|---|---|
| Bcl-2 | 5-ATCGTCGCCTTCTTCGAGTT-3 | 5-ATCCCATCCTCCGTTGTCCT-3 | NM_205339.2 | 61 | 78 |
| Atg5 | 5-GATGAAATAACTGAAAGGGAAGC-3 | 5-TGAAGATCAAAGAGCAAACCAA-3 | NM_001006409.1 | 52 | 124 |
| Atg7 | 5-TCAGATTCAAGCACTTCAGA-3 | 5-GAGGAGATACAACCACAGAG-3 | NM_001030592.1 | 55 | 62 |
| Beclin-1 | 5-CAGACACGCTGCTGGACC-3 | 5-TCTCCTTGTCATCCTCGTTCA-3 | NM_001006332.1 | 60 | 84 |
| β-actin | 5-CCGCTCTATGAAGGCTACGC-3 | 5-CTCTCGGCTGTGGTGGTGAA-3 | NM_204313.1 | 60 | 127 |

### 4.8. Western Blot Analysis

The refrigerated livers were washed with pre-cold PBS twice and centrifugation at 3000× *g* for 5 min at 4 °C, then removed the supernatant. Total protein extracts were obtained by homogenizing liver in RIPA lysis buffer (Sigma Aldrich) supplemented with protease inhibitor cocktail and phosphatase inhibitors. After centrifugation, the supernatant was collected and stored at −80 °C. Protein concentration was determined by the BCA protein detection kit (Sangon Biotech, Shanghai, China). Western blot analysis was performed as previously described by Han et al. The primary antibodies were used: caspase-3 (ZenBio, Chengdu, China), caspase-9 (ZenBio), β-actin (Abcam, Cambridge, MA, USA), Bax (ZenBio), Bcl-2 (Santa Cruz, Heidelberg, Germany), LC3B (Sigma), P62 (Santa Cruz), beclin-1 (Sigma), PI3K/Akt/mTOR/70S6K protein and phosphorylated antibody were purchased from Bioss Biotechnology Co. Ltd. (Bioss, Beijing, China). The secondary antibodies used were as follows: mouse anti-rabbit (Sigma), goat anti-rabbit (Sigma), mouse anti-rabbit horseradish peroxidase (HRP) (Zenbio). The enhanced chemiluminescence (ECL) kit (Beyotime, Jiangsu, China) was used to capture the bands via a CanoScan LiDE 100 scanner (Canon, Tokyo, Japan), and western blots were analyzed by Image J software (Bethesda, MD, USA, 2007).

### 4.9. Cytochrome C Release

The cytoplasm was first isolated from the mitochondria using the cytochrome C release apoptosis kit (BioVision, Mountain View, CA, USA). After treatment with E2 for 24 h, the cells were lysed by homogenizing in the cytosol extraction solution provided by the kit and then centrifuged at 700× *g* for 10 min. Cells were then centrifuged at 12,000× *g* for 30 min to separate cytoplasmic and mitochondrial components. Determination of cytoplasmic and mitochondrial cytochrome C abundance was performed by western blot using mouse monoclonal antibodies provided in the kit.

### 4.10. Transmission Electron Microscopy (TEM) Observations

Hepatocytes were fixed in 2.5% glutaraldehyde phosphate buffer saline (Sigma, St. Louis, MO, USA) and post-fixed in 1% osmium tetroxide (Sigma). The samples were dehydrated in graded ethanol solutions, and cells were embedded in the stimulating resin. Sections (60 nm) were cut using ultramicrobody (Leica Microsystems, Milan, Italy). The divided grid has a saturated solution of uranyl acetate and lead citric acid. Samples were examined by electron microscopy (FEI, Milan, Italy).

### 4.11. Intracellular Reactive Oxygen Species (ROS) Detection

Production of intracellular ROS production was measured using the fluorescent dye substrate 2′,7′-dichlorofluorescin-diacetate (DCFH-DA; Procell, Wuhan, China) as a substrate. Cells were incubated for 60 min at 37 °C with 10 μM DCFH-DA and then harvested and suspended in Hank's Balanced Salt Solution (D-HBSS; Procell). The generation of ROS was analyzed using FACSCanto II flow cytometry (BD Bioscience, New York, NJ, USA).

### 4.12. Antioxidative Enzymes and Malondialdehyde Detection

The activities of superoxide dismutase (SOD), glutathione peroxidase (GPX-Px) and catalase (CAT) and malondialdehyde (MDA) level were determined by commercial assay kits (Jiancheng, Nanjing, China) according to the manufacturer's instructions. After mixing the liver cell homogenate with the reagents, the cells were incubated at 37 °C overnight for multi-scan spectroscopy detection.

### 4.13. Immunofluorescence and Confocal Microscopy

Hepatocytes grown on 24-well plates were fixed with 4% paraformaldehyde (Jianke Biotech, Guangzhou, China) for 10 min. After washing with PBS twice, cells were blocked using 3% bovine serum albumin (BSA; Thermo Fischer Scientific; former Savant, MA, USA) and 0.2% Triton X-100 (Thermo Fischer Scientific, Waltham, MA, USA) in PBS for 10 min at 37 °C. The samples were incubated with the relevant antibodies in PBS/10% FSC for 1 h and then stained with the appropriate fluorescent secondary antibody. Fluorescence intensities were captured by an Olympus FluoView FV1000 confocal microscope (Olympus, Melville, NY, USA). To block or induce autophagy, cells were treated with 3-methyladenine (10 mM; Sigma, St. Louis, MO, USA) or rapamycin (4 μM; Sigma), respectively, for 6 h.

### 4.14. Statistical Analysis

Statistical analyses were performed using SPSS 19.0 software (SPSS Inc., Chicago, IL, USA, 2000). Data are shown as least squares means ± standard error of the mean (SEM). Differences between groups were assessed using t-test, and values were considered significant difference at $p < 0.05$.

**Author Contributions:** Conceptualization, Y.C.; data curation, S.H.; formal analysis, S.H., and D.L.; funding acquisition, Q.Z. and H.Y.; investigation, S.H., and Y.C.; project administration, Y.W. and H.Y.; resources, H.Y.; supervision, H.Y.; writing—original draft, S.H. and H.Y.; writing—review and editing, Q.Z. All authors read and approved the final manuscript.

**Funding:** This work was financially supported by the China Agriculture Research System (CARS-40), Sichuan Science and Technology Program (2016NYZ0050).

**Acknowledgments:** We thank Liwen Bianji, Edanz Editing China (www.liwenbianji.cn/ac), for polishing the English text of this manuscript.

**Conflicts of Interest:** The authors declare no conflicts of interest.

## References

1. Chen, F.; Ma, Y.; Xue, C.; Ma, J.; Xie, Q.; Wang, G.; Bi, Y.; Cao, Y. The combination of deoxynivalenol and zearalenone at permitted feed concentrations causes serious physiological effects in young pigs. *J. Vet. Sci.* **2008**, *9*, 39–44. [CrossRef]
2. World Health Organization. *Selected Mycotoxins: Ochratoxins, Trichothecenes, Ergot-Environmental Health Criteria 105*; World Health Organization: Geneva, Switzerland, 1990.
3. Smith, J.E.; Solomons, G.; Lewis, C.; Anderson, J.G. Role of mycotoxins in human and animal nutrition and health. *Nat. Toxins* **1995**, *3*, 187–192. [CrossRef] [PubMed]
4. Rocha, O.; Ansari, K.; Doohan, F. Effects of trichothecene mycotoxins on eukaryotic cells: A review. *Food Addit. Contam.* **2005**, *22*, 369–378. [CrossRef]
5. Shinozuka, J.; Suzuki, M.; Noguchi, N.; Sugimoto, T.; Uetsuka, K.; Nakayama, H.; Doi, K. T-2 toxin-induced apoptosis in hematopoietic tissues of mice. *Toxicol. Pathol.* **1998**, *26*, 674–681. [CrossRef] [PubMed]
6. Ihara, T.; Sugamata, M.; Sekijima, M.; Okumura, H.; Yoshino, N.; Ueno, Y. Apoptotic cellular damage in mice after T-2 toxin-induced acute toxicosis. *Nat. Toxins* **1997**, *5*, 141–145. [CrossRef] [PubMed]
7. Li, G.; Shinozuka, J.; Uetsuka, K.; Nakayama, H.; Doi, K. T-2 toxin-induced apoptosis in intestinal crypt epithelial cells of mice. *Exp. Toxicol. Pathol.* **1997**, *49*, 447–450. [CrossRef]
8. Boonchuvit, B.; Hamilton, P.; Burmeister, H. Interaction of T-2 toxin with Salmonella infections of chickens. *Poult. Sci.* **1975**, *54*, 1693–1696. [CrossRef] [PubMed]

9. Yang, L.; Tu, D.; Zhao, Z.; Cui, J. Cytotoxicity and apoptosis induced by mixed mycotoxins (T-2 and HT-2 toxin) on primary hepatocytes of broilers in vitro. *Toxicon* **2017**, *129*, 1–10. [CrossRef]
10. Maiuri, M.C.; Zalckvar, E.; Kimchi, A.; Kroemer, G. Self-eating and self-killing: crosstalk between autophagy and apoptosis. *Nat. Rev. Mol. Cell Biol.* **2007**, *8*, 741. [CrossRef] [PubMed]
11. Galbenu-Morvay, P.L.; Alexandra, T.; Damiescu, L.; Simion, G. T-2 Toxin Occurrence in Cereals and Cereal-Based Foods. *Bull. Univ. Agric. Sci. Vet. Med. Cluj-Napoca. Agric.* **2011**, *68*, 274–280.
12. Li, Y.; Wang, Z.; Beier, R.C.; Shen, J.; Smet, D.D.; De Saeger, S.; Zhang, S. T-2 toxin, a trichothecene mycotoxin: Review of toxicity, metabolism, and analytical methods. *J. Agric. Food Chem.* **2011**, *59*, 3441–3453. [CrossRef]
13. Chi, M.; Mirocha, C.; Kurtz, H.; Weaver, G.; Bates, F.; Shimoda, W. Subacute toxicity of T-2 toxin in broiler chicks. *Poult. Sci.* **1977**, *56*, 306–313. [CrossRef] [PubMed]
14. Weber, M.; Fodor, J.; Balogh, K.; Wagner, L.; Erdelyi, M.; Mézes, M. Effect of vitamin E supplementation on immunity against Newcastle disease virus in T-2 toxin challenged chickens. *Acta Vet. Brno* **2008**, *77*, 45–49. [CrossRef]
15. Raju, M.; Devegowda, G. Esterified-glucomannan in broiler chicken diets-contaminated with aflatoxin, ochratoxin and T-2 toxin: Evaluation of its binding ability (in vitro) and efficacy as immunomodulator. *Asian-Australas. J. Anim. Sci.* **2002**, *15*, 1051–1056. [CrossRef]
16. Chen, B.; Li, D.; Li, M.; Li, S.; Peng, K.; Shi, X.; Zhou, L.; Zhang, P.; Xu, Z.; Yin, H. Induction of mitochondria-mediated apoptosis and PI3K/Akt/mTOR-mediated autophagy by aflatoxin B2 in hepatocytes of broilers. *Oncotarget* **2016**, *7*, 84989. [CrossRef] [PubMed]
17. Li, Y.; Zhang, J.; Mao, X.; Wu, Y.; Liu, G.; Song, L.; Li, Y.; Yang, J.; You, Y.; Cao, X. High-sensitivity chemiluminescent immunoassay investigation and application for the detection of T-2 toxin and major metabolite HT-2 toxin. *J. Sci. Food Agric.* **2017**, *97*, 818–822. [CrossRef]
18. Rachitha, P.; Khanum, F. T-2 Mycotoxin induced toxicity: A review. *Int. J. Curr. Res.* **2014**, *12*, 10798–10806.
19. Moosavi, M.; Rezaei, M.; Kalantari, H.; Behfar, A.; Varnaseri, G. l-carnitine protects rat hepatocytes from oxidative stress induced by T-2 toxin. *Drug Chem. Toxicol.* **2016**, *39*, 445–450. [CrossRef]
20. Yang, L.; Yu, Z.; Hou, J.; Deng, Y.; Zhou, Z.; Zhao, Z.; Cui, J. Toxicity and oxidative stress induced by T-2 toxin and HT-2 toxin in broilers and broiler hepatocytes. *Food Chem. Toxicol.* **2016**, *87*, 128–137. [CrossRef]
21. Albarenque, S.M.; Doi, K. T-2 toxin-induced apoptosis in rat keratinocyte primary cultures. *Exp. Mol. Pathol.* **2005**, *78*, 144–149. [CrossRef]
22. Smith, T. Recent advances in the understanding of Fusarium trichothecene mycotoxicoses. *J. Anim. Sci.* **1992**, *70*, 3989–3993. [CrossRef] [PubMed]
23. Guerre, P.; Eeckhoutte, C.; Burgat, V.; Galtier, P. The effects of T-2 toxin exposure on liver drug metabolizing enzymes in rabbit. *Food Addit. Contam.* **2000**, *17*, 1019–1026. [CrossRef] [PubMed]
24. Meissonnier, G.; Laffitte, J.; Raymond, I.; Benoit, E.; Cossalter, A.-M.; Pinton, P.; Bertin, G.; Oswald, I.; Galtier, P. Subclinical doses of T-2 toxin impair acquired immune response and liver cytochrome P450 in pigs. *Toxicology* **2008**, *247*, 46–54. [CrossRef] [PubMed]
25. Ok, S.; Yu, J.; Lee, Y.; Cho, H.; Shin, I.; Sohn, J. Lipid emulsion attenuates apoptosis induced by a toxic dose of bupivacaine in H9c2 rat cardiomyoblast cells. *Hum. Exp. Toxicol.* **2016**, *35*, 929–937. [CrossRef] [PubMed]
26. Wong, W.W.L.; Puthalakath, H. Bcl-2 family proteins: The sentinels of the mitochondrial apoptosis pathway. *Iubmb Life* **2008**, *60*, 390–397. [CrossRef]
27. Haddad, J.J. The role of Bax/Bcl-2 and pro-caspase peptides in hypoxia/reperfusion-dependent regulation of MAPKERK: Discordant proteomic effect of MAPKp38. *Protein Pept. Lett.* **2007**, *14*, 361–371. [CrossRef]
28. Mu, P.; Xu, M.; Zhang, L.; Wu, K.; Wu, J.; Jiang, J.; Chen, Q.; Wang, L.; Tang, X.; Deng, Y. Proteomic changes in chicken primary hepatocytes exposed to T-2 toxin are associated with oxidative stress and mitochondrial enhancement. *Proteomics* **2013**, *13*, 3175–3188. [CrossRef]
29. Wu, J.; Jing, L.; Yuan, H.; Peng, S.-Q. T-2 toxin induces apoptosis in ovarian granulosa cells of rats through reactive oxygen species-mediated mitochondrial pathway. *Toxicol. Lett.* **2011**, *202*, 168–177. [CrossRef]
30. Fang, H.; Wu, Y.; Guo, J.; Rong, J.; Ma, L.; Zhao, Z.; Zuo, D.; Peng, S. T-2 toxin induces apoptosis in differentiated murine embryonic stem cells through reactive oxygen species-mediated mitochondrial pathway. *Apoptosis* **2012**, *17*, 895–907. [CrossRef]
31. Mizushima, N.; Komatsu, M. Autophagy: Renovation of cells and tissues. *Cell* **2011**, *147*, 728–741. [CrossRef]
32. Shang, Y.; Lu, X. The relationship between apoptosis and autophagy in tumor therapy. *Prog. Mod. Biomed.* **2010**, *10*, 766–769.

33. Marquez, R.T.; Xu, L. Bcl-2: Beclin 1 complex: multiple, mechanisms regulating autophagy/apoptosis toggle switch. *Am. J. Cancer Res.* **2012**, *2*, 214.
34. Pattingre, S.; Tassa, A.; Qu, X.; Garuti, R.; Liang, X.H.; Mizushima, N.; Packer, M.; Schneider, M.D.; Levine, B. Bcl-2 antiapoptotic proteins inhibit Beclin 1-dependent autophagy. *Cell* **2005**, *122*, 927–939. [CrossRef]
35. Wang, Y.; Zheng, W.; Bian, X.; Yuan, Y.; Gu, J.; Liu, X.; Liu, Z.; Bian, J. Zearalenone induces apoptosis and cytoprotective autophagy in primary Leydig cells. *Toxicol. Lett.* **2014**, *226*, 182–191. [CrossRef] [PubMed]
36. Wu, J.; Zhou, Y.; Yuan, Z.; Yi, J.; Chen, J.; Wang, N.; Tian, Y. Autophagy and Apoptosis Interact to Modulate T-2 Toxin-Induced Toxicity in Liver Cells. *Toxins* **2019**, *11*, 45. [CrossRef] [PubMed]
37. Saiki, S.; Sasazawa, Y.; Imamichi, Y.; Kawajiri, S.; Fujimaki, T.; Tanida, I.; Kobayashi, H.; Sato, F.; Sato, S.; Ishikawa, K.-I. Caffeine induces apoptosis by enhancement of autophagy via PI3K/Akt/mTOR/p70S6K inhibition. *Autophagy* **2011**, *7*, 176–187. [CrossRef]
38. Li, Y.-C.; He, S.-M.; He, Z.-X.; Li, M.; Yang, Y.; Pang, J.-X.; Zhang, X.; Chow, K.; Zhou, Q.; Duan, W. Plumbagin induces apoptotic and autophagic cell death through inhibition of the PI3K/Akt/mTOR pathway in human non-small cell lung cancer cells. *Cancer Lett.* **2014**, *344*, 239–259. [CrossRef]
39. Xu, G.; Zhang, W.; Bertram, P.; Zheng, X.F.; McLeod, H. Pharmacogenomic profiling of the PI3K/PTEN-AKT-mTOR pathway in common human tumors. *Int. J. Oncol.* **2004**, *24*, 893–900. [CrossRef]
40. Zhang, G.-L.; Song, J.-L.; Ji, C.-L.; Feng, Y.-L.; Yu, J.; Nyachoti, C.M.; Yang, G.-S. Zearalenone exposure enhanced the expression of tumorigenesis genes in donkey granulosa cells via the PTEN/PI3K/AKT signaling pathway. *Front. Genet.* **2018**, *9*, 293. [CrossRef]
41. Xing, X.; Wang, J.; Xing, L.X.; Li, Y.H.; Yan, X.; Zhang, X.H. Involvement of MAPK and PI3K signaling pathway in sterigmatocystin-induced G2 phase arrest in human gastric epithelium cells. *Mol. Nutr. Food Res.* **2011**, *55*, 749–760. [CrossRef]
42. Kim, S.-H.; Son, K.-M.; Kim, K.-Y.; Yu, S.-N.; Park, S.-G.; Kim, Y.-W.; Nam, H.-W.; Suh, J.-T.; Ji, J.-H.; Ahn, S.-C. Deoxypodophyllotoxin induces cytoprotective autophagy against apoptosis via inhibition of PI3K/AKT/mTOR pathway in osteosarcoma U2OS cells. *Pharmacol. Rep.* **2017**, *69*, 878–884. [CrossRef]

*toxins*

MDPI

*Article*

# Comparison of Apoptosis and Autophagy in Human Chondrocytes Induced by the T-2 and HT-2 Toxins

**Fang-Fang Yu [1], Xia-Lu Lin [2], Xi Wang [2], Zhi-Guang Ping [1] and Xiong Guo [2,*]**

1 Department of Epidemiology and Biostatistics, College of Public Health, Zhengzhou University, Zhengzhou 45001, China; yufangfang@zzu.edu.cn (F.-F.Y.); pingzhg@zzu.edu.cn (Z.-G.P.)

2 NHC Key Laboratory of Trace Elements and Endemic Diseases, Institute of Endemic Diseases, School of Public Health of Health Science Center, Xi'an Jiaotong University, Xi'an 710061, China; summer2047@stu.xjtu.edu.cn (X.-L.L.); wn18andlife@xjtu.edu.cn (X.W.)

* Correspondence: guox@mail.xjtu.edu.cn; Tel.: +86-029-8265-5091; Fax: +86-029-8265-5032

Received: 31 March 2019; Accepted: 7 May 2019; Published: 8 May 2019

**Abstract:** In this report, we have investigated the apoptosis and autophagy of chondrocytes induced by the T-2 and HT-2 toxins. The viability of chondrocytes was measured by the MTT assay. Malondialdehyde (MDA) and superoxide dismutase (SOD) kits were used to measure the oxidative stress of chondrocytes. The apoptosis of chondrocytes was measured using flow cytometry. Hoechst 33258 and MDC staining agents were introduced to analyze apoptosis and autophagy induction in chondrocytes, respectively. Protein expression of Bax, caspase-9, caspase-3, and Beclin1 was examined by western blotting analysis. The T-2 and HT-2 toxins significantly decreased the viability of chondrocytes in a time-dependent manner. The level of oxidative stress in chondrocytes induced by the T-2 toxin was significantly higher when compared with that of the HT-2 toxin. The apoptosis rate of chondrocytes induced by the T-2 toxin increased from 3.26 ± 1.03%, 18.38 ± 1.28%, 34.5 ± 1.40% to 49.67 ± 5.31%, whereas apoptosis rate of chondrocytes induced by the HT-2 toxin increased from 3.82 ± 1.03%, 11.61 ± 1.27%, 25.72 ± 2.95% to 36.28 ± 2.81% in 48 h incubation time. Hoechst 33258 staining confirmed that apoptosis of chondrocytes induced by the T-2 toxin was significantly higher than that observed when the chondrocytes were incubated with the HT-2 toxin. MDC staining revealed that the autophagy rate of chondrocytes induced by the T-2 toxin increased from 6.38% to 63.02%, whereas this rate induced by the HT-2 toxin changed from 6.08% to 53.33%. The expression levels of apoptosis and autophagy related proteins, Bax, caspase-9, caspase-3, and Beclin1 in chondrocytes induced by the T-2 toxin were significantly higher when compared with those levels induced by the HT-2 toxin.

**Keywords:** T-2 toxin; HT-2 toxin; apoptosis; autophagy

**Key Contribution:** The T-2 and HT-2 toxins can significantly induce apoptosis and autophagy of chondrocytes; and apoptosis and autophagy of chondrocytes induced by T-2 toxin were much higher when compared with that of the HT-2 toxin.

## 1. Introduction

Kashin–Beck disease (KBD) is an endemic, chronic, and deformed osteoarthropathic disease. There are 0.64 million KBD patients distributed from northeast to southwest regions of China. KBD patients suffer from joint pain, morning stiffness, limited motion, and joint enlargement [1,2]. Three underlying risk factors are considered to be responsible for KBD: mycotoxin (T-2 toxin) in grain, selenium deficiency, and organic acid in drinking water [3,4]. Recently, research effort has focused on apoptosis of human chondrocytes induced by the T-2 toxin [5]. Previous epidemiologic studies have confirmed the presence of higher concentrations of the T-2 toxin in grains from endemic areas [6]. The T-2 toxin has been showed to exert various toxin effects on experimental animals and human chondrocytes, including the dysplasia tibial growth plate cartilage in chicken, and induction of apoptosis of human chondrocytes, which involves p53, Bcl-xL, Bcl-2, Bax, and caspase-3 signaling pathways [7].

T-2 toxin is hydrolyzed to the HT-2 toxin in nature. For example, the T-2 toxin is rapidly metabolized to the HT-2 toxin in microsomes of liver, kidney, and spleen with conversion rates of 80%. The T-2 toxin detected in grains can be rapidly converted in vivo to the HT-2 toxin after consuming the contaminated food. The T-2 toxin rapidly combines with proteins in the blood and is delivered to organs through the mouth, skin, and respiratory tract [8]. The T-2 toxin is metabolized to the HT-2 toxin in the liver after entering enterohepatic circulation. Rats treated with T-2 toxin for 8 h, were found to convert the toxin at different rates in various tissues with conversion rates ranging from 68.20% to 90.70%, and the T-2 and HT-2 toxins were both detected in the skeletal system (thighbone, knee joint, and costal cartilage) [9]. The T-2 toxin in cultured chondrocytes is metabolized into the HT-2 toxin. The concentration of the T-2 toxin in the cell medium was found to decrease from 20 to 6.67 ng/mL during 48 h incubation period, while the concentration of the HT-2 toxin increased from 0 to 6.88 ng/mL over the same period [10]. Metabolism of the T-2 toxin to the HT-2 toxin in the liver and digestive systems can directly affect the human skeletal system. However, the toxic effects of the HT-2 toxin on human chondrocytes remain poorly understood.

In this study, human chondrocytes were cultured in fetal bovine serum (FBS) media. The chondrocytes were exposed to the T-2 and HT-2 toxins for 48 h, and the resulting apoptotic and autophagic effects were monitored.

## 2. Results

### 2.1. Viability of Chondrocytes Induced by the T-2 and HT-2 Toxins

Chondrocytes were incubated with the T-2 and HT-2 toxins (20 ng/mL) for 48 h. As shown in Figure 1, the T-2 and HT-2 toxins decreased the viability of chondrocytes significantly in a time-dependent manner, and the toxic effect of the T-2 toxin on the viability of chondrocytes was significantly higher than that of the HT-2 toxin after 24 h and 48 h incubation time. Therefore, the toxic effect of the T-2 toxin on the viability of chondrocytes was significantly higher when compared with that of the HT-2 toxin.

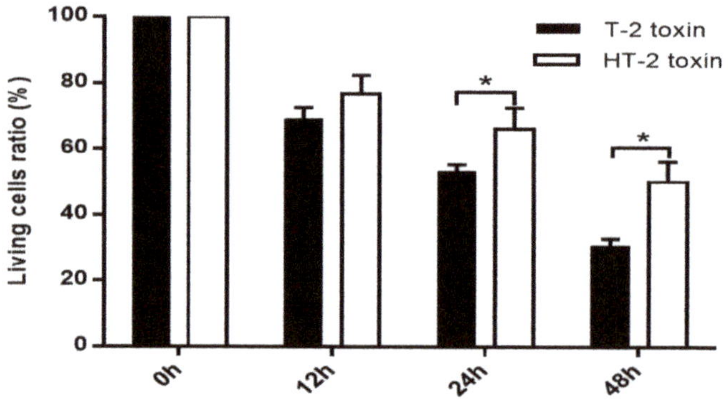


**Figure 1.** Effects of same concentration of the T-2 and HT-2 toxins on the cellular viability of chondrocytes were estimated by MTT reduction. * $p < 0.05$ was considered as significant difference between the two groups.

### 2.2. Oxidative Stress of Chondrocytes Induced by the T-2 and HT-2 Toxins

MDA is an important indicator of lipid peroxidation damage in tissue and cells. As shown in Figure 2a, the chondrocytes were treated with the T-2 and HT-2 toxins (20 ng/mL) for 48 h.

The MDA content in the chondrocytes increased as the incubation time in the presence of the two toxins increased. At the same dose and incubation period (12 h and 48 h), the MDA content in the chondrocytes induced by the T-2 toxin was significantly higher than the chondrocytes exposed to HT-2 toxin ($p < 0.05$).

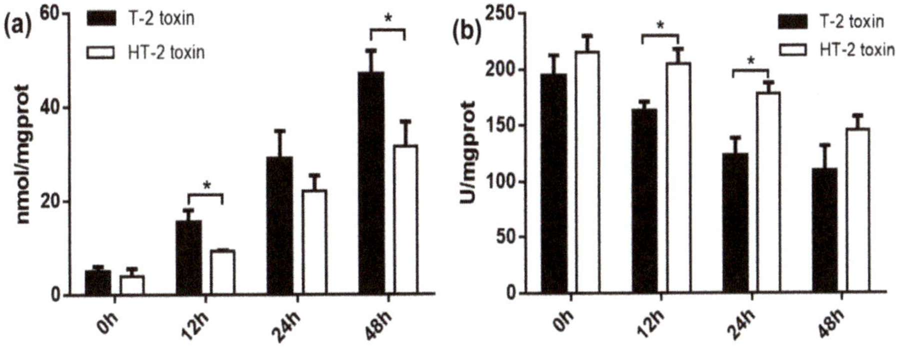


**Figure 2.** The malondialdehyde (MDA) (**a**) and superoxide dismutase (SOD) (**b**) content in the chondrocytes were induced by the T-2 and HT-2 toxins. * $p < 0.05$ was considered as significant difference between the two groups.

SOD is an important antioxidant defense enzyme in humans. As shown in Figure 2b, the SOD content in the chondrocytes decreased as the incubation period of the T-2 and HT-2 toxins increased. At the same dose and incubation period (12 h and 24 h), the SOD content in the chondrocytes incubated with the T-2 toxin was significantly lower when compared with the SOD content present in chondrocytes cultured with the HT-2 toxin ($p < 0.05$).

### 2.3. *Apoptosis of Chondrocytes Induced by the T-2 and HT-2 Toxins*

Flow cytometry was used to analyze apoptosis of chondrocytes induced by the T-2 and HT-2 toxins (20 ng/mL). Apoptosis of chondrocytes increased gradually as the incubation period with the toxins increased (Figure 3); the apoptosis of chondrocytes induced by the T-2 toxin increased in the range 3.26 ± 1.03%, 18.38 ± 1.28%, 34.5 ± 1.40%, and 49.67 ± 5.31% after incubation for 0, 12, 24, and 48 h, respectively, whereas apoptosis of chondrocytes induced by HT-2 toxin increased in the range 3.82 ± 1.03%, 11.61 ± 1.27%, 25.72 ± 2.95%, and 36.28 ± 2.81% over the same time. At the same dose and incubation period, the apoptosis of chondrocytes induced by the T-2 toxin was significantly higher than that induced by the HT-2 toxin, and the difference was statistically significant ($p < 0.05$).

Hoechst 33258 staining was used to analyze apoptosis of chondrocytes induced by the T-2 and HT-2 toxins. Cell nuclei that stained white and thick dense were considered to be positive apoptosis cells. As shown in Figure 4, the apoptosis rate of chondrocytes incubated with the T-2 toxin increased from 3.94% to 60.67%, whereas the apoptosis rate of chondrocytes incubated with the HT-2 toxin increased from 3.74% to 40.75%. Therefore, the apoptosis of chondrocytes induced by the T-2 toxin was significantly higher when compared with that of HT-2 toxin, and the difference was statistically significant between two groups ($p < 0.05$).

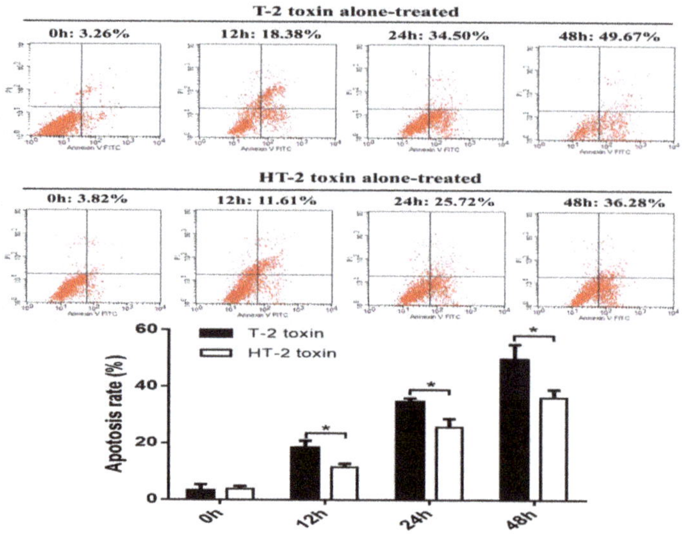


**Figure 3.** Apoptosis of chondrocytes was induced by the T-2 and HT-2 toxins using flow cytometry analysis. * $p < 0.05$ was considered as significant difference between two groups.

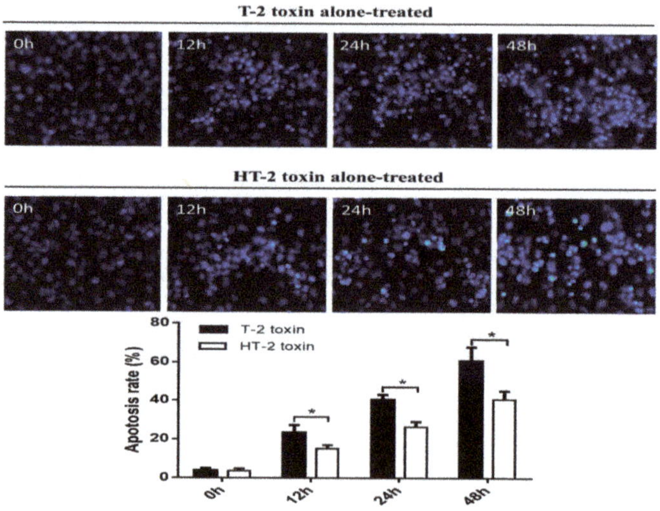


**Figure 4.** Apoptosis of chondrocytes was induced by the T-2 and HT-2 toxins using Hoechst 33258 staining. The cell nucleus with a white, thick dense cells were considered to be positive apoptosis cells under the fluorescence microscope (×400). * $p < 0.05$ was considered as significant difference between two groups.

## *2.4. Apoptosis-Related Proteins in Chondrocyte Induced by T-2 and HT-2 Toxins*

As shown in Figure 5, chondrocytes incubated with the T-2 and HT-2 toxin (20 ng/mL) for 48 h shown an increased expression level of Bax (Figure 5a), caspase-9 (Figure 5b), and caspase-3 (Figure 5c), and the increases in protein levels were dependent on the incubation period. The relative expression level of Bax, caspase-9, and caspase-3 proteins in chondrocytes induced by the T-2 toxin was 1.29 fold, 0.99 fold, and 1.32 fold, respectively. The relative expression level of Bax, caspase-9, and caspase-3 proteins in chondrocytes induced by the HT-2 toxin was 0.91 fold, 0.68 fold, and 1.12 fold, respectively. The increased expression levels of Bax, caspase-9, and caspase-3 in chondrocytes induced by the T-2 toxin were statistically significant when compared with that of the HT-2 toxin ($p < 0.05$).

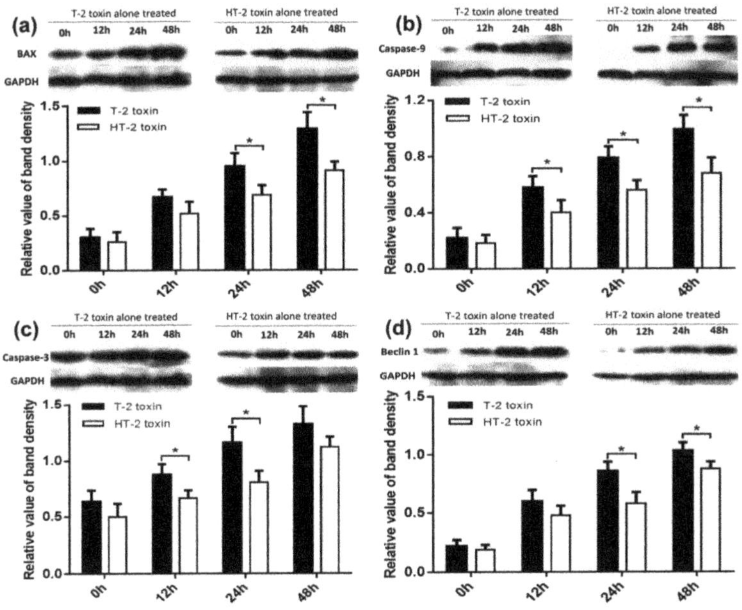


**Figure 5.** Apoptosis and autophagy related with proteins (**a**) Bax, (**b**) caspase-9, (**c**) caspase-3, and (**d**) Beclin1 of chondrocytes were induced by the T-2 and HT-2 toxins. The expression levels of Bax, caspase-9, caspase-3, and Beclin1 referred to the GAPDH (load control) were calculated in the T-2 toxin group and HT-2 toxin group. And then the expression levels of Bax, caspase-9, caspase-3, and Beclin1 were compared between two groups. * $p < 0.05$ was considered as significant difference between two groups.

### *2.5. Autophagy of Chondrocytes Induced by the T-2 and HT-2 Toxins*

As shown in Figure 6, the MDC kit was used to analyze autophagy of chondrocytes induced by the T-2 and HT-2 toxins (20 ng/mL). Cell nuclei stained cyan-green were positive for an acidic autophagosome. The autophagy rate of chondrocytes induced by the T-2 toxin increased from 6.38% to 63.02%, and the autophagy rate of chondrocytes induced by the HT-2 toxin increased from 6.08% to 53.33%. Therefore, the autophagy rate of chondrocytes induced by the T-2 toxin was significantly higher than that caused by the HT-2 toxin, and the difference was statistically significant ($p < 0.05$).

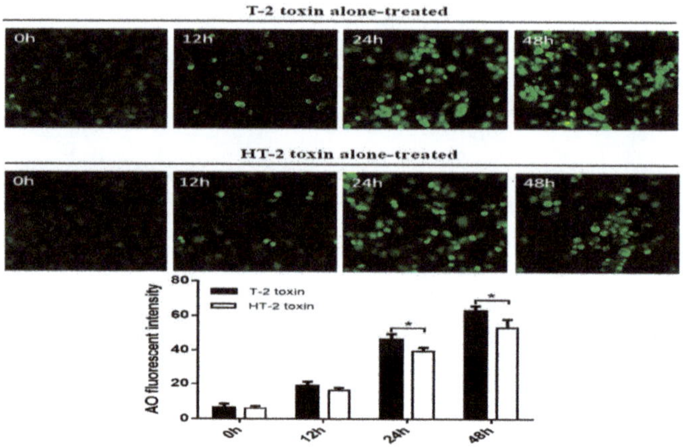


**Figure 6.** Autophagy of chondrocytes was induced by the T-2 and HT-2 toxins using MDC staining, cell nuclei stained cyan-green were positive for an acidic autophagosome under the fluorescence microscope (×400). * $p < 0.05$ was considered as significant difference between two groups.

### *2.6. Autophagy-Related Proteins in Chondrocytes Induced by the T-2 and HT-2 Toxins*

As shown in Figure 5d, the relative expression level of Beclin1 was observed to increase gradually as the incubation period increased. The relative expression level of Beclin1 in chondrocytes induced by the T-2 toxin was increased 1.03 fold, and the relative expression level of Beclin1 in chondrocytes induced by the HT-2 toxin was increased 0.88 fold after an incubation of 48 h. The increased expression level of Beclin1 in chondrocytes induced by the T-2 toxin was significantly higher when compared with that of the HT-2 toxin (24 h and 48 h), and the difference was statistically significant ($p < 0.05$).

## 3. Discussion

Currently, research efforts have focused mainly on T-2 toxin contamination in grains for the etiology of KBD. However, it remains unclear that whether the T-2 toxin in grains specifically damages articular cartilage of children KBD, and that the expression levels of apoptotic and autophagic proteins in chondrocytes are exposed to the T-2 toxin during the early stages of the disease. Based on our previous experiments [9,10], the T-2 toxin is metabolized to the HT-2 toxin after entering into the skeletal system of rats. The T-2 toxin levels were observed to decrease in chondrocytes over a 48 h period concomitant with the significant increase in the concentration of the HT-2 toxin. In contrast, there is a paucity of data describing the toxicity of the HT-2 toxin on chondrocytes, and there is no comparative study describing the toxicity of the T-2 and HT-2 toxins toward chondrocytes. Therefore, in this study, chondrocytes were incubated with the same concentration of the T-2 and HT-2 toxins to explore the apoptotic and autophagic affects induced by these toxins.

In this study, chondrocytes were incubated with the T-2 and HT-2 toxins for 48 h. MTT analysis revealed that the toxicity of the toxins on chondrocytes is time-dependent. The T-2 and HT-2 toxins increased oxidative stress in chondrocytes significantly. Flow cytometry analysis showed that the T-2 toxin induced an increase from 3.26% to 49.67% in the apoptosis rate of chondrocytes, whereas the apoptosis rate of chondrocytes induced by the HT-2 toxin increased significantly from 3.82% to 36.28%. Immunofluorescence analysis also confirmed that the apoptosis rate of chondrocytes induced by the two toxins increased significantly. Western blot analysis showed that the relative expression levels of Bax, caspase-3, and caspase-9 in chondrocytes incubated with the T-2 and HT-2 toxins increased significantly. The oxidative stress level, apoptosis rate, and apoptosis-related proteins for chondrocytes induced by the T-2 toxin were significantly higher than those observed when these cells were incubated with the HT-2 toxin. Nonetheless, the oxidative stress of chondrocytes incubated with both toxins increased significantly, which caused a change to the mitochondrial membrane potential and mitochondrial membrane osmosis, release of mitochondrial pro-apoptotic protein Bax, and the subsequent release of cytochrome C related proteins (caspase-9 and caspase-3). All these factors eventually resulted in apoptosis of the chondrocytes.

Autophagy of the chondrocytes was induced by both toxins, and immunofluorescence analysis showed that the autophagy rate of chondrocytes induced by the T-2 toxin increased from 3.94% to 60.67%, whereas the autophagy rate of chondrocytes induced by the HT-2 toxin increased from 3.74% to 40.75%. Western blot analysis revealed that the expression levels of Beclin1 increased significantly in chondrocytes incubated with the T-2 and HT-2 toxins. Autophagy of chondrocytes induced by the T-2 toxin was also significantly higher than that induced by the HT-2 toxin. Recent studies have reported that the T-2 and HT-2 toxins induce autophagy and apoptosis of porcine and mouse oocytes, rat brain, primary cardiomyocyte, liver cells, and mouse primary leydig cells. Two studies [11,12] showed an increase in the ROS levels of porcine and mouse oocytes when incubated with the HT-2 toxin, indicating an increase in oxidative stress. ROS levels in the treated group were also higher, confirming that the HT-2 toxin caused oxidative stress, which induced apoptosis and autophagy. A previous study [13] reported autophagy in the brain and apoptosis in the pituitary, suggesting that the T-2 toxin may induce different acute reactions in different tissues. Three studies [14–16] also confirmed that incubation of the T-2 toxin with mouse primary leydig cells, liver cells, and primary cardiomyocyte caused up-regulation of LC3-II and Beclin1, suggesting that the T-2 toxin promotes a high level of autophagy. Pretreatment of these cells with chloroquine and rapamycin was shown to increase and decrease the rate of apoptosis, respectively. Therefore, autophagy may prevent apoptosis of cells by reducing T-2 toxin-induced cytotoxicity. The T-2 toxin is also an environmental risk factor of the KBD, and our results showed that the T-2 and HT-2 toxins can significantly induce apoptosis and autophagy of chondrocytes, and these observations were consistent with previous studies [11–17]. The apoptosis and autophagy rates of chondrocytes induced by the T-2 toxin were much higher than those rates induced when the chondrocytes were incubated with the HT-2 toxin, and such an observation has not been reported previously.

The results showed an increase of both apoptosis and autophagy in chondrocytes treated with the T-2 and HT-2 toxins, which is in agreement with previous studies. Autophagy is a normal physiological activity of cells, which was activated in chondrocytes treated with the T-2 and HT-2 toxins, to avoid further cell damage. There is a complex relationship between autophagy and apoptosis. When cells are exposed to low environmental pressures, activation of autophagy can prevent apoptosis and subsequent cell death. When cells are subjected to strong or prolonged environmental stress, the process of autophagy consumes excessive levels of intracellular proteins or organelles, leading to cell survival failure that promotes programmed cell death [18–20].

## 4. Conclusions

In conclusion, our results showed that the T-2 and HT-2 toxins induce apoptosis and autophagy of chondrocytes, and that the level of oxidative stress plays an important role in autophagy activation. The activation of autophagy can reduce oxidative damage and therefore functions in protecting chondrocytes from apoptosis through capture, elimination, and degradation of damaged mitochondria.

## 5. Methods and Materials

### 5.1. Reagents and Antibodies

Fetal bovine serum (FBS), dimethyl sulfoxide (DMSO), and Hoechst 33258 were purchased from Sigma-Aldrich (St. Louis, MO, USA). The T-2 and HT-2 toxins were purchased from J&K Chemical Ltd (Beijing, China). The thiazolyl blue tetrazolium bromide (MTT) was purchased from Amresco (Solon, OH, USA). The malondialdehyde (MDA) kit and the superoxide dismutase (SOD) kit were purchased from the Nanjing Jiancheng Bioengineering Institute (Nanjing, China). The Bicinchoninic Acid

(BCA) Protein Assay kit was purchased from TianGen Biotech (Beijing, China). Anti-Bax, anti-Caspase 9, anti-Caspase 3, and anti-Beclin1 antibodies were purchased from Cell Signaling Technology, Inc. (Danvers, MA, USA).

### 5.2. Cell Culture and Treatment

The human chondrocytes cell line (C28/I2) was cultured in DMEM/F12 medium with 9% FBS at 37 °C and 5% $CO_2$ in a humidified atmosphere. Once the chondrocytes had reached a steady state of the exponential growth phase, these cells were seeded at a density of $1.0 \times 10^4$ per well in 96-well plates and grown overnight. The cells were then cultured in a medium containing either the T-2 toxin or the HT-2 toxin (20 ng/mL) for 0, 12, 24, and 48 h. The T-2 and HT-2 toxins (1 mg) were freshly dissolved in 1 mL DMSO and protected from light. In the T-2 toxin and HT-2 toxin treatment group, the cellular viability, oxidative stress, apoptosis, and autophagy of chondrocyte were determined.

### 5.3. MTT Assay

Human chondrocytes in the logarithmic phase were suspended in 0.1% EDTA trypsin. Two hundred microliter cell suspensions were seeded into individual 96-well plates at a density of $1 \times 10^4$ cells per well. The experiments were carried out in the toxin group and control group. Complete medium with either the T-2 toxin or HT-2 toxin (20 ng/mL) was added and the cells were incubated for 0, 12, 24, and 48 h. Twenty microliters of MTT was added into the toxin and control groups to a final concentration of 0.5 mg/mL at each incubation time point. After 4 h at 37 °C, the medium containing MTT was aspirated and replaced with 150 μL DMSO and incubated for a further 1 h. Following this incubation, the absorbance was measured using an automatic microplate reader at 510 nm. The calculation of the viability rate at different concentrations and time points is as follows (1):

$$\begin{aligned} &\text{Viability rate (\%)} = \{[(\text{control group} - \text{blank control group}) \\ &- (\text{toxin group} - \text{blank toxin group})]/(\text{control group} - \text{blank control group})\} \times 100\% \end{aligned} \quad (1)$$

### 5.4. Oxidative Stress

Sample pretreatment: The supernatant of cell culture was discarded, and the pellet was digested with 0.25% trypsin for 2 min. Then, the culture medium was added to stop digestion by gentle micropipetting, and transferred into an EP tube and centrifuged at 3500–4000 rpm for 10 min. The supernatant was discarded and the precipitated cells were broken into suspension using ultrasonic wave. Their protein concentration was determined using bicinchoninic acid (BCA) protein assay kit. A volume of 0.2 mL of the suspension in a centrifuge tube (1.5 mL) was used for the assay.

The MDA assay kit was purchased from Nanjing Jiancheng Bioengineering Institute and used to measure oxidative stress damage. The centrifuge tubes were divided into four groups: standard tubes (0.2 mL 10 nmon/mL standards + 0.2 mL reagent 1 + 1.5 mL reagent 2 + 1.5 mL reagent 3), standard blank tubes (0.2 mL absolute ethyl alcohol + 0.2 mL reagent 1 + 1.5 mL reagent 2 + 1.5 mL reagent 3), measure tubes (0.2 mL measure sample + 0.2 mL reagent 1 + 1.5 mL reagent 2 + 1.5 mL reagent 3), and measure blank tubes (0.2 mL measure sample + 0.2 mL reagent 1 + 1.5 mL reagent 2 + 1.5 mL 50% glacial acetic acid). A spiral vortex mixer was used to mix samples in the standard tubes, standard blank tubes, measure tubes, and measure blank tubes. Test tubes were placed in a water bath for 40 min at 95 °C, cooled with a water cooling tube, and centrifuged at 3500–4000 rpm for 10 min.

The supernatant was collected and the absorbance value (OD) of samples in each tube was measured at 532 nm with 1 cm optical path (2).

$$\begin{aligned} \text{MDA (nmol/mgprot)} = {} & [(\text{OD measure tube} - \text{OD measure blank tube})/(\text{OD standard tube} \\ & - \text{OD standard blank tube})] \times \text{concentration of standard sample (10 nmol/mL)} \\ & \div \text{protein concentration of measure sample (mgprot/mL)} \end{aligned} \tag{2}$$

The SOD assay kit was also purchased from Nanjing Jiancheng Bioengineering Institute and used to determine the activity of SOD using the WST-1 method. The centrifuge tubes were divided into four groups: control tubes (20 μL double distilled water + 20 μL enzyme working solution + 200 μL substrate application solution), control blank tubes (20 μL double distilled water + 20 μL enzyme diluents solution + 200 μL substrate application solution), measure tubes (20 μL measure sample + 20 μL enzyme working solution + 200 μL substrate application solution), and measure blank tubes (20 μL measure sample + 20 μL enzyme diluents solution + 200 μL substrate application solution). A spiral vortex mixer was used to mix samples in the control tubes, control blank tubes, measuring tubes, and measuring blank tubes, and then samples were incubated at 37 °C for 20 min. The absorbance value (OD) of samples was measured at 450 nm. The SOD activity is then measured by the degree of inhibition of this reaction. One unit of SOD was defined as the amount of enzyme needed to produce 50% dismutation of superoxide radical. The calculation of SOD activity is as below (3):

$$\begin{aligned} \text{(U/mgprot)} = {} & \text{inhibition rate of SOD (\%)} \div 50\% \times [\text{reaction system (0.24 mL)}/ \\ & \text{dilution ratio (0.02 mL)}] \div \text{protein concentration of measuring sample (mgprot/mL)} \end{aligned} \tag{3}$$

### 5.5. *Flow Cytometry of AV/PI*

The apoptosis assay kit was used to measure apoptosis using Annexin V and PI double staining. Chondrocytes were incubated with either the T-2 or HT-2 toxin (20 ng/mL) for 0, 12, 24, and 48 h. Chondrocytes were washed with PBS twice and 250 μL binding buffer was added to resuspend chondrocytes at a density of $1.0 \times 10^6$/mL. The cell suspension (100 μL), PI solution (10 mL, 20 μg/mL), and Annexin V/FITC (5 μL) were added to the 5 mL flow tube. The flow tube was mixed and incubated for 15 min in the dark at room temperature. Then 400 μL PBS was added to the reaction tube for flow cytometry analysis. As Annexin V and PI double staining were used to measure the apoptosis rate, automatic compensation regulation was used to avoid overlapping of two fluorescein wavelengths in the flow cytometry. When obtaining data from flow cytometric analysis, the gating was set using the combination of Forward Scatter (FSC) and Side Scatter (SSC), to establish FSC versus SSC dot diagram. By setting FSC threshold according to the size and granularity of chondrocytes, it can distinguish different cell populations, and remove from cell fragments, dead cells, and adhesion cells. The early apoptotic cells had been quantified using the Gated% data, the calculation of early apoptosis rate was Lower Right/(Upper Left + Upper Right + Lower Left + Lower Right).

### 5.6. *Fluorescence Intensity Analysis*

Hoechst 33258 was used to detect apoptosis of the chondrocytes. Chondrocytes were cultured in a 12-well plate. After the cells absorbed to the plate, the supernatant was discarded and the chondrocytes were fixedwith 4% formaldehyde for 30 min. The fixed chondrocytes were stained using a Hoechst 33258 working solution for 1 h at 37 °C with 5% $CO_2$ in a humidified atmosphere. The maximum excitation and emission wavelength of Hoechst-DNA were 352 and 461 nm, respectively. Nuclei of normal chondrocytes fluoresced blue under the fluorescence microscope, whereas pale, dense, and hyperchromatic nuclei represented apoptotic cells.

Monodansylcadaverine (MDC) can be used to specifically mark the formation of autophagosomes. The chondrocytes were treated with the T-2 and HT-2 toxins in 24-well plates, and the medium was absorbed. One hundred microliters of the MDC staining solution was added to each well and staining was carried out for 30 min at room temperature in the presence of light. The culture medium was discarded, and the cells were washed three times with 1× wash buffer (300 μL). The cell slide was covered with the collection buffer (100 μL). The wavelengths of stimulation and blocking filters of the fluorescence microscope were of 355 and 512 nm, respectively. Cell nuclei stained cyan-green were positive for an acidic autophagosome. When the cells were photographed using the fluorescence microscope, we identified four microscope fields of every replication microscopic picture (×400) and the cells were counted. Then the apoptosis rate was calculated as number of apoptotic cells/number of apoptotic cells and normal cells. Finally, the results were presented by mean ± standard deviations.

### 5.7. Protein Extraction and Western Blot Analysis

The chondrocytes were lysed using RIPA (Trizol method) and total protein in cell lysates was harvested by centrifugal separation according to the manufacturer's instructions. The concentration of extracted protein was quantified by the BCA assay kit (Beijing Tiangen Biotech Company, Beijing, China). Equal amounts (50 μg) of extracted protein were subjected to 10% (w/v) sodium dodecyl sulfate-polyacrylamide gel electrophoresis (SDS-PAGE) and electrophoretically transferred onto PVDF membrane. They were pre-incubated in blocking buffer containing 5% (w/v) non-fat milk with Tween 20 for 60 min at room temperature, rinsed three times with TBST for 5 min. The membranes were incubated with different primary antibodies against Bax, caspase-9, caspase-3, and Beclin1 (Cell Signaling Technology, Boston, MA, USA) overnight at 4 °C; all primary antibodies were used at a 1:1000 dilution. After being washed three times in TBS, the membrane was incubated with an appropriately diluted horseradish peroxidase-labeled secondary antibody (1:5000) in blotting buffer for 30 min. The blots were visualized by enhanced chemiluminescent (ECL). Western blot signals were exposed to X-ray films and the bands were quantified by Quantity One software. The protein levels were standardized by comparison with anti-GAPDH antibody.

### 5.8. Statistical Analysis

All experiments were performed in three independent trials, each of which included three replications. Experimental data were presented as the mean and standard deviations. SPSS18.0 software (IBM, Armonk, NY, USA) was used to analyze the experimental data, and the *t*-test was used to compare the differences between two groups. $p < 0.05$ was considered to be statistically significant between two groups.

**Author Contributions:** The conception and design of the study: F.-F.Y., X.-L.L. Collection, analysis and interpretation of the data entry as described above: F.-F.Y., X.-L.L. and X.W. Draft of the article and critical revision of the article for important intellectual content: F.-F.Y., Z.-G.P. and X.G.

**Funding:** This research was funded by the National Natural Scientific Foundation of China (81620108026), General Financial Grant from the China Postdoctoral Science Foundation (2019M652595) and Cultivating grand for youth key teacher in Higher Education Institutions of Henan province (2017GGJS012).

**Acknowledgments:** We thank Liwen Bianji, Edanz Editing China for editing the English text of a draft of our manuscript.

**Conflicts of Interest:** The authors declare no competing financial interests.

## References

1. Guo, X.; Ma, W.J.; Zhang, F.; Ren, F.L.; Qu, C.J.; Lammi, M.J. Recent advances in the research of an endemic osteochondropathy in China: Kashin-Beck disease. *Osteoarthr. Cartil.* **2014**, *22*, 1774–1783. [CrossRef] [PubMed]
2. Xiong, G. Diagnostic, clinical and radiological characteristics of Kashin-Beck disease in Shaanxi Province, PR China. *Int. Orthop.* **2001**, *25*, 147–150. [CrossRef] [PubMed]
3. Yu, F.F.; Han, J.; Wang, X.; Fang, H.; Liu, H.; Guo, X. Salt-rich selenium for prevention and control children with Kashin–Beck disease: A meta-analysis of community-based trial. *Biol Trace Elem. Res.* **2016**, *170*, 25–32. [CrossRef] [PubMed]

4. Chen, J.; Chu, Y.; Cao, J.; Yang, Z.; Guo, X.; Wang, Z. T-2 toxin induces apoptosis, and selenium partly blocks, T-2 toxin induced apoptosis in chondrocytes through modulation of the Bax/Bcl-2 ratio. *Food Chem. Toxicol.* **2006**, *44*, 567–573. [CrossRef] [PubMed]
5. Li, S.Y.; Cao, J.L.; Shi, Z.L.; Chen, J.H.; Zhang, Z.T.; Hughes, C.E.; Caterson, B. Promotion of the articular cartilage proteoglycan degradation by T-2 toxin and selenium protective effect. *J. Zhejiang Univ. Sci. B.* **2008**, *9*, 22–33. [CrossRef] [PubMed]
6. Wang, X.; Liu, X.; Liu, J.; Wang, G.; Wan, K. Contamination level of T-2 and HT-2 toxin in cereal crops from Aba area in Sichuan Province, China. *Bull Environ. Contam. Toxicol.* **2012**, *88*, 396–400. [CrossRef]
7. Chen, J.H.; Cao, J.L.; Chu, Y.L.; Wang, Z.L.; Yang, Z.T.; Wang, H.L. T-2 toxin-induced apoptosis involving Fas, p53, Bcl-xL, Bcl-2, Bax and caspase-3 signaling pathways in human chondrocytes. *J. Zhejiang Univ. Sci. B.* **2008**, *9*, 455–463. [CrossRef] [PubMed]
8. Wu, Q.; Huang, L.; Liu, Z.; Yao, M.; Wang, Y.; Dai, M.; Yuan, Z. A comparison of hepatic in vitro metabolism of T-2 toxin in rats, pigs, chickens, and carp. *Xenobiotica.* **2011**, *41*, 863–873. [CrossRef]
9. Yu, F.F.; Lin, X.L.; Lei, Y.; Huan, L.; Xi, W.; Hua, F.; Lammi, Z.J.; Xiong, G. Comparison of T-2 toxin and HT-2 Toxin distributed in the skeletal system with that in other tissues of rats by acute toxicity test. *Biomed. Environ. Sci.* **2017**, *30*, 851–854.
10. Yu, F.F.; Lin, X.L.; Wang, X.; Liu, H.; Yang, L.; Goldring, M.B.; Lammi, Z.J.; Guo, X. Selenium promotes metabolic conversion of T-2 toxin to HT-2 toxin in cultured human chondrocytes. *J. Trace Elem. Med. Biol.* **2017**, *44*, 218–224. [CrossRef] [PubMed]
11. Zhu, C.C.; Zhang, Y.; Duan, X.; Han, J.; Sun, S.C. Toxic effects of HT-2 toxin on mouse oocytes and its possible mechanisms. *Arch. Toxicol.* **2016**, *90*, 1495–1505. [CrossRef] [PubMed]
12. Zhang, Y.; Han, J.; Zhu, C.C.; Tang, F.; Cui, X.S.; Kim, N.H.; Sun, S.C. Exposure to HT-2 toxin causes oxidative stress induced apoptosis/autophagy in porcine oocytes. *Sci. Rep.* **2016**, *6*, 33904. [CrossRef] [PubMed]
13. Guo, P.; Liu, A.; Huang, D.; Wu, Q.; Fatima, Z.; Tao, Y.; Cheng, G.; Wang, X.; Yuan, Z. Brain damage and neurological symptoms induced by T-2 toxin in rat brain. *Toxicol. Lett.* **2018**, *286*, 96–107. [CrossRef] [PubMed]
14. Chen, X.; Xu, J.; Liu, D.; Sun, Y.; Qian, G.; Xu, S.; Gan, F.; Pan, C.; Huang, K. The aggravating effect of selenium deficiency on T-2 toxin-induced damage on primary cardiomyocyte results from a reduction of protective autophagy. *Chem. Biol. Interact.* **2019**, *300*, 27–34. [CrossRef] [PubMed]
15. Wu, J.; Zhou, Y.; Yuan, Z.; Yi, J.; Chen, J.; Wang, N.; Tian, Y. Autophagy and Apoptosis Interact to Modulate T-2 Toxin-Induced Toxicity in Liver Cells. *Toxins* **2019**, *11*, 45. [CrossRef] [PubMed]
16. Yang, J.Y.; Zhang, Y.F.; Meng, X.P.; Kong, X.F. Delayed effects of autophagy on T-2 toxin-induced apoptosis in mouse primary Leydig cells. *Toxicol. Ind. Health* **2019**, *35*, 256–263. [CrossRef] [PubMed]
17. Wu, Q.; Wang, X.; Nepovimova, E.; Miron, A.; Liu, Q.; Wang, Y.; Su, D.; Yang, H.; Li, L.; Kuca, K. Trichothecenes: Immunomodulatory effects, mechanisms, and anti-cancer potential. *Arch. Toxicol.* **2017**, *91*, 3737–3785. [CrossRef]
18. Gump, J.M.; Thorburn, A. Autophagy and apoptosis: What is the connection? *Trends Cell Biol.* **2011**, *21*, 387–392. [CrossRef]
19. Thorburn, A. Apoptosis and autophagy: regulatory connections between two supposedly different processes. *Apoptosis* **2008**, *13*, 1–9. [CrossRef]
20. Gordy, C.; He, Y.W. The crosstalk between autophagy and apoptosis: where does this lead? *Protein cell* **2012**, *3*, 17–27. [CrossRef] [PubMed]

*toxins*

MDPI

*Article*

# Reduced Toxicity of Trichothecenes, Isotrichodermol, and Deoxynivalenol, by Transgenic Expression of the *Tri101* 3-*O*-Acetyltransferase Gene in Cultured Mammalian FM3A Cells

**Nozomu Tanaka [1], Ryo Takushima [2], Akira Tanaka [2], Ayaki Okada [1], Kosuke Matsui [3], Kazuyuki Maeda [3], Shunichi Aikawa [4], Makoto Kimura [3] and Naoko Takahashi-Ando [1,2,4,*]**

1 Graduate School of Science and Engineering, Toyo University, 2100 Kujirai, Kawagoe, Saitama 350-8585, Japan; tnknzmjudo@gmail.com (N.T.); berry.wing1418@gmail.com (A.O.)

2 Graduate School of Engineering, Toyo University, 2100 Kujirai, Kawagoe, Saitama 350-8585, Japan; souldout33@hotmail.co.jp (R.T.); word_of_the_world@yahoo.co.jp (A.T.)

3 Department of Biological Mechanisms and Functions, Graduate School of Bioagricultural Sciences, Nagoya University, Furo-cho, Chikusa-ku, Nagoya, Aichi 464-8601, Japan; matsuik.toyo@gmail.com (K.M.); kmaeda@meiji.ac.jp (K.M.); mkimura@agr.nagoya-u.ac.jp (M.K.)

4 Research Institute of Industrial Technology, Toyo University, 2100 Kujirai, Kawagoe, Saitama 350-8585, Japan; s-aikawa@toyo.jp

* Correspondence: ando_n@toyo.jp; Tel.: +81-49-239-1384

Received: 14 September 2019; Accepted: 7 November 2019; Published: 10 November 2019

**Abstract:** In trichothecene-producing fusaria, isotrichodermol (ITDol) is the first intermediate with a trichothecene skeleton. In the biosynthetic pathway of trichothecene, a 3-*O*-acetyltransferase, encoded by *Tri101*, acetylates ITDol to a less-toxic intermediate, isotrichodermin (ITD). Although trichothecene resistance has been conferred to microbes and plants transformed with *Tri101*, there are no reports of resistance in cultured mammalian cells. In this study, we found that a 3-*O*-acetyl group of trichothecenes is liable to hydrolysis by esterases in fetal bovine serum and FM3A cells. We transfected the cells with *Tri101* under the control of the MMTV-LTR promoter and obtained a cell line G3 with the highest level of C-3 acetylase activity. While the wild-type FM3A cells hardly grew in the medium containing 0.40 μM ITDol, many G3 cells survived at this concentration. The $IC_{50}$ values of ITDol and ITD in G3 cells were 1.0 and 9.6 μM, respectively, which were higher than the values of 0.23 and 3.0 μM in the wild-type FM3A cells. A similar, but more modest, tendency was observed in deoxynivalenol and 3-acetyldeoxynivalenol. Our findings indicate that the expression of *Tri101* conferred trichothecene resistance in cultured mammalian cells.

**Keywords:** trichothecene; biosynthetic pathway; acetyltransferase; deacetylase; deoxynivalenol; 3-acetyldeoxynivalenol; isotrichodermol; isotrichodermin

**Key Contribution:** This is the first study to demonstrate that transfection of *Tri101* encoding trichothecene 3-*O*-acetyltransferase confers resistance to trichothecenes in mammalian cells. As the C-3 acetyl group of trichothecenes is liable to be digested by esterases present in cell culture, the toxicities of 3-*O*-acetyltrichothecenes may have been overestimated in previous studies.

## 1. Introduction

Trichothecenes are a group of mycotoxins produced by several filamentous fungi including *Fusarium*. They have a trichothecene skeleton of 12,13-epoxytrichothec-9-ene in common, but their side chain modification greatly varies, resulting in a large difference in their toxicity [1,2]. They exert toxicity mainly through the inhibition of protein synthesis in eukaryotes [3]. Some fusaria are notorious fungi, known to cause *Fusarium* head blight in important crops.

Based on the biosynthetic pathways, trichothecenes are largely divided into two groups: t-type trichothecenes, with a modifying group at C-3 position, and d-type trichothecenes, without a modifying group [4,5]. In the early biosynthetic pathway of trichothecenes, trichodiene is first synthesized through the cyclization of farnesyl pyrophosphate by Tri5p [6]. Trichodiene is then oxygenated to isotrichotriol, followed by spontaneous cyclization to produce the following t-type trichothecenes: *Fusarium graminearum* produces deoxynivalenol (DON), nivalenol, and their acetylated forms; *Fusarium sporotrichioides* produces T-2 toxin, neosalaniol, and diacetoxyscirpenol. On the other hand, in non-fusaria, including *Myrothecium*, *Trichoderma*, *Trichothecium*, *Stachybotrys*, and *Spicellum* [7], trichodiene is oxygenated to isotrichodiol followed by spontaneous cyclization to produce d-type trichothecenes. There is another classification method of dividing trichothecenes into four types (A–D) based on their chemical structures [8]. Type B group is distinguished from type A group by the presence of a ketone at C-8, and either type is synthesized by both t-type and d-type trichothecene producers. Type C group, which contains a 7,8-epoxide, and type D group, which contains a macrocyclic ring between C-4 and C-15, are exclusively produced by d-type trichothecene producers.

In fusaria, the first trichothecene produced is isotrichodermol (ITDol), which is immediately acetylated at the C-3 position by 3-*O*-acetyltransferase, Tri101p, into isotrichodermin (ITD) [5,9]. It has been reported that a 3-acetylated trichothecene is generally less toxic than its corresponding 3-hydroxy form [10–13]. Hence, it was suggested that Tri101p confers self-resistance to trichothecene produced in fusaria; indeed, *Schizosaccharomyces pombe* transformed with the *Tri101* gene has been found to be more resistant to T-2 toxin than the wild type (WT) [5]. So far, *Tri101* has been isolated from fusaria, including *F. graminearum* and *F. sporotrichioides*, and their enzyme kinetics have been evaluated extensively [14].

Trichothecenes are phytotoxins and may play a role as a virulence factor that contributes toxin producers to infect host plants [15–17]. Therefore, in order to combat *Fusarium* head blight, researchers have made extensive efforts to examine the effect of the transgenic expression of *Tri101* on trichothecene resistance and *Fusarium* infection in host cereals [18]. These studies have unequivocally proved that transgenic tobacco and rice showed improved trichothecene resistance [19,20]. In wheat, moderate tolerance to *Fusarium* infection was observed in a field trial [21]. On the contrary, in barley, deoxynivalenol may not be a virulence factor, and no effect on infection was observed in a field trial [22]. Thus, the gene manipulation of *Tri101* has been effective to confer tolerance to trichothecenes in some host plants, although the effect might be limited.

In contrast to the case with microbes and plants, the effects of trichothecene acetylation at the C-3 position and the transfection of *Tri101* into cultured mammalian cells are complicated to understand. Although there is approximately a 100-fold difference in terms of the in vitro inhibition of protein synthesis in rabbit reticulocytes between 3-acetylated trichothecenes and their corresponding 3-hydroxy forms, this difference was reduced to tenfold in terms of the in vivo inhibition of glycoprotein synthesis in BGK-21 cells [5]. Although it has been reported that a 3-acetyl trichothecene has lower toxicity than its corresponding 3-hydroxy form [2], there is a conflicting report of 3-acetyl T-2 toxin being as toxic as T-2 toxin in human cell cultures [23], and, so far, no reports have shown that improved resistance to trichothecenes is conferred by *Tri101* transfection in cultured mammalian cells. Moreover, it has been reported that the acetyl group at the C-3 position of trichothecene is easily removed in animal systems [24]. In this way, the toxicity of a C-3 acetyl trichothecene has tended to be inaccurately estimated by measuring the toxicity of a mixture of C-3 acetyl and C-3 hydroxy trichothecenes. Therefore, in this study, we attempted to maintain the 3-*O*-acetyl group attached to the trichothecene skeleton by the transgenic expression of *Tri101* in murine FM3A cells, resulting in a more accurate evaluation of the toxicity of 3-acetyl trichothecenes. We also examined whether *Tri101* transfection into mammalian cultured cells improves their resistance to 3-hydorxytrichothecenes.

## 2. Results and Discussion

### 2.1. Deacetylation of 3-Acetyldeoxynivalenol (3-ADON) and ITD

Assuming that the acetyl group of 3-acetyltrichothecenes was cleaved to produce more-toxic 3-hydroxytrichothecenes in cytotoxicity and animal studies, we first verified the extent of the deacetylation of two trichothecenes, 3-ADON, which is an acetylated form of the most common trichothecene DON, and, ITD, the first acetylated trichothecene produced by Tri101p in trichothecene biosynthesis.

First, 3-ADON or ITD was added to $H_2O$, 125 mM Tris-HCl buffer (pH 6.5), and RPMI medium (without any additive), and the solutions were incubated in a $CO_2$ incubator for 48 h. Neither DON nor ITDol was detected in $H_2O$ containing its corresponding 3-acetyltrichothecene, but some deacetylated forms were detected in both the buffer and the RPMI medium after incubation (Supplementary Table S1), which suggests that non-enzymatic deacetylation of these 3-acetylated trichothecenes occurred in them. Next, the actual culture medium for FM3A cells was examined. RPMI medium was supplemented with antibiotics, sodium pyruvate, β-mercaptoethanol, and deactivated fetal bovine serum (FBS). Considering the possibility that FBS contained contaminating esterases, we prepared the culture medium supplemented with non-boiled FBS (designated as N-medium) and boiled FBS (designated as B-medium). When 3-ADON or ITD was added to the media, the deacetylation rates of these trichothecenes were much higher in N-medium than B-medium, with ITD being deacetylated more efficiently than 3-ADON. While up to 96% of ITD was deacetylated to ITDol in the N-medium, only 4.6% of ITD was deacetylated in the B-medium. These results suggest that FBS contained broad-substrate-specificity esterases that could be deactivated by boiling, and ITD was more efficiently deacetylated than 3-ADON by these esterases.

FM3A cells were confirmed to grow in B-medium as normally as in N-medium; thus, the cells were incubated in B-medium containing 3-ADON or ITD in order to examine the stability of 3-*O*-acetyl group of these trichothecenes in a cell culture environment. As shown in Supplementary Table S1, 4.9% and 10.3% of 3-ADON was deacetylated to DON in 3 mL of cell culture medium containing $1 \times 10^5$ cells and $6 \times 10^5$ cells, respectively, while 17.0% and 39.1% ITD was deacetylated to ITDol, respectively. These results suggest that FM3A cells themselves contained esterases acting on C-3 of the trichothecene skeleton.

### 2.2. Transfection of FM3A Cells and Screening Cell Lines with High Expression of *Tri101*

First, we confirmed that the growth of FM3A WT cells was completely suppressed in the N-medium containing 30 μg/mL of blasticidin S and in the B-medium containing 0.1 μg/mL (0.40 μM) of ITDol. The growth of FM3A transfected with an empty vector was also completely suppressed in the B-medium containing 0.40 μM of ITDol. Thus, just after transfection of the vector carrying *Tri101*, the transformants were screened in N-medium with 60 μg/mL of blasticidin S and, subsequently, with increasing concentrations of the antibiotic (up to 250 μg/mL). Next, we transferred the screened cells into B-medium with 0.40 μM of ITDol, followed by B-medium with 0.80 μM of ITDol, in order to screen the transformants with a high Tri101p activity. Over 100 cell lines that survived the screening process were then cloned in B-medium containing 0.16 μM of ITDol by limiting dilution. Crude enzyme was prepared from each clone and the Tri101p activity toward ITDol or DON was initially evaluated by TLC, followed by HPLC. We selected one cell line, designated as G3, which showed the highest Tri101p activity. In the absence of the drugs, the growth rate of G3 was comparable to that of the WT cells.

### 2.3. Acetylase and Deacetylase Activities of Crude Cell Extracts from WT and G3 Cells

Next, we measured the in vitro acetylase activities of WT and the transformant G3 cells by HPLC. We added 169 μM DON or 200 μM ITDol at a final concentration to the reaction mixture, in order to measure the approximate $V_{max}$, as these concentrations were much higher than the $K_m$ values for DON and ITDol, 11.7 and 10.2 μM, respectively [14]. The crude enzymes from the WT cells showed no acetylase activities toward either substrate, with or without induction by dexamethasone (DEX; an inducer of transgene expression) (Figure 1, right). In contrast, the crude enzymes from the G3 cells showed acetylase activities toward both DON and ITDol. As expected, significantly higher acetylase activities were observed in the crude enzymes from G3 cells pretreated with DEX than in those without DEX ($p < 0.05$). This result is consistent with the previous observation that DEX resulted in a two- to fivefold increase in the levels of expression of a luciferase gene from the mouse mammary tumor virus-long terminal repeat (MMTV-LTR) promoter in FM3A cells [25]. All the crude enzyme prepared here showed deacetylase activities toward both 3-ADON and ITD (Figure 1, left).

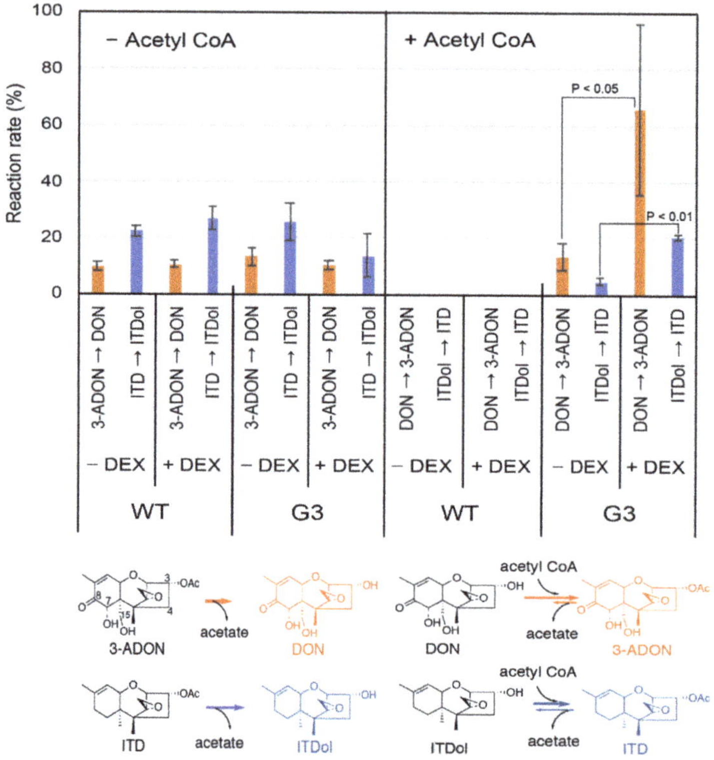


**Figure 1.** Acetylase and deacetylase activities of crude enzymes from FM3A cells. Wild-type (WT) and the transformant (G3) cells were pretreated with or without DEX (dexamethasone) and the crude enzyme was prepared from the harvested cells. The enzyme reaction was carried out in 200 μL reaction mixture, with (**right**) or without (**left**) 1 mM acetyl CoA, and 10 μg of a trichothecene as a substrate; 148 μM 3-ADON (3-acetyldeoxynivalenol), 171 μM ITD (isotrichodermin), 169 μM DON (deoxynivalenol), or 200 μM ITDol (isotrichodermol) at a final concentration. The trichothecene denoted at the root of the arrows represents the substrate, while the trichothecene at the tip of the arrow is the product. The percentage reaction rate (%) represents the initial molar ratio of the product over the added substrate per protein (1.0 mg/mL) in the reaction mixture. The values represent the average ± standard deviation (SD) ($n = 3$).

### 2.4. Acquired Trichothecene Resistance in the Cells Transfected with *Tri101*

After the WT and G3 cells were seeded in the B-medium, the vehicle or ITDol was added to the culture medium, and the cell numbers were counted on day 3, 5, or 7 (Figure 2). Both WT and G3 cells grew normally until day 3 in the medium containing the vehicle, after which they underwent apoptosis. In contrast, in B-medium containing 0.40 μM ITDol, almost all the WT cells underwent apoptosis by day 3, but G3 cells continued to grow until day 5, after which the cell numbers decreased. In B-medium containing 0.80 μM ITDol, the G3 cells slowly continued to grow until day 5–7. In the medium containing a higher concentration of ITDol, even the G3 cells struggled to grow. Thus, it was concluded that G3 cells had acquired resistance to ITDol. This is the first study reporting that the transfection of *Tri101* into mammalian cells confers resistance to trichothecenes.

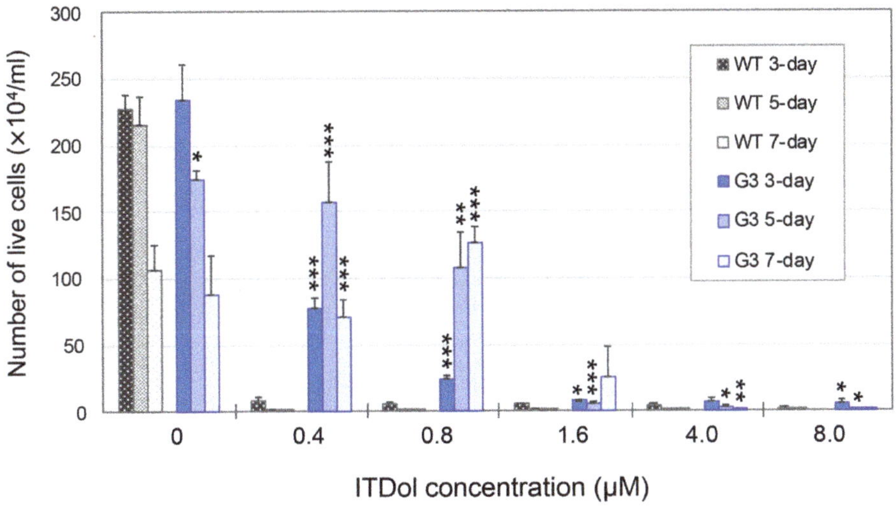


**Figure 2.** Growth of WT and the transformant G3 cells in B-medium containing ITDol. After pretreatment with DEX, the cells were seeded in 24-well plates, and ITDol solution was added to the cells. On day 3, 5, and 7, the cells were harvested and diluted with trypan blue solution, and the number of the live cells were counted. The values represent the average ± SD ($n = 3$). The numbers of live cells of G3 which showed statistical differences from those of their corresponding WT are marked with asterisks (* $p < 0.05$; ** $p < 0.01$; *** $p < 0.001$).

*2.5. Cytotoxicity Evaluation of Each Trichothecene in WT and G3 Cells*

We performed a water-soluble tetrazolium salts (WST) assay to evaluate the cytotoxicity of DON, 3-ADON, ITDol, and ITD more accurately, based on the assumption that the cytotoxicity of 3-acetyltrichothecenes had been overestimated in previous studies. First, the half maximal inhibitory concentration ($IC_{50}$) values of ITDol and ITD in WT cells were determined using N-medium or B-medium (Supplementary Figure S1). The observed $IC_{50}$ values of ITDol and ITD were close when WT cells were incubated in N-medium (0.19 ± 0.01 and 0.26 ± 0.01 μM, respectively), however, a large difference was evident when assayed in B-medium (0.20 ± 0.01 and 2.14 ± 0.06 μM, respectively). The higher sensitivity of cultured mammalian cells to ITD in N-medium seems to be attributed to the contaminating esterases that act on ITD (Supplementary Table S1), resulting in the formation of much more toxic ITDol. This observation strongly suggests that without an elaboration to keep the 3-acetyl group attached to the ITDol ring, the toxicity of 3-acetyltrichothecene tends to be overestimated. Although the apparent $IC_{50}$ value of 2.14 μM observed for ITD in B-medium could be closer to the actual $IC_{50}$ value of intact ITD, this value may in fact be lower than the actual value, as an acetyl group may not remain attached to the C-3 position of the trichothecene skeleton due to the presence of intrinsic esterases hydrolyzing the 3-*O*-acetyl group in cultured mammalian cells (Figure 1, chemical reactions). Thus, we attempted to measure the concentration of ITDol possibly produced from ITD in the cell culture medium in this assay; however, ITDol was not detected in our HPLC analysis (limit of detection; 1.2 μM). As the $IC_{50}$ value of FM3A cells against ITDol was as low as 0.22 μM (Figure 3),

ITDol levels below the detection limit possibly affected cell growth. The higher toxicity of ITD may be explained by the C-3 deacetylation of ITD during the assay.

Next, in order to evaluate cytotoxicity of 3-ADON and ITD more accurately, we determined their $IC_{50}$ values using G3 cells expressing *Tri101*. Figure 3A shows the dose–response cytotoxicity curves of DON and 3-ADON using WT and G3 cells. In WT cells, the difference in the $IC_{50}$ values between DON and 3-ADON was around 12-fold. In G3 cells, all the $IC_{50}$ values were increased significantly compared to their corresponding values in WT cells. The $IC_{50}$ value in G3 cells pretreated with DEX was slightly higher than that without DEX, and the values were significantly different in DON, but not in 3-ADON. No significant difference was observed in the $IC_{50}$ value of these trichothecenes in WT cells with and without DEX pretreatment. These results indicate that the transformant G3 cells were more resistant to both DON and 3-ADON than WT cells due to the expression of *Tri101* in G3 cells. As it is likely that the more accurate $IC_{50}$ of 3-ADON was that of G3 cells treated with DEX (11.68 μM), this value was significantly higher than that of WT cells (7.09 μM without DEX, 6.45 μM with DEX) suggesting that cytotoxicity of 3-ADON might be overestimated in previous studies. Here, the $IC_{50}$ of 3-ADON was at least 21-fold higher than that of DON (0.56 μM) obtained in WT.

The effect of the transgenic expression of *Tri101* in G3 was more obvious in the $IC_{50}$ values of ITDol and ITD than in those of DON and 3-ADON. Figure 3B presents the result of the WST assay of ITDol and ITD in WT and G3 cells. In WT cells, the difference of the $IC_{50}$ values between ITDol and ITD was 13–16 fold. In G3 cells, without DEX induction, the $IC_{50}$ values of ITDol and ITD were almost doubled compared to those in the WT cells. Moreover, with DEX induction, the $IC_{50}$ values of ITDol and ITD were three- to fourfold compared with those in the WT cells. This indicates that DEX induced *Tri101* expression, which resulted in the increased acetylation of ITDol to ITD. Thus, the $IC_{50}$ values of both ITDol and ITD were almost doubled in G3 cells treated with DEX compared to those without DEX, and the values were significantly higher in both ITDol and ITD by DEX pretreatment. In WT cells, no significant increase was observed in the $IC_{50}$ value of these trichothecenes by DEX pretreatment. Similar to DON and 3-ADON, a more accurate $IC_{50}$ of ITD was likely to be that of G3 cells treated with DEX (9.58 μM), thus, this value was significantly higher than that of WT cells (2.78 μM without DEX, 3.59 μM with DEX), suggesting that cytotoxicity of ITD in previous studies might be overestimated. It represented an at least 44-fold increase of $IC_{50}$ value of ITD (9.58 μM), which is supposedly to be more accurate, compared to that of ITDol obtained in WT (0.21–0.22 μM).

In this study, the level of *Tri101* expression was found to affect the $IC_{50}$ values of trichothecenes in mammalian transformants. However, the *Tri101* expression level may not be sufficient to fully compete with the C-3 deacetylation activity of strong endogenous esterases. Nevertheless, this study clearly showed that the 3-acetyl group of 3-*O*-acetyltrichothecenes could be hydrolyzed enzymatically in mammalian cells and that their cytotoxicities were overestimated in other studies. The $IC_{50}$ of trichothecenes were much lower than the $K_m$ of Tri101p against them, making it difficult to completely acetylate the C-3 of the trichothecenes added to the culture.

This is the first report to unambiguously demonstrate the acquired trichothecene resistance of cultured mammalian cells transformed with *Tri101*. These results strongly support the theory that C-3 acetylation blocks the toxicity of t-type trichothecenes, which serves as a self-defense mechanism of the producing organisms [5]. In contrast to fungi and plants, the strong C-3 deacetylase activity of mammalian cells activates 3-acetyltrichothecenes, the toxicity of which has been overestimated in previous studies.

(A)

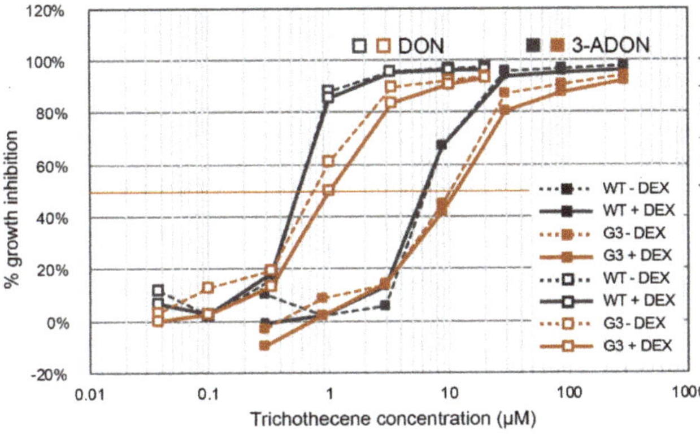


$IC_{50}$ (μM)

| | toxin | - DEX | + DEX |
|---|---|---|---|
| WT | DON | 0.56 ± 0.03 | 0.56 ± 0.02 |
| | 3-ADON | 7.09 ± 0.31 | 6.45 ± 0.20 |
| G3 | DON | 0.80 ± 0.05 | 1.06 ± 0.05 |
| | 3-ADON | 9.88 ± 0.59 | 11.68 ± 0.73 |

(B)

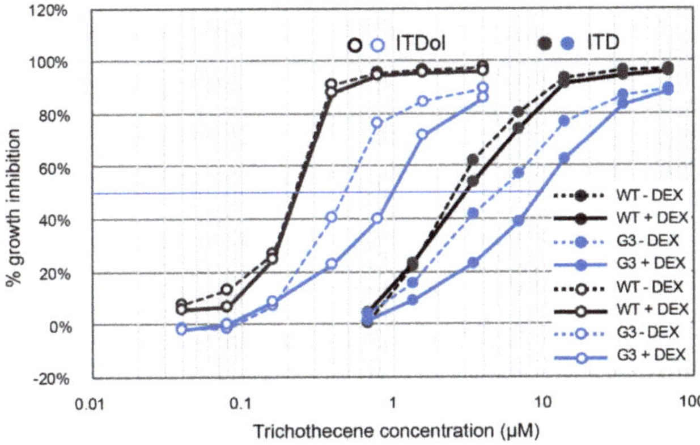


$IC_{50}$ (μM)

| | toxin | - DEX | + DEX |
|---|---|---|---|
| WT | ITDmol | 0.21 ± 0.01 | 0.22 ± 0.01 |
| | ITD | 2.78 ± 0.11 | 3.59 ± 0.38 |
| G3 | ITDmol | 0.50 ± 0.02 | 0.97 ± 0.06 |
| | ITD | 5.12 ± 0.33 | 9.58 ± 0.33 |

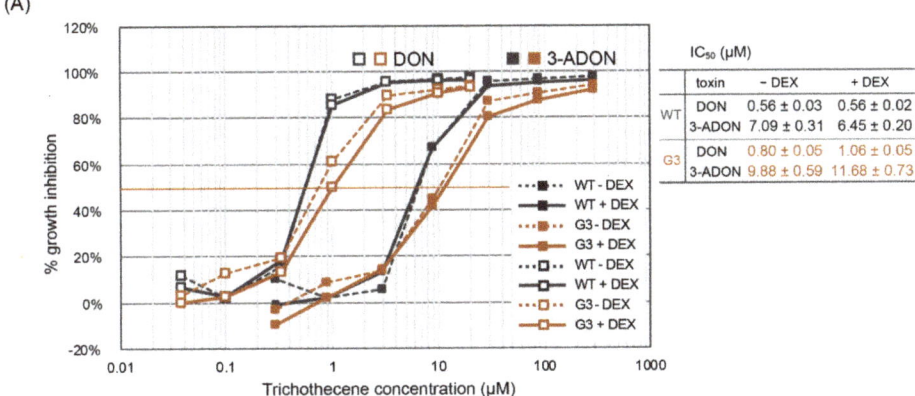

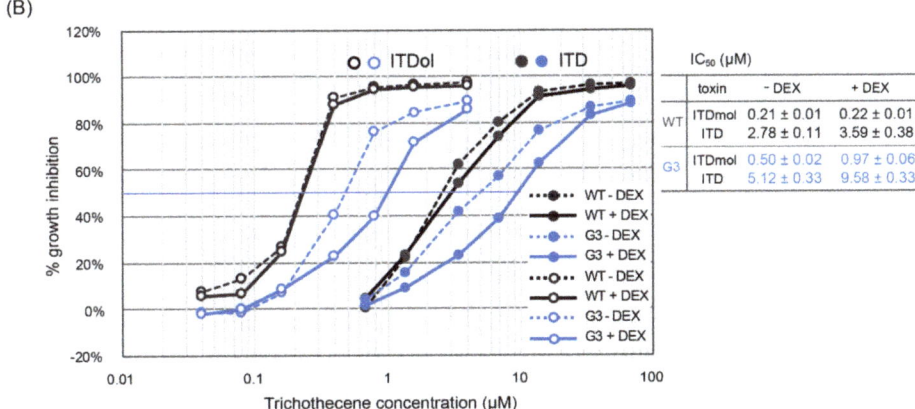

**Figure 3.** The dose–response cytotoxicity curves of the trichothecenes. (**A**) DON or 3-ADON and (**B**) ITDol or ITD was used as a toxin. Cytotoxicity assay of trichothecenes on FM3A cells was carried out using Cell Counting Kit 8 (CCK-8) reagent in 96-well plates. Cells were pretreated with or without 50 μM DEX. One microliter of a toxin or vehicle was added to 99 μL of cell culture, which was seeded ($5 \times 10^4$/mL) one day before. After two days of incubation with a toxin or vehicle, a WST assay was performed. Growth inhibition (%) was calculated as follows: $100 \times \{(OD_{450}$ of vehicle control − $OD_{450}$ of background) − ($OD_{450}$ of trichothecene added − $OD_{450}$ of background)}/($OD_{450}$ of vehicle control − $OD_{450}$ of background). The $IC_{50}$ values represent the average ± standard error.

## 3. Materials and Methods

### 3.1. Production and Purification of Trichothecenes

Each trichothecene was obtained from rice medium [26] or rice flour liquid medium [27] inoculated with *F. graminearum*: *Gibberella zeae* JCM 9873 for DON [28] and *F. graminearum* DSM 4528 for 3-acetyldeoxynivalenol (3-ADON) [29]. Isotrichodermin was obtained from the culture medium of *F. graminearum* MAFF 111233 *Fgtri11* disruptant (*Fgtri11*$^-$, NBRC 113181) [27], while ITDol was obtained by the deacetylation of ITD in 2.8% ammonium solution. For purification, the ethyl acetate extract was applied to Purif-Rp2 equipped with Purif-Pack SI 30 μm SIZE (Shoko Scientific, Kanagawa, Japan), and the fraction containing a target trichothecene was concentrated. The concentrate was dissolved in ethanol and applied to preparative HPLC (UV detection at 254 nm for DON and 3-ADON, and at

195 nm for ITD and ITDol) equipped with a $C_{18}$ column (Pegasil ODS SP100 10 φ × 250 mm, Senshu Scientific Co., Ltd., Tokyo, Japan). The concentration of each purified trichothecene was measured by HPLC equipped with a $C_{18}$ column (Pegasil ODS SP100 4.6 φ × 250 mm) based on the standard curve previously obtained. The purity of each trichothecene used for the assays was confirmed to be >99%.

### 3.2. *Maintenance of Cultured Cells*

FM3A WT cells which were originally established from mammary carcinoma in C3H/He mouse were purchased from RIKEN BRC (Tsukuba, Japan). Cells were grown in RPMI1640 medium (Nacalai Tesque Co., Inc. Kyoto, Japan) with 10% FBS (Biowest, Nuaillé, France), penicillin/streptomycin (1000 units/mL each), 1 mM sodium pyruvate, and 50 μM 2-mercaptoethanol, denoted "N (non-boiled)-medium." In order to deactivate any contaminating esterases in FBS, we prepared the same medium with FBS boiled at 100 °C for 5 min beforehand, denoted "B (boiled)-medium." Cultured cells were incubated in a $CO_2$ incubator (5% $CO_2$, 37 °C).

### 3.3. *Evaluation of Stability of 3-Acetyl Trichothecenes*

Twenty micrograms of 3-ADON (59.1 nmol) or ITD (68.4 nmol) in ethanol was added into a 6 cm dish containing 3 mL of water, 125 mM Tris-HCl buffer (pH 6.8), and RPMI1640 medium without any supplements. Each solution was incubated in a $CO_2$ incubator (5% $CO_2$, 37 °C) for 48 h. Similarly, 3 mL of the N-medium and B-medium containing 10 μg of 3-ADON (29.6 nmol) or ITD (34.2 nmol) was incubated in a $CO_2$ incubator for 48 h. We also prepared FM3A WT cells ($3.3 \times 10^4$/mL or $2 \times 10^5$/mL) in 3 mL B-medium supplemented with 10 μg of 3-ADON or ITD. After 48 h, each solution or medium was extracted with the same volume of ethyl acetate twice. The extract was dried up under an $N_2$ stream and resuspended in 200 μL ethanol. These concentrating steps were necessary for detection of the mycotoxins. The filtered samples were subjected to HPLC.

### 3.4. *Plasmid Construction*

*Tri101* was excised from pCold-His-TRI101 [30] by double digestion with *Nde*I and *Eco*RI. The *Nde*I–*Eco*RI fragment was cloned into the corresponding sites of pColdIII-NFH (Supplementary Figure S2). The *Tri101* sequence, *N*-terminally fused with a FLAG-HA tag, was amplified by PCR from the resulting plasmid using primers FLAG-HA-Tri101F_NheI (5′-AAAAGCTAGCATGGACTACAAGGACGACGAT-3′) and FLAG-HA-Tri101R_XhoI (5′-AAAACTCGAGCTAACCAACGTACTGCGCATA-3′). After double digestion with *Nhe*I and *Xho*I, the PCR product was inserted between these sites downstream of a MMTV-LTR promoter in pMAM2BSD [25], yielding a DEX-inducible *Tri101* expression vector, pMAM2BSD_FH_Tri101.

### 3.5. *Transfection of FM3A Cells and Selection of Transformants*

The plasmid pMAM2BSD_FH_Tri101 or pMAM2BSD was transfected into FM3A cells using Lipofectamine® 2000 reagent (Thermo Fisher Scientific, Waltham, MA, USA) following the manufacturer's instructions. Plasmid DNA (5 μg) was diluted in 100 μL Opti-MEM medium without FBS. Five microliters of Lipofectamine® 2000 was diluted in 100 μL of Opti-MEM medium and left for 5 min. Diluted plasmid DNA and Lipofectamine were mixed gently and left for 20 min and added to FM3A cells ($7 \sim 10 \times 10^5$/3 mL).

Transfected cells were incubated for one day before being transferred to N-medium containing 60 μg/mL of blasticidin S (Fujifilm Wako Pure Chemical Co., Osaka, Japan). During selection, the concentration of blasticidin S was increased to 250 μg/mL over one month. For the next selection step, the cells were transferred to B-medium containing 50 μM DEX and 0.1 μg/mL (0.4 μM) ITDol. The ITDol concentration was increased to 0.2 μg/mL (0.8 μM) over three weeks. The selected transformants (>100 cell lines) were cloned using limited dilution methods in B-medium containing 50 μM DEX and 0.04 μg/mL ITDol (0.16 μM). After limited dilution, both DEX and ITDol were removed from the medium. Among the survived transformants in this condition, the cell line whose crude enzyme showed the highest 3-*O*-acetyltransferase activity was chosen and designated as G3. Measurement of activities of prepared crude enzymes was performed as described below.

### *3.6. Preparation and Reaction of Crude Enzymes from Cultured Cells*

Wild-type FM3A cells and the selected transformants were seeded (10 mL aliquots of cell suspension at 1 × $10^4$/mL). After a three-day incubation period, DEX (50 μM at final concentration) was added for the induction of *Tri101* expression in the transformed cells, and for comparison, in WT cells. In parallel, the carrier solvent (10% dimethylsulfoxide [DMSO]; 0.1% DMSO at a final concentration) was added to these cells. Once the cells became semi-confluent, these were harvested and washed twice in 2 mL PBS. The washed cells were suspended in 500 μL of 125 mM Tris-HCl buffer (pH 6.8) and sonicated. After centrifugation (13,000 rpm at 4 °C for 5 min), the supernatant was subjected to a protein quantitation assay (Pierce$^{TM}$ BCA protein assay kit, Thermo Fisher Scientific). The resulting crude enzyme fraction was assayed for modification activity against C-3 of the trichothecene skeleton.

To initiate the reaction, 100 μL of the crude enzyme (with a protein concentration around 1.0 mg/mL) was mixed with 100 μL of substrate solution, which contained a 3-hydroxy (169 μM DON or 200 μM ITDol) or 3-acetyl (148 μM 3-ADON or 171 μM ITD) trichothecene in 125 mM Tris-HCl buffer (pH 6.5), respectively, with or without 1 mM acetyl CoA. We used rTRI101 from *Escherichia coli* (BL21 (DE3)-pColdIII-*Tri101*) (1 mg/mL) [30] as a positive control and boiled rTRI101 as a negative control. Each enzyme assay was performed in triplicate. The mixture was incubated for 3 h at 37 °C and the reaction was terminated by adding 200 μL of ethyl acetate. Trichothecenes were extracted with ethyl acetate three times, concentrated under $N_2$, resuspended in the appropriate amount of ethanol, and subjected to TLC and HPLC analysis.

### *3.7. TLC and HPLC Analysis*

The trichothecenes in each sample were detected roughly by TLC and the concentration of each trichothecene was precisely measured by HPLC. The samples dissolved in ethanol were applied to TLC plates (Merck, Darmstadt, Germany) and developed with ethyl acetate/toluene (3:1). Trichothecenes on TLC plates were visualized using the 4-(p-nitrobenzyl)pyridine-tetraethylenepentamine method [31].

For HPLC analysis, the samples dissolved in ethanol were filtered, and 10 μL was applied to HPLC (LC-2000 plus; Jasco, Tokyo, Japan) loaded with a $C_{18}$ reverse-phase column (4.6 φ × 250 mm, PEGASIL ODS SP100). Trichothecenes were eluted with a mobile phase of acetonitrile and water, according to the following steps: for DON and 3-ADON, 20% acetonitrile for 6 min, a linear gradient of 20%–50% acetonitrile for 9 min, 50% acetonitrile held for 6 min, then 20% acetonitrile held for 10 min; for ITDol and ITD, 20% acetonitrile for 6 min, a linear gradient of 20%–100% acetonitrile for 16 min, 100% acetonitrile held for 3 min, then 20% acetonitrile held for 10 min. Deoxynivalenol and 3-ADON were detected at 254 nm, while ITDol and ITD were detected at 195 nm. The molar concentration of each trichothecene was calculated from the peak area, based on the previously obtained standard curve.

### *3.8. Toxicity Evaluation of Trichothecenes*

In order to evaluate the effect of *Tri101* gene transfection into FM3A cells, we counted the number of live WT and G3 cells, to which ITDol had been added beforehand. First, the cells were seeded at 5 × $10^4$/mL in B-medium and were treated with 50 μM DEX. After one day of incubation, 1 mL of the cells were transferred to a 24-well plate and ITDol (0, 0.4, 0.8, 1.6, 4.0, or 8.0 μM ITDol in 0.1% DMSO at a final concentration) was added and incubated for 3, 5, or 7 days in a $CO_2$ incubator at 37 °C. The cells were carefully harvested and centrifuged (300× *g*, 5 min, 25 °C). The precipitated cells were then tapped gently, and the appropriate amount of medium was added. The cell suspension was diluted twofold with 0.5% trypan blue (Nacalai Tesque) and only the live cells were counted.

For the cytotoxicity evaluation, colorimetric cell viability assays using WST-8 were performed. Each trichothecene was prepared in 50% DMSO as follows: for DON, 0, 0.0034, 0.010, 0.034, 0.10, 0.34, 1.0, or 2.0 mM (0, 0.001, 0.003, 0.01, 0.03, 0.1, 0.3, or 0.6 mg/mL); for 3-ADON, 0, 0.030, 0.089, 0.30,

0.89, 3.0, 8.9, or 30 mM (0, 0.01, 0.03, 0.1, 0.3, 1.0, 3.0, or 10.0 mg/mL); for ITDol, 0, 0.004, 0.008, 0.016, 0.040, 0.080, 0.16, or 0.40 mM (0, 0.001, 0.002, 0.004, 0.01, 0.02, 0.04, or 0.10 mg/mL); for ITD, 0, 0.0068, 0.014, 0.034, 0.068, 0.14, 0.34, 0.68, 1.4, 3.4, or 6.8 mM (0, 0.002, 0.004, 0.01, 0.02, 0.04, 0.1, 0.2, 0.4, 1.0, or 2.0 mg/mL). Wild-type or G3 cells were suspended at a cell density of $5 \times 10^4$/mL in B-medium with or without 50 μM DEX and incubated for one day. Into each well of 96-well plates, 99 L of cell suspension was seeded and 1 μL of each trichothecene prepared above or 50% DMSO (vehicle) was added in triplicate. The cells were incubated for 48 h in a $CO_2$ incubator. Into each well, 10 μL of Cell Counting Kit (CCK)-8 solution (Dojindo Molecular Technologies, Inc., Kumamoto, Japan) was added, and the microtiter plate was incubated for 3 h at 37 °C. $OD_{450}$ was measured using a Multiskan$^{TM}$ FC plate reader (Thermo Fisher Scientific), and growth inhibition (%) caused by each trichothecene was calculated.

### 3.9. Statistical Analysis

Statistical analysis was performed using Student's *t*-test. Regarding the calculation and statistical analysis of $IC_{50}$ values, log-logistic model was applied using R version 3.5.0 (R project for statistical computing).

**Supplementary Materials:** The following are available online at http://www.mdpi.com/2072-6651/11/11/654/s1, Table S1: The rate of deacetylation of 3-ADON and ITD under various conditions, Figure S1: The dose–response cytotoxicity curves of trichothecenes, Figure S2: Construction of pMAM2BSD_FH_Tri101.

**Author Contributions:** N.T., R.T., and A.T. performed the cell culture experiments and analyses. A.O., K.M. (Kosuke Matsui), and S.A. produced, purified and identified each trichothecene. K.M. (Kazuyuki Maeda) produced the plasmid. M.K. and N.T.-A. designed the experiments and discussed the draft manuscript. N.T.-A. wrote the paper.

**Funding:** This study was supported by the Tojuro Iijima Foundation for Food Science and Technology (H27-Kyodo-11, H25-Kojin-37), Grant-in-Aid for Scientific Research (KAKENHI 15K07459), and the Science Research Promotion Fund (the Promotion and Mutual Aid Corporation for Private School of Japan, 2018 and 2019).

**Acknowledgments:** We greatly acknowledge T. Sagawa, Y. Yashiro, and Y. Higuchi for their technical assistance, and T. Matsumura, a professional statistician, in WAKARA (Tokyo Japan) for his technical support with statistical analysis. We are also very thankful to D. Yamanaka and S. Takahashi from the University of Tokyo for their invaluable advice.

**Conflicts of Interest:** The authors declare no conflict of interest.

## References

1. Kimura, M.; Tokai, T.; Takahashi-Ando, N.; Ohsato, S.; Fujimura, M. Molecular and genetic studies of *Fusarium* trichothecene biosynthesis: Pathways, genes, and evolution. *Biosci. Biotechnol. Biochem.* **2007**, *71*, 2105–2123. [CrossRef] [PubMed]
2. Wu, Q.; Dohnal, V.; Kuca, K.; Yuan, Z. Trichothecenes: Structure-toxic activity relationships. *Curr. Drug Metab.* **2013**, *14*, 641–660. [CrossRef] [PubMed]
3. Pestka, J.J. Deoxynivalenol: Toxicity, mechanisms and animal health risks. *Anim. Feed Sci. Technol.* **2007**, *137*, 283–298. [CrossRef]
4. McCormick, S.P.; Stanley, A.M.; Stover, N.A.; Alexander, N.J. Trichothecenes: From simple to complex mycotoxins. *Toxins* **2011**, *3*, 802–814. [CrossRef]
5. Kimura, M.; Kaneko, I.; Komiyama, M.; Takatsuki, A.; Koshino, H.; Yoneyama, K.; Yamaguchi, I. Trichothecene 3-*O*-acetyltransferase protects both the producing organism and transformed yeast from related mycotoxins. Cloning and characterization of *Tri101*. *J. Biol. Chem.* **1998**, *273*, 1654–1661. [CrossRef]
6. Tokai, T.; Koshino, H.; Takahashi-Ando, N.; Sato, M.; Fujimura, M.; Kimura, M. *Fusarium Tri4* encodes a key multifunctional cytochrome P450 monooxygenase for four consecutive oxygenation steps in trichothecene biosynthesis. *Biochem. Biophys. Res. Commun.* **2007**, *353*, 412–417. [CrossRef]
7. Proctor, R.H.; McCormick, S.P.; Kim, H.S.; Cardoza, R.E.; Stanley, A.M.; Lindo, L.; Kelly, A.; Brown, D.W.; Lee, T.; Vaughan, M.M.; et al. Evolution of structural diversity of trichothecenes, a family of toxins produced by plant pathogenic and entomopathogenic fungi. *PLoS Pathog.* **2018**, *14*, e1006946. [CrossRef]

8. Ueno, Y.; Nakajima, M.; Sakai, K.; Ishii, K.; Sato, N. Comparative toxicology of trichothec mycotoxins: Inhibition of protein synthesis in animal cells. *J. Biochem.* **1973**, *74*, 285–296.
9. McCormick, S.P.; Alexander, N.J.; Trapp, S.E.; Hohn, T.M. Disruption of *TRI101*, the gene encoding trichothecene 3-*O*-acetyltransferase, from *Fusarium sporotrichioides*. *Appl. Environ. Microbiol.* **1999**, *65*, 5252–5256.
10. Thompson, W.L.; Wannemacher, R.W., Jr. Structure-function relationships of 12,13-epoxytrichothecene mycotoxins in cell culture: Comparison to whole animal lethality. *Toxicon* **1986**, *24*, 985–994. [CrossRef]
11. Eriksen, G.S.; Pettersson, H.; Lundh, T. Comparative cytotoxicity of deoxynivalenol, nivalenol, their acetylated derivatives and de-epoxy metabolites. *Food Chem. Toxicol.* **2004**, *42*, 619–624. [CrossRef] [PubMed]
12. Desjardins, A.E.; McCormick, S.P.; Appell, M. Structure-activity relationships of trichothecene toxins in an *Arabidopsis thaliana* leaf assay. *J. Agric. Food Chem.* **2007**, *55*, 6487–6492. [CrossRef] [PubMed]
13. Abbas, H.K.; Yoshizawa, T.; Shier, W.T. Cytotoxicity and phytotoxicity of trichothecene mycotoxins produced by *Fusarium* spp. *Toxicon* **2013**, *74*, 68–75. [CrossRef] [PubMed]
14. Garvey, G.S.; McCormick, S.P.; Rayment, I. Structural and functional characterization of the *TRI101* trichothecene 3-*O*-acetyltransferase from *Fusarium sporotrichioides* and *Fusarium graminearum*: Kinetic insights to combating *Fusarium* head blight. *J. Biol. Chem.* **2008**, *283*, 1660–1669. [CrossRef]
15. Jansen, C.; von Wettstein, D.; Schafer, W.; Kogel, K.H.; Felk, A.; Maier, F.J. Infection patterns in barley and wheat spikes inoculated with wild-type and trichodiene synthase gene disrupted *Fusarium graminearum*. *Proc. Natl. Acad. Sci. USA* **2005**, *102*, 16892–16897. [CrossRef]
16. Kazan, K.; Gardiner, D.M.; Manners, J.M. On the trail of a cereal killer: Recent advances in *Fusarium graminearum* pathogenomics and host resistance. *Mol. Plant Pathol.* **2012**, *13*, 399–413. [CrossRef]
17. McLaughlin, J.E.; Bin-Umer, M.A.; Widiez, T.; Finn, D.; McCormick, S.; Tumer, N.E. A lipid transfer protein increases the glutathione content and enhances *Arabidopsis* resistance to a trichothecene mycotoxin. *PLoS ONE* **2015**, *10*, e0130204. [CrossRef]
18. Karlovsky, P. Biological detoxification of the mycotoxin deoxynivalenol and its use in genetically engineered crops and feed additives. *Appl. Microbiol. Biotechnol.* **2011**, *91*, 491–504. [CrossRef]
19. Muhitch, M.J.; McCormick, S.P.; Alexander, N.J.; Hohn, T.M. Transgenic expression of the *TRI101* or *PDR5* gene increases resistance of tobacco to the phytotoxic effects of the trichothecene 4,15-diacetoxyscirpenol. *Plant Sci.* **2000**, *157*, 201–207. [CrossRef]
20. Ohsato, S.; Ochiai-Fukuda, T.; Nishiuchi, T.; Takahashi-Ando, N.; Koizumi, S.; Hamamoto, H.; Kudo, T.; Yamaguchi, I.; Kimura, M. Transgenic rice plants expressing trichothecene 3-*O*-acetyltransferase show resistance to the *Fusarium* phytotoxin deoxynivalenol. *Plant Cell Rep.* **2007**, *26*, 531–538. [CrossRef]
21. Okubara, P.A.; Blechl, A.E.; McCormick, S.P.; Alexander, N.J.; Dill-Macky, R.; Hohn, T.M. Engineering deoxynivalenol metabolism in wheat through the expression of a fungal trichothecene acetyltransferase gene. *Theor. Appl. Genet.* **2002**, *106*, 74–83. [CrossRef] [PubMed]
22. Manoharan, M.; Dahleen, L.S.; Hohn, T.M.; Neate, S.M.; Yu, X.H.; Alexander, N.J.; McCormick, S.P.; Bregitzer, P.; Schwarz, P.B.; Horsley, R.D. Expression of 3-OH trichothecene acetyltransferase in barley (*Hordeum vulgare* L.) and effects on deoxynivalenol. *Plant Sci.* **2006**, *171*, 699–706. [CrossRef]
23. Chanh, T.C.; Hewetson, J.F. Structure/function studies of T-2 mycotoxin with a monoclonal antibody. *Immunopharmacology* **1991**, *21*, 83–89. [CrossRef]
24. Eriksen, G.S.; Pettersson, H.; Lindberg, J.E. Absorption, metabolism and excretion of 3-acetyl DON in pigs. *Arch. Tierernahr.* **2003**, *57*, 335–345. [CrossRef] [PubMed]
25. Kimura, M.; Takatsuki, A.; Yamaguchi, I. Blasticidin S deaminase gene from *Aspergillus terreus* (BSD): A new drug resistance gene for transfection of mammalian cells. *Biochim. Biophys. Acta* **1994**, *1219*, 653–659. [CrossRef]
26. Tanaka, A.; Shinkai, K.; Maeda, K.; Nakajima, Y.; Ishii, S.; Yoshida, Y.; Kimura, M.; Takahashi-Ando, N. Comparison of HPLC-UV and LC-MS methods for evaluating the amount of deoxynivalenol-type trichothecenes in axenic solid culture of *Fusarium graminearum*. *JSM Mycotoxins* **2019**, *69*, 15–17. [CrossRef]
27. Maeda, K.; Tanaka, A.; Sugiura, R.; Koshino, H.; Tokai, T.; Sato, M.; Nakajima, Y.; Tanahashi, Y.; Kanamaru, K.; Kobayashi, T.; et al. Hydroxylations of trichothecene rings in the biosynthesis of *Fusarium* trichothecenes: Evolution of alternative pathways in the nivalenol chemotype. *Environ. Microbiol.* **2016**, *18*, 3798–3811. [CrossRef]

28. Sugiura, Y.; Watanabe, Y.; Tanaka, T.; Yamamoto, S.; Ueno, Y. Occurrence of *Gibberella zeae* strains that produce both nivalenol and deoxynivalenol. *Appl. Environ. Microbiol.* **1990**, *56*, 3047–3051.
29. Altpeter, F.; Posselt, U.K. Production of high quantities of 3-acetyldeoxynivalenol and deoxynivalenol. *Appl. Microbiol. Biotechnol.* **1994**, *41*, 384–387. [CrossRef]
30. Nakajima, Y.; Kawamura, T.; Maeda, K.; Ichikawa, H.; Motoyama, T.; Kondoh, Y.; Saito, T.; Kobayashi, T.; Yoshida, M.; Osada, H.; et al. Identification and characterization of an inhibitor of trichothecene 3-*O*-acetyltransferase, *TRI101*, by the chemical array approach. *Biosci. Biotechnol. Biochem.* **2013**, *77*, 1958–1960. [CrossRef]
31. Takahashi-Ando, N.; Tokai, T.; Yoshida, M.; Fujimura, M.; Kimura, M. An easy method to identify 8-keto-15-hydroxytrichothecenes by thin-layer chromatography. *Mycotoxins* **2008**, *58*, 115–117. [CrossRef]

*toxins*

MDPI

*Article*

# Twenty-Eight Fungal Secondary Metabolites Detected in Pig Feed Samples: Their Occurrence, Relevance and Cytotoxic Effects In Vitro

**Barbara Novak [1,*], Valentina Rainer [1], Michael Sulyok [2], Dietmar Haltrich [3], Gerd Schatzmayr [1] and Elisabeth Mayer [1]**

1 BIOMIN Research Center, Technopark 1, 3430 Tulln, Austria; valentina.rainer@biomin.net (V.R.); gerd.schatzmayr@biomin.net (G.S.); e.mayer@biomin.net (E.M.)

2 Institute of Bioanalytics and Agro-Metabolomics, University of Natural Resources and Life Sciences, Konrad-Lorenz-Straße 20, 3430 Tulln, Austria; michael.sulyok@boku.ac.at

3 Food Biotechnology Laboratory, Department of Food Science and Technology, University of Natural Resources and Life Sciences, Muthgasse 11, 1190 Vienna, Austria; dietmar.haltrich@boku.ac.at

* Correspondence: barbara.novak@biomin.net; Tel.: +43-2272-81166-13480

Received: 27 August 2019; Accepted: 11 September 2019; Published: 14 September 2019

**Abstract:** Feed samples are frequently contaminated by a wide range of chemically diverse natural products, which can be determined using highly sensitive analytical techniques. Next to already well-investigated mycotoxins, unknown or unregulated fungal secondary metabolites have also been found, some of which at significant concentrations. In our study, 1141 pig feed samples were analyzed for more than 800 secondary fungal metabolites using the same LC-MS/MS method and ranked according to their prevalence. Effects on the viability of the 28 most relevant were tested on an intestinal porcine epithelial cell line (IPEC-J2). The most frequently occurring compounds were determined as being cyclo-(L-Pro-L-Tyr), moniliformin, and enniatin B, followed by enniatin B1, aurofusarin, culmorin, and enniatin A1. The main mycotoxins, deoxynivalenol and zearalenone, were found only at ranks 8 and 10. Regarding cytotoxicity, apicidin, gliotoxin, bikaverin, and beauvericin led to lower $IC_{50}$ values, between 0.52 and 2.43 μM, compared to deoxynivalenol ($IC_{50}$ = 2.55 μM). Significant cytotoxic effects were also seen for the group of enniatins, which occurred in up to 82.2% of the feed samples. Our study gives an overall insight into the amount of fungal secondary metabolites found in pig feed samples compared to their cytotoxic effects in vitro.

**Keywords:** *Fusarium*; *Aspergillus*; *Penicillium*; *Alternaria*; fungi; emerging mycotoxin; in vitro; IPEC-J2; occurrence data

**Key Contribution:** Less investigated fungal compounds were found more frequently and in higher concentrations in pig feed samples than regulated mycotoxins. Furthermore, some of them cause stronger cytotoxic effects than deoxynivalenol in vitro.

## 1. Introduction

Mycotoxins are described as secondary fungal metabolites produced by filamentous fungi in the field, and during storage and transportation under appropriate conditions. The main fungal species *Fusarium*, *Alternaria*, *Aspergillus*, and *Penicillium* possess a remarkable potential to produce a wide range of metabolites. Researchers assume that around 38% of the known 22,630 microbial products are of fungal origin; however, the exact number is the still subject of research [1].

The European Food Safety Authority (EFSA) set maximum allowed concentration levels or guidance values for some of these metabolites called "regulated mycotoxins" [2]. These include aflatoxins, deoxynivalenol, HT-2/T-2 toxins, zearalenone, fumonisins, and ochratoxin A, which have been proven to cause detrimental effects in humans and animals. Some other fungal metabolites are so-called "emerging mycotoxins" and are claimed to be metabolites for which no guidance values exist yet. Scientific opinions and risk assessments have only been published for aflatoxin precursors (such as sterigmatocystin), ergot alkaloids, enniatins, beauvericin, and moniliformin so far [3–6]. However, for many other fungal metabolites, only a few, contradictory studies are available [7–9]. One reason for the underestimation of their potential threat might be the limited knowledge about their prevalence. Because of the continuous development of LC-MS/MS (liquid chromatography tandem mass spectroscopy) methods, a more sensitive detection of a wide range of secondary fungal metabolites in feed and food matrixes is now available [10]. Furthermore, studies indicate that climatic change might affect mycotoxin production patterns, leading to an increase in the emerging mycotoxin level [11,12]. In 2013, Streit et al. [13] published data on the *Fusarium* metabolites beauvericin, enniatins, aurofusarin, and moniliformin, which occur in 98%, 96%, 84%, and 76% of 83 analyzed feed samples, respectively. In the same study, the well-investigated mycotoxins deoxynivalenol (89%), zearalenone (87%), and fumonisins (22%) were additionally found in the analyzed samples. Besides, metabolites produced by *Alternaria* spp. were detected in many of the analyzed feed samples (e.g., alternariol, 80%; alternariol monomethyl ether, 82%; tenuazonic acid, 65%; and tentoxin, 80%). Although further publications revealed higher occurrences and concentrations of uncommon mycotoxins, they were limited to specific geographic regions and feed commodities [14–18].

The aim of this study was, first, to provide a complete picture of the effects of 28 chemically diverse fungal metabolites on the cell viability of an intestinal porcine epithelial cell line (IPEC-J2), and second, to compare the tested concentrations with the actual values found in pig feed samples worldwide. The cell line IPEC-J2 was chosen as an optimal test model since the intestine is the first target after ingesting mycotoxin-contaminated feed and most of the metabolites are absorbed in the jejunum [19]. The selection of fungal metabolites to be tested was mainly based on their relevance and occurrence in pig feed samples obtained from the BIOMIN mycotoxin survey program, conducted in the years 2014 to 2019. Here, the most relevant metabolites were *Fusarium*-derived compounds, such as enniatins, beauvericin, moniliformin, culmorin, fusaric acid, etc., but also many compounds produced by the genera *Alternaria*, *Penicillium*, and *Aspergillus* were evaluated. Cytotoxicity studies for selected metabolites are available for different cell types [9,20–23], but here we compared, for the first time, the in vitro effects of 28 metabolites taken from occurrence data of 1141 pig feed samples analyzed with the same analytical method [18].

## 2. Results

### *2.1. Occurrence Data*

The challenge of collecting and analyzing manifold feed samples from all over the world is not only a logistical one, but is mainly found in trying to measure the samples with the same analytical method, limits of detection (LOD), and performance parameters at the same instrument [11] to achieve comparable results. Therefore, BIOMIN started a unique global mycotoxin survey including samples from 44 countries, obtained between February 2014 and February 2019, where 4978 feed samples were analyzed for more than 800 different metabolites using a multi-analyte LC-MS/MS-based method [24]. For our study, we selected 1141 out of the 4978 feed samples that were only intended for swine nutrition.

#### Secondary Fungal Metabolites in Finished Pig Feed Samples

Analyzed pig feed samples were taken as described in Section 5.3.2. and evaluated according to the method of Malachová et al. [24]. The list of analytes in this method has increased over recent years and covers now more than 800 metabolites. The most frequently occurring secondary fungal metabolites of 34 emerging and masked mycotoxins, as well as regulated mycotoxins in samples from 44 different countries, are summarized in Table 1. Twenty-eight metabolites, which are not regulated yet or are defined as an "emerging mycotoxin" [25], were selected to be tested for their effects on the viability of an intestinal porcine epithelial cell line (IPEC-J2). Gliotoxin and patulin were added to these tests because of their previously described harmful effects, making novel data beneficial for the scientific community [26,27]. The uncommon metabolites 15-hydroxy-culmorin, infectopyron, and asperglaucide could not be tested because authentic analytical standards were not commercially available. The prevalence (%), mean, median, and maximum concentrations (in µg/kg) for each compound are summarized in Table 1. In the following section, the focus lies only on the median and maximum concentrations for better legibility.

A ranking according to the prevalence of the main 34 secondary fungal metabolites as shown in Table 1 indicates that the cyclic dipeptide cyclo-(L-Pro-L-Tyr) was most frequently found with an occurrence of 87.6% and a maximum concentration of 34,910 µg/kg; followed by moniliformin (82.6%) and enniatin B (82.2%). Even though the median concentrations of the latter two were only 17 and 30 µg/kg, individual samples reached levels of up to 2053 µg/kg and 1514 µg/kg, respectively. In 82.1% of all pig feed samples, enniatin B1 had similar concentrations as enniatin B (max. 1846 µg/kg; median 34 µg/kg). Two other common enniatins, enniatin A1 and A, were found in 77.4% and 49.5% of all samples, albeit at lower concentrations compared to the B analogues (B and B1). Additionally, samples were vastly contaminated with the *Fusarium* metabolites aurofusarin and culmorin, which were identified in approximately 909 feed samples (79%), with median concentrations of 210 µg/kg and 118 µg/kg, which was comparable to the median concentration of deoxynivalenol (DON) with 193 µg/kg measured in 879 feed samples (77%). This contrasts with the maximum measured concentrations found for aurofusarin (85,360 µg/kg) and culmorin (157,114 µg/kg), while only 34,862 µg/kg for DON was detected. The second regulated mycotoxin on our list was zearalenone (ZEN), which was found at rank 10 with a prevalence of 73.3% and a median concentration of 18 µg/kg. Another uncommon metabolite, which was determined in 75.4% of all samples, was tryptophol, which was thus positioned before ZEN in the ranking according to prevalence. About 69% of the samples were positive for the hexadepsipeptide beauvericin (BEA) with a median concentration of only 6 µg/kg. Individual samples were contaminated with a maximum concentration of 413 µg/kg BEA.

Mainly unexpected compounds, such as emodin, brevianamid F, equisetin (EQUI), and cyclo-(L-Pro-L-Val), were found at the prevalence ranking positions of 13, 15, 16 and 34, respectively. These were nevertheless detected in about 70, 69, 64 and 62% of all feed samples, respectively, relating to 799, 787, 730 and 707 feed samples, respectively, out of a total of 1141. Compounds found to a lesser extent were *Alternaria* metabolites, such as tenuazonic acid (55.0%), alternariol (50.7%), alternariol monomethyl ether (40.3%), and tentoxin (37.3%). Another group of detected metabolites was produced by *Aspergillus* and/or *Penicillium* spp., but also by some *Fusarium* species, and these included 3-nitropropionic acid (3-NP), apicidin (API), kojic acid, bikaverin, fusaric acid, and mycophenolic acid. While 3-NP and API were found in 56.5% and 52.2% of samples, respectively, the others were detected in ≤33.7% feed samples.

Other regulated mycotoxins, such as fumonisin B1, ochratoxin A, and aflatoxin B1, did not occur frequently or in high concentrations in pig feed samples. These metabolites were determined in only 43% (median 82.7 µg/kg), 5% (median 2.6 µg/kg), and 3% (median 2.0 µg/kg) of all samples, respectively (data not shown). The mycotoxins gliotoxin and patulin, relevant due to their toxicity, scarcely occurred (0.2%) or could not be detected (<LOD) in these pig feed samples.

**Table 1.** Summary of 34 secondary fungal metabolites ranked according to their prevalence with mean, median, and maximum concentration, measured in 1141 finished feed samples for swine obtained from February 2014 to February 2019 using a multi-analyte LC-MS/MS-based method.

| Rank | Metabolite | Mean Concentration | Median Concentration | Maximum Concentration | Prevalence |
|---|---|---|---|---|---|
| 1 | Cyclo-(L-Pro-L-Tyr) | 321 | 105 | 34,910 | 87.6% |
| 2 | Moniliformin, *t* > 2.0 ppb | 66 | 17 | 2053 | 82.6% |
| 3 | Enniatin B | 73 | 30 | 1514 | 82.2% |
| 4 | Enniatin B1 | 78 | 34 | 1846 | 82.1% |
| 5 | Aurofusarin | 932 | 210 | 85,360 | 80.7% |
| 6 | Culmorin | 905 | 118 | 157,114 | 79.7% |
| 7 | Enniatin A1 | 30 | 14 | 549 | 77.4% |
| 8 | Deoxynivalenol, *t* > 1.5 ppb | 634 | 193 | 34,862 | 77.0% |
| 9 | Tryptophol | 291 | 138 | 10,270 | 75.4% |
| 10 | Zearalenone* | 126 | 18 | 9905 | 73.3% |
| 11 | 15-Hydroxy-culmorin* | 468 | 152 | 19,320 | 73.2% |
| 12 | Beauvericin, *t* > 2.0 ppb | 17 | 6 | 413 | 68.7% |
| 13 | Emodin | 17 | 4 | 591 | 69.3% |
| 14 | Infectopyron* | 983 | 294 | 66,094 | 65.9% |
| 15 | Brevianamid F | 44 | 25 | 1170 | 65.2% |
| 16 | Equisetin | 50 | 11 | 6120 | 64.2% |
| 17 | Cyclo-(L-Pro-L-Val) | 187 | 71 | 5042 | 62.1% |
| 18 | DON-3-glucoside*, *t* > 15.0 ppb | 74 | 22 | 2741 | 62.8% |
| 19 | Asperglaucide* | 113 | 31 | 6232 | 61.8% |
| 20 | Nivalenol*, *t* > 15.0 ppb | 65 | 31 | 1143 | 56.7% |
| 21 | 3-Nitro-propionic acid | 16 | 6 | 509 | 56.5% |
| 22 | Tenuazonic acid | 255 | 82 | 9910 | 55.0% |
| 23 | Apicidin | 22 | 8 | 1568 | 52.2% |
| 24 | Alternariol | 17 | 4 | 2508 | 50.7% |
| 25 | Enniatin A | 7 | 3 | 307 | 49.5% |
| 26 | Alternariol monomethyl ether | 6 | 3 | 208 | 40.3% |
| 27 | Tentoxin | 8 | 3 | 157 | 37.3% |
| 28 | Kojic acid | 192 | 78 | 3030 | 33.7% |
| 29 | Bikaverin | 58 | 19 | 1564 | 29.8% |
| 30 | Fusaric acid | 333 | 81 | 5566 | 13.0% |
| 31 | Mycophenolic acid | 39 | 8 | 1178 | 13.1% |
| 32 | Rubrofusarin | 199 | 38 | 1696 | 2.3% |
| 33 | Gliotoxin | 5 | 5 | 6 | 0.2% |
| 34 | Patulin | <LOD | <LOD | <LOD | n.a. |

Concentrations in µg/kg. * = not tested in vitro (lack of availability or known as regulated or masked mycotoxin). If not otherwise stated, a threshold (t) of >1.0 µg/kg or >LOD (limit of detection) was established.

As seen in Figure 1, 77.7% of the obtained samples had their origin in Europe, mainly from Germany (22.4%), Denmark (15.3%), and Austria (14.1%). Few samples came from other parts of the world, such as Central and South America (9%), Russia and Asian countries (5.6%), North America (3.5%), and Africa (2.4%). The analyzed feed samples obtained from Australia (0.6%) were marginal. Thirteen samples (1.1%) could not be assigned to a specific country. It can thus be stated that the picture of the occurrence primarily reflected the situation of Central Europe, since no major changes were seen in the ranking when samples from the other countries were excluded from the analysis.

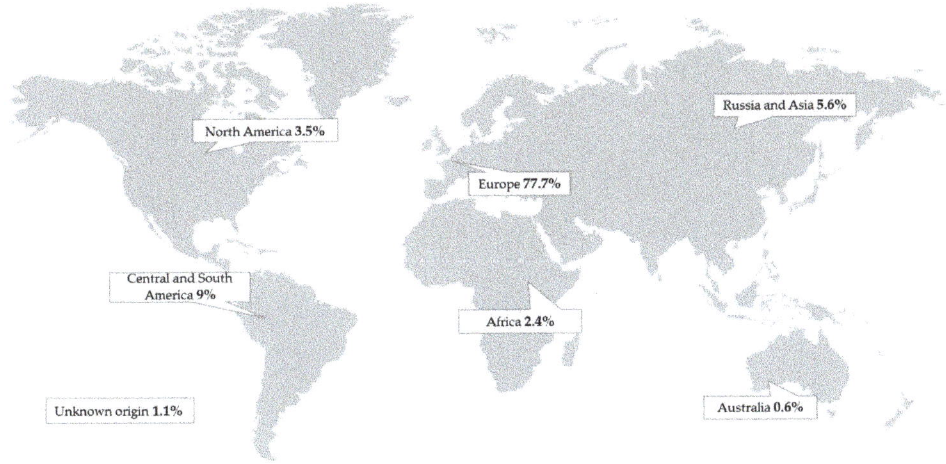


**Figure 1.** Origin of 1141 pig feed samples obtained from different parts of the world.

## 2.2. *Cell Viability after 48 h Toxin Treatment*

The cell viability of intestinal porcine epithelial cells (IPEC-J2) was assessed after an incubation of 48 h with the respective metabolite in concentrations of up to 150 μM. Absolute and relative $IC_{50}$ values were calculated. Deoxynivalenol (DON) (Figure 2A) was included in the test system as an internal standard to have comparable values representing a well-investigated mycotoxin. DON had already reduced the cell viability to 78.8% at 1.25 μM, resulting in absolute and relative $IC_{50}$ values of 2.55 μM and 1.88 μM, respectively. The 28 tested fungal metabolites are listed according to their calculated absolute $IC_{50}$ value, starting from the strongest (for 11 metabolites, relative and absolute $IC_{50}$ value could be calculated) over moderate (for 5 metabolites, only a relative $IC_{50}$ value could be calculated) to no cytotoxicity (for 12 metabolites, $IC_{50}$ calculation was not possible). Apicidin was the metabolite that showed the strongest cytotoxic effect with an absolute $IC_{50}$ value of 0.52 μM (relative 0.49 μM), followed by gliotoxin, bikaverin, beauvericin, and patulin. For all tested metabolites except enniatin B, the calculated relative $IC_{50}$ value was lower than the absolute $IC_{50}$ value (Figure 2).

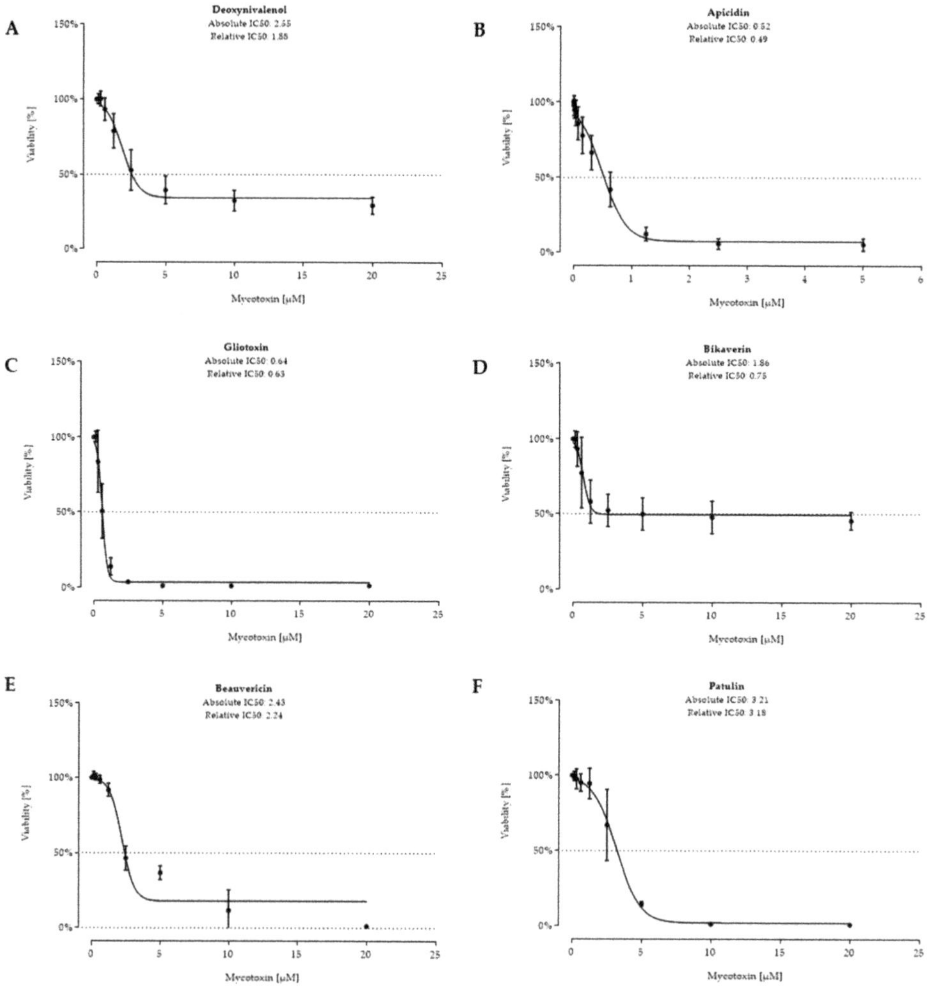


**Figure 2.** Viability (%) after 48 h of incubation with deoxynivalenol (**A**), apicidin (**B**), gliotoxin (**C**), bikaverin (**D**), beauvericin (**E**), and patulin (**F**) (tested at (0.156–20 µM)); except for apicidin (0.0049–5 µM)) of confluent intestinal porcine epithelial cells (IPEC-J2). Data represent mean ± standard deviation.

The next six fungal metabolites that showed a strong cytotoxic effect are presented in Figure 3. The four enniatins B, A, B1, and A1 showed similar absolute $IC_{50}$ values of 3.25 µM, 3.40 µM, 3.67 µM, and 4.15 µM, respectively. Aurofusarin was less toxic, resulting in an absolute $IC_{50}$ value of 11.86 µM. Although emodin was tested at higher concentrations, viability did not further decrease at concentrations >50 µM. Hence, $IC_{50}$ values of 18.71 µM (absolute) and 13.09 µM (relative) were calculated.

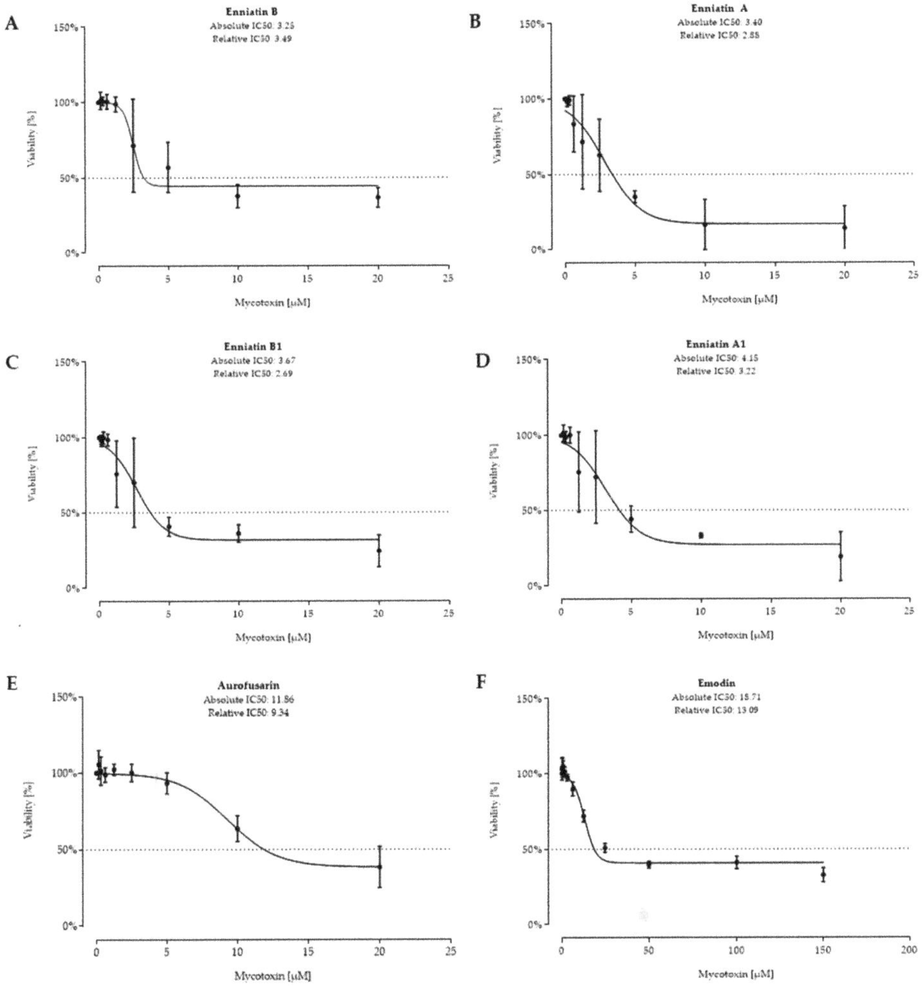


**Figure 3.** Viability (%) after 48 h of incubation of enniatin B (**A**), enniatin A (**B**), enniatin B1 (**C**), enniatin A1 (**D**), aurofusarin (**E**), and emodin (**F**) (tested at (0.156–20 µM), except for emodin (0.625–150 µM)) of confluent intestinal porcine epithelial cells (IPEC-J2). Data represent mean ± standard deviation.

Assessment of the following five fungal metabolites resulted in moderate cytotoxicity on IPEC-J2, as relative, but no absolute, $IC_{50}$ values could be calculated (Figure 4). Examination of the effects of equisetin was only possible up to a concentration of 20 µM, leading to a decreased viability of 64.0% (±7.6%). The other fungal metabolites seen in Figure 4 (B–E) were tested in a concentration range of 0.625 to 150 µM. The *Alternaria* metabolites tenuazonic acid (B) and alternariol (C) showed similar effects of reducing cell viability starting at 20 µM (76.2% and 76.3%), resulting in relative $IC_{50}$ values of 20.88 µM and 20.26 µM. However, despite increased concentrations being used, viability remained around 50%. Rubrofusarin (D) reduced viability started at 50 µM (64.0 ± 8.7%) with a calculated relative $IC_{50}$ value of 21.54 µM. Interestingly, mycophenolic acid (E) led to an abrupt decreased viability (26.1% ± 12.1%) at very low concentrations (0.156 to 1.25 µM), but no further loss in viability was determined at concentrations from 2.5 to 150 µM.

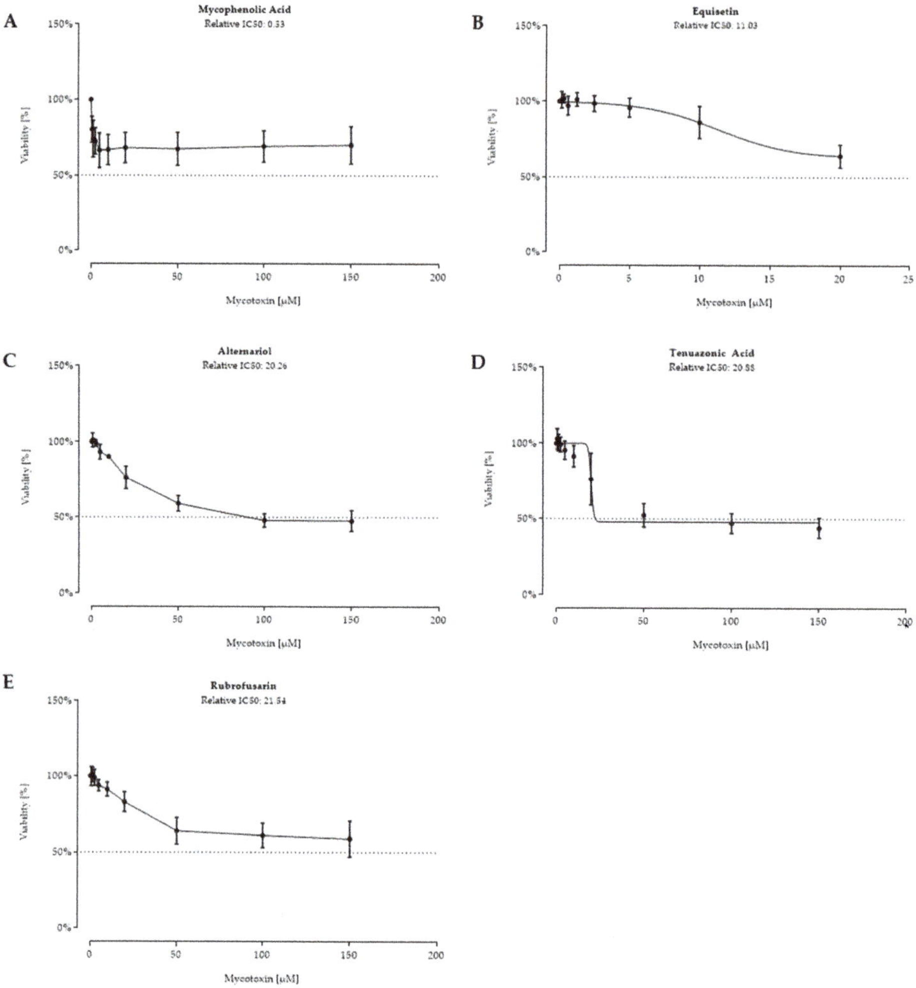


**Figure 4.** Viability (%) after 48 h of incubation with mycophenolic acid (**A**) (0.156–150 µM), equisetin (**B**) (0.156–20 µM), alternariol (**C**), tenuazonic acid (**D**), and rubrofusarin (**E**) ((0.156–150 µM) for C–E) of confluent intestinal porcine epithelial cells (IPEC-J2). Data represent mean ± standard deviation.

For the following twelve fungal secondary metabolites, shown in Figures 5 and 6, no reduced cell viability was seen, and hence, no $IC_{50}$ calculation was possible.

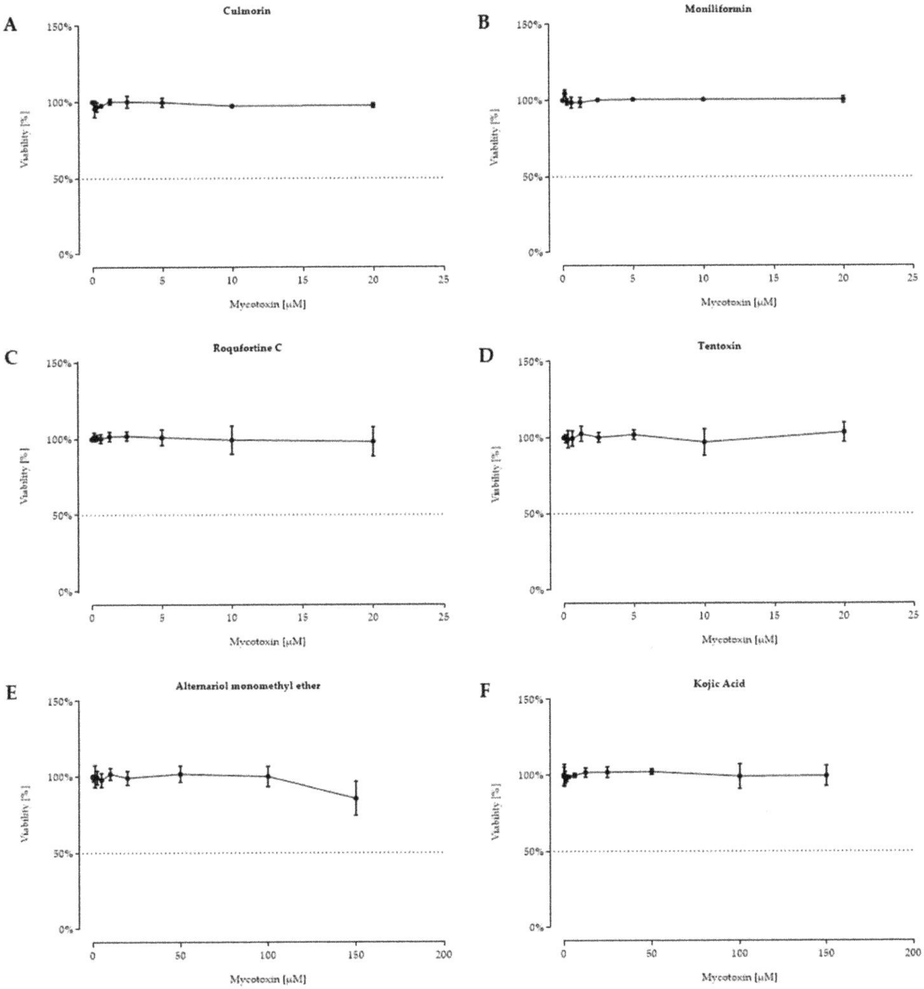


**Figure 5.** Viability (%) after 48 h of incubation with culmorin (**A**), moniliformin (**B**), roquefortine C (**C**), tentoxin (**D**) ((0.156–20 µM) for A–D), alternariol monomethyl ether (**E**), and kojic acid (**F**) ((0.625–150 µM) for E–F) of confluent intestinal porcine epithelial cells (IPEC-J2). Data represent mean ± standard deviation.

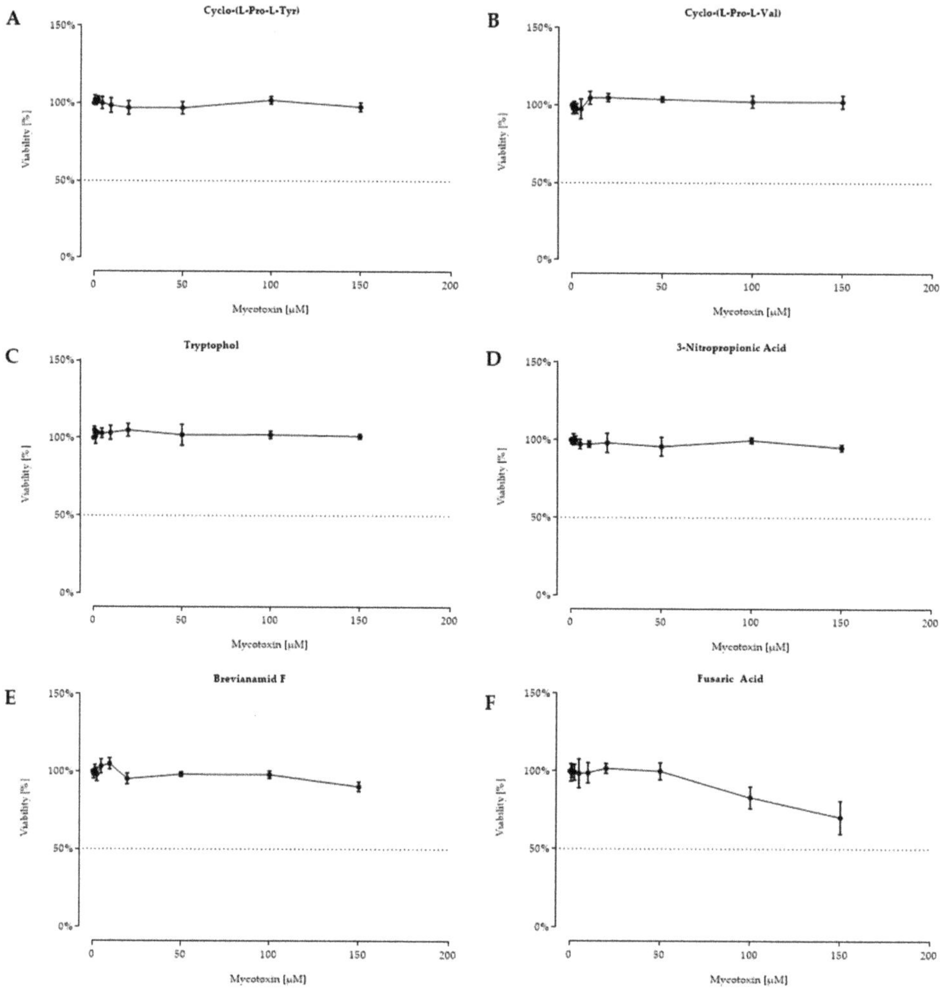


**Figure 6.** Viability (%) after 48 h of incubation with cyclo-(L-Pro-L-Tyr) (**A**), cyclo-(L-Pro-L-Val) (**B**), tryptophol (**C**), 3-nitropropionic acid (**D**), and brevianamid F (**E**), and fusaric acid (**F**) ((0.625–150 µM) for A–F) of confluent intestinal porcine epithelial cells (IPEC-J2). Data represent mean ± standard deviation.

An overview of the obtained $IC_{50}$ values (in µM and µg/kg) for the 16 secondary fungal metabolites with strong and moderate effects on viability is presented in Table 2, together with their median and maximum concentrations in µg/kg found in 1141 pig feed samples.

**Table 2.** List of absolute and relative $IC_{50}$ values in μM (left columns) and in μg/kg (middle columns), compared to median and maximum concentration in μg/kg (right columns) ranked according their cytotoxicity.

| Rank | Fungal Metabolite | $IC_{50}$ Value (μM) | | $IC_{50}$ Value (μg/kg) | | Occurrence | |
|---|---|---|---|---|---|---|---|
| | | Absolute | Relative | Absolute | Relative | Median (μg/kg) | Maximum (μg/kg) |
| 1 | API | 0.52 | 0.49 | 324 | 306 | 8 | 1568 |
| 2 | GLIO | 0.64 | 0.63 | 209 | 206 | 5 | 6 |
| 3 | BIK | 1.86 | 0.75 | 711 | 287 | 19 | 1564 |
| 4 | BEA | 2.43 | 2.24 | 1905 | 1756 | 6 | 413 |
| Control | DON | 2.55 | 1.88 | 756 | 557 | 193 | 34,862 |
| 5 | PAT | 3.21 | 3.18 | 495 | 490 | <LOD | <LOD |
| 6 | EnnB | 3.25 | 3.49 | 2079 | 2233 | 30 | 1514 |
| 7 | EnnA | 3.40 | 2.88 | 2319 | 1964 | 3 | 307 |
| 8 | EnnB1 | 3.67 | 2.69 | 2400 | 1759 | 34 | 1846 |
| 9 | EnnA1 | 4.15 | 3.22 | 2772 | 2151 | 14 | 549 |
| 10 | AUR | 11.86 | 9.34 | 6766 | 5329 | 210 | 85,360 |
| 11 | EMO | 18.71 | 13.09 | 5056 | 3537 | 4 | 591 |
| 12 | MPA | nc | 0.53 | nc | 170 | 8 | 1178 |
| 13 | EQUI | nc | 11.03 | nc | 4120 | 11 | 6120 |
| 14 | ALT | nc | 20.26 | nc | 5232 | 4 | 2508 |
| 15 | TeA | nc | 20.88 | nc | 4761 | 82 | 9910 |
| 16 | RUB | nc | 21.54 | nc | 5865 | 38 | 1696 |

nc = not calculable.

## 3. Discussion

Twenty-eight fungal metabolites plus DON were assessed for their effects on the viability of intestinal porcine epithelial cells (IPEC-J2) in comparison to their prevalence in 1149 analyzed pig feed samples. The strength of our study is that analytical measurements were performed by using one single LC-MS/MS multi-mycotoxin method, as well as the same cell line and viability assay, for all samples to achieve comparable data [24]. A general problem with global mycotoxin occurrence data is usually the difference in methodologies, which make a comparison of concentrations challenging due to different limits of detection (LODs), sample extractions, and performance parameters [11]. Research on toxicology and occurrence of emerging mycotoxins is still scarce, although it has been steadily rising during the past few decades. This can partly be explained by the fact that the sensitivity and potential of LC-MS-based methods have been improved by analyzing hundreds of metabolites simultaneously, as well as by lower detection limits [24]. Furthermore, tremendous climatic abnormalities in some parts of the world favor an increasing formation of uncommon fungal metabolites [12]. Even though not all the detected metabolites might be relevant regarding food and feed safety, the abundance and co-occurrence of those compounds in different feed matrixes might pose a certain risk to susceptible animals. IPEC-J2 provides an optimal in vitro model, as swine is considered as the most sensitive species regarding mycotoxicosis [28]. This non-transformed cell line is isolated out of jejunal epithelial cells, in which the absorption of nutrients and other compounds mainly takes place. Furthermore, it possesses strong morphological and functional similarity to intestinal epithelial cells in vivo [29,30] compared to cancer cell lines such as Caco-2 and HT-29 cells. For in vitro experiments, we decided to test concentrations of up to 150 μM or, in order not to exceed a solvent concentration of 1%, the highest possible test concentration. A solvent concentration of 1% did not negatively influence viability in our test system (data not shown). For our study, we have chosen to discuss the absolute $IC_{50}$ value, as this value is representative for the concentration, where the half-maximal inhibitory concentration was calculated. As described by Sebaugh [31], when the response of more than two assay concentrations is above 50%, the calculation of the relative $IC_{50}$ value would be ambiguous. Furthermore, the calculation of the relative $IC_{50}$ value uses the top and bottom plateau, even when values do not reach 50% viability. Therefore, those $IC_{50}$ values would result in false positive results. Mycophenolic acid (MPA) is a representative example, as viability was never lower than 66%; however, a relative $IC_{50}$ value of 0.543 was calculated, making this toxin one of the most toxic in our ranking. The calculation for the absolute $IC_{50}$ value was not possible for this toxin, and therefore, the calculation of the absolute $IC_{50}$ values was used, first, because it was more accurate, second, only with this value were we able to rank these fungal metabolites according to their toxicity, and third, for reflecting a realistic scenario. For the sake of completeness, both $IC_{50}$ values are shown if calculation was possible. For comparison with the occurrence data, maximum and median concentrations are used, as the median concentration seems to be a more accurate measure of central tendency because of a generally skewed data distribution.

Deoxynivalenol (DON) was included in our study as a comparable internal reference toxin since it is well investigated and manifold deleterious effects of DON are known, as summarized in the review by Pestka [32]. For DON, an $IC_{50}$ concentration of 2.55 µM (= 756 µg/kg) was calculated, whereas a median concentration of 193 µg/kg was found in swine feed. Although the detected concentration was lower than the determined $IC_{50}$ value, it is known that in particular chronic low doses of DON lead to immune dysregulation, growth retardation, and impaired reproduction [32]. This is of increased importance because the bioavailability for DON after oral administration is 98.6% ± 23.6% in pigs [33]. This might also be true for other metabolites, but neither feeding trial nor bioavailability studies have been conducted for most of them. Therefore, the choice of in vitro concentrations is challenging. Stability and retention time in the gastrointestinal tract (GIT) have not been sufficiently researched. Thus, an accumulation of metabolites in the GIT by ingesting chronic low concentrations is very likely and we tried to test a broad concentration range up to 150 µM, if possible.

Apicidin (API), only discovered in the year 1996 and isolated from *Fusarium* spp., showed the strongest cytotoxicity in our test system ($IC_{50}$ of 0.52 µM = 324 µg/kg). This is in accordance with a study on other cell lines, reporting an $IC_{50}$ concentration of 0.16 to 3.8 µM on cell proliferation [34]. Furthermore, this compound possesses antiprotozoal activity [35] and causes toxic effects in rats leading to death at levels of 0.05 and 0.1% [36]. Although the measured median concentration in feed samples was rather low (8 µg/kg), API was found in more than half of the samples and individual samples reached concentrations of up to 1568 µg/kg. Streit et al. [13] detected a maximum concentration of 160 µg/kg in 66% positively tested samples, but additional occurrence studies are missing. The second-ranked cytotoxic compound was gliotoxin (GLIO) with an $IC_{50}$ value of 0.64 µM (= 209 µg/kg). This *Aspergillus fumigatus* metabolite hardly occurs in swine feed, but was detected in corn silage used as cattle feedstuff [37]. GLIO has been reported to cause immunosuppressive, genotoxic, apoptotic, and cytotoxic effects determined in a rat intestinal cell line (IEC-6), in hamster ovary cells (CHO), and in mouse macrophages (RAW264.7) [38,39], and might pose a risk for other animal species that are frequently exposed to this mycotoxin. Literature about the effects and occurrence of our third-ranked toxic compound bikaverin (BIK) is scarce. It is reported as a red pigment produced by different *Fusarium* spp. with antibiotic and antibacterial properties [40,41]. A study from 1975 reported its cytotoxicity against three different cancer cell lines, leading to $ED_{50}$ values of 0.5–4.2 µg/mL (1.31–10.99 µM) [42], which is comparable with our $IC_{50}$ value of 1.86 µM. Furthermore, we found BIK in almost 30% of the feed samples with a maximum concentration of 1564 µg/kg, whereas another study reported contaminations of up to 51,130 µg/kg [13]. Our in vitro data give the first evidence of its cytotoxic effects on epithelial cells, and considering an $IC_{50}$ value of only 1.86 µM (= 711 µg/kg), the high contamination level might be alarming. We would like to point out that for this toxin, viability did not further decrease below 50% after applying higher concentrations, which has also been observed for other metabolites such as enniatin B, emodin, and tenuazonic acid. More research has been carried out for the cyclic hexadepsipeptides beauvericin (BEA) and the group of enniatins (ENNs; A, A1, B, B1). Their cytotoxicity was demonstrated in a variety of cell culture models [7,9,43–46] and is attributed to their ionophoric properties. A recently published study from Fraeyman et al. [46] revealed that proliferating IPEC-J2 are more sensitive to BEA, but not to the ENNs. Differentiated cells seem to be more robust against their detrimental effects, which was already shown by Springler and Broekaert et al. [47,48]. According to Fraeyman's study, the overall cytotoxicity after 24 h of incubation was ranked as BEA > ENN A >> ENN A1 > ENN B1 >>> ENN B. This contrasts with our results that led to the following ranking: BEA > ENN B > ENN A > ENN B1 > ENN A1 in proliferating

IPEC-J2. This discrepancy could be due to different incubation time points (24 h vs. 48 h) and different measured endpoints (flow cytometry vs. Sulforhodamine B assay). Additionally, more data about their occurrence are available. We mostly found ENN B and B1 (≈82% positive); however, 77.4%, 68.7%, and 49.5% of the feed samples were also contaminated with ENN A, BEA, and ENN A1, respectively. The maximum detected concentrations varied between 1514, 1846, 307, 413 and 549 μg/kg, respectively. Considering that those compounds usually co-occur, the total amount can exceed a level of 4500 μg/kg or even 5543 μg/kg, as described in Kovalsky et al. [18]. A high prevalence of BEA and ENNs in cereal grains was already described in other peer-reviewed studies [14,15,18,49]. Additionally, a high oral bioavailability, particularly seen for ENN B1, has been reported [50,51], which turn them into a potential risk factor for exposed animals.

For patulin (PAT), a low $IC_{50}$ value of 3.21 μM (= 495 μg/kg) was determined as well, but since not a single sample was contaminated with PAT, it does not seem to be relevant regarding porcine health. PAT is better known as a feed contaminant in fruits, especially apples and vegetables, and its toxicity was demonstrated in different animal species [52,53]. Other conclusions have to be drawn regarding the *Fusarium* metabolite aurofusarin (AURO), which led to an $IC_{50}$ value of 11.86 μM (= 6766 μg/kg) and was detected in a median and maximum concentration of 210 μg/kg and 85,360 μg/kg, respectively. An interference of AURO with antioxidants and fatty acids in the eggs and embryos of quails has already been reported [54,55], as well as its negative effect on the growth performance in red tilapia [56] and cytotoxicity in mammalian cells [23,57,58]. Our results are comparable with a study from Jarolim et al. [23], reporting a significant decrease in viability of HT29 and HCEC-1CT cells starting at 5 μM AURO after 48 h. Even though the calculated $IC_{50}$ value of 6766 μg/kg seems to be high in our approach, when considering the maximum found concentration of 85,360 μg/kg, a critical risk assessment is urgently required. The last metabolite where an $IC_{50}$ calculation was possible was emodin (EMO), which is claimed to be a therapeutic agent of various diseases used in traditional Chinese medicine for centuries. As EMO is produced by a range of different plant families, and found ubiquitously in herbs, trees, and shrubs [59], a potential risk to animal health seems very unlikely.

Five out of the tested metabolites, mycophenolic acid (MPA), equisetin (EQUI), alternariol (ALT), tenuazonic acid (TeA), and rubrofusarin (RUB) led to a slight decrease in viability, and relative $IC_{50}$ values could be determined. Despite increasing concentrations, a reduction of more than 50% was not found; therefore, absolute $IC_{50}$ values could not be calculated. We have chosen the SRB assay to measure the protein content because this cell target was the most sensitive one in preliminary studies. However, it seems that for other compounds, a different cell target might be more suitable. As described in an study from 2017 [60], different endpoint analyses can lead to a different outcomes. Especially for MPA, a study about its cytotoxicity has been published where the mitochondrial activity of Caco-2 cells was only decreased by 45% at 780 μM MPA after 48 h of incubation, but no effect was seen in THP-1 monocytes [61]. These results vary from ours since we determined a constant decline of 20.0 to 33.6% viability already starting from 1.25 to 150 μM MPA by measuring the cellular protein content. Interestingly, similar results about ALT were published, in which the cell viability of HepG2 cells did not decrease in a concentration-dependent manner up until a concentration of 100 μM [62,63].

None of the other compounds, culmorin (CUL), moniliformin (MON), roquefortine C, tentoxin, alternariol monomethyl ether, kojic acid, cyclo-(L-Pro-L-Tyr), cyclo-(L-Pro-L-Val), tryptophol, 3-nitropropionic acid, brevianamid F, and fusaric acid (FA) showed negative effects in the tested concentration range on IPEC-J2. However, we would like to refer to four of them: although the metabolite culmorin (CUL) elucidated no cytotoxic effect in our tests, it was found in 79.7% of all samples, with remarkable concentrations of 157,114 μg/kg. Interestingly, its natural occurrence is always correlated to the occurrence of DON. A recent study showed that CUL is able to inhibit the glucuronidation of DON in human liver microsomes, and thus, its detoxification process [64,65]. These findings make the compound highly relevant regarding synergistic effects, not only for the detoxification of DON, but also for other toxins. MON was already described as a hazardous contaminant for poultry, and therefore, a risk assessment has been recently published by EFSA [6,66]. Finally, although being non-cytotoxic in our experimental approach, cyclo-(L-Pro-L-Tyr) was found to be the most frequently detected compound in our survey program with 87.6% positive samples. Only a few publications described its antibacterial activity against two gram-negative bacteria, as well as its cytotoxic and genotoxic effects in lymphocytes and various cell lines to date [67–69]. However, due to its high occurrence, along with its high concentration, further studies are needed. Furthermore, we would like to stress that other metabolites, such as aflatoxin B1 and fumonisin B1, are also known for their non-cytotoxic effects in vitro and their detrimental effect in animals. Thus, a lack of cytotoxicity in vitro does not necessarily indicate a complete harmlessness.

## 4. Conclusions

Taken together, our study focused on the occurrence data and concentrations of 28 secondary fungal metabolites without regulatory guidelines and their effect on the viability of an intestinal porcine cell line. In the majority of the analyzed pig feed samples, low median concentrations (15 of 28 metabolites gave median concentrations of <20 μg/kg) were determined; however, some individual samples were contaminated with high concentration levels, which might be relevant for animal health. The maximum occurrence values exceeded the absolute $IC_{50}$ concentrations for apicidin, bikaverin, and aurofusarin. Moreover, even if acute exposure to most of the metabolites is low, concerns regarding chronic exposure at lower levels are rising. An important factor that needs to be considered for further investigations comprise the absorption, distribution, metabolism, and excretion (ADME) of the substances and their ability to enter the target cell. Therefore, cytotoxicity studies provide a first overall picture of the relevance of the detected compounds and serve as a suitable alternative and prerequisite to animal testing. For a qualified risk assessment, however, reliable combination studies to investigate synergistic, additive, and antagonistic effects are needed due to the frequent co-occurrence of toxic compounds, especially with the regulated main mycotoxins. Finally, data from feeding trials in productive livestock with chronic exposure of those compounds have to be the logical target for the testing process within the next few years.

## 5. Materials and Methods

### 5.1. Cell Culture

The porcine jejunal intestinal epithelial cell line, IPEC-J2 (ACC 701; Leibnitz Institute DSMZ, German Collection of Microorganisms and Cell Cultures, Braunschweig, Germany), originated from a neonatal, unsuckled piglet. These non-transformed cells were continuously maintained in complete cultivation medium consisting of Dulbecco's modified eagle medium (DMEM/Ham's F12 (1:1), Biochrom AG, Berlin, Germany), supplemented with 5% fetal bovine serum, 1% insulin-transferrin-selenium, 5 ng/mL epidermal growth factor, 2.5 mM Glutamax (all GibcoTM, Life Technologies, Carlsbad, CA, USA), and 16 mM 4-(2-hydroxyethyl)-1-piperazineethanesulfonic acid (Sigma-Aldrich, St. Louis, MO, USA), and grown at 39 °C in a humidified atmosphere of 5% $CO_2$. IPEC-J2 between passages 1–15 were routinely seeded at $1 \times 10^6$ cells/mL in 150 $cm^2$ tissue culture flasks (Starlab, Hamburg, Germany) with 28 mL complete cultivation medium and subcultured upon confluence every 3–4 days. For assays, confluent cells were detached using Trypsin (0.25%)-ethylenediaminetetraacetic acid (EDTA, 0.5 mM, Sigma-Aldrich, St. Louis, MO, USA). Cell culture was regularly tested and found to be free of mycoplasma contamination via PCR (Venor®GeM Mycoplasma Detection Kit; Minvera Biolabs GmbH, Berlin, Germany).

### 5.2. Material

All tested chemicals are listed in Table 3 and were dissolved either in dimethylsulfoxid (DMSO, Sigma-Aldrich, St. Louis, MO, USA), ethanol (EtOH absolut, VWR International, Radnor, PA, USA), acetonitrile (ACN, Sigma-Aldrich, St. Louis, MO, USA), or distilled water.

**Table 3.** List of chemicals.

| Chemical | Purity | Solvent | Highest Tested Concentration (μM) | Company |
|---|---|---|---|---|
| Alternariol (*Alternaria* sp.) | ≈96% | DMSO | 150 | Sigma-Aldrich |
| Alternariol monoethyl ether (*Alternaria alternata)* | ≥98% | DMSO | 150 | Sigma-Aldrich |
| Apicidin (*Fusarium* sp.) | ≥95% | DMSO | 5 | Santa Cruz |
| Aurofusarin (*Fusarium graminearum)* | ≥97% | DMSO | 20 | AdipoGen Life Sciences |
| Beauvericin (*Beauveria* sp.) | ≥95% | DMSO | 20 | AdipoGen Life Sciences |
| Bikaverin (*Fusarium* sp.) | 95% | DMSO | 20 | Santa Cruz |
| Brevianamid F | >98% | DMSO | 150 | MedChem Express |
| Cyclo(L-Pro-L-Tyr) | >98% | DMSO | 150 | BioAustralis |
| Cyclo(L-Pro-L-Val) | >98% | DMSO | 150 | BioAustralis |
| Culmorin | 100% | ACN | 20 | Generous gift from Dr. Fruhmann |
| Deoxynivalenol (*Fusarium* sp.) | ≥95% | Distilled water | 20 | Biopure |
| Emodin | ≥97% | DMSO | 150 | Sigma-Aldrich |
| Enniatin A, A1, B, B1 (*Gnomonia errabunda)* | ≥95% | DMSO | 20 | Sigma-Aldrich |
| Equisetin (*Fusarium equiseti)* | >99% | DMSO | 20 | Santa Cruz |
| Fusaric acid (*Gibberella fujikuroi)* | ≥98% | 96% EtOH | 150 | Sigma-Aldrich |
| Gliotoxin (*Gladiocladium fimbriatum)* | ≥97% | DMSO | 20 | Santa Cruz |
| Kojic acid | ≥99% | Distilled water | 150 | Sigma-Aldrich |
| Moniliformin (*Fusarium moniliforme)* | ≥99% | Distilled water | 20 | BioAustralis |
| Mycophenolic acid (*Penicillium brevicompactum)* | ≥98% | DMSO | 150 | Sigma-Aldrich |
| Patulin | 98% | DMSO | 20 | Santa Cruz |
| Roquefortine C (*Penicillium* sp.) | ≥98% | DMSO | 20 | AdipoGen Life Sciences |
| Tentoxin (*Alternaria tenuis*) | ≥95% | 70% EtOH | 20 | Sigma-Aldrich |
| Tenuazonic acid (*Alternaria alternata)* | ≥98% | DMSO | 150 | AdipoGen Life Sciences |
| Tryptophol | >98% | DMSO | 150 | AdipoGen Life Sciences |
| 3-Nitropropionic acid | ≥97% | 70% EtOH | 150 | Sigma-Aldrich |

Adipogen Life Sciences, Switzerland; BioAustralis, Australia; Biopure, Austria; MedChem Express, Sweden; Santa Cruz, Germany; Sigma-Aldrich, USA.

### 5.3. Method

#### 5.3.1. Cell Viability Assay

For the measurement of cell viability, $3 \times 10^4$ cells/well were seeded into a flat-bottom, cell-culture-treated 96-well microplate (Eppendorf) in 200 μL cultivation media and grown for 24 hours at 39 °C and 5% $CO_2$. After reaching confluence, IPEC-J2 were treated with a broad range of concentrations of all chemicals (listed in Table 3).

A sulforhodamine B (SRB) assay (Xenometrix, Allschwil, Switzerland) was used to determine cellular protein content and was performed according to the manual. Briefly, the supernatant was discarded and the cell layer was washed with 300 μL SRB I solution per well. Then, 100 μL SRB II fixing solution was added to each well and the plate was incubated for 1 h at 4 °C. After the incubation time, cells were washed three times with 200 μL distilled water. Cells were stained with 50 μL SRB III labelling solution/well for 15 min, and afterwards, cells were washed again two times with 400 μL SRB IV rinsing solution. Then, bound SRB was solubilized with 200 μL SRB V and after 15–60 min, absorbance was measured at 540 nm and a reference wavelength of 690 nm using a microplate reader (Synergy HT, Biotek, Bad Friedrichshall, Germany).

5.3.2. LC-MS/MS Multi-Analyte Method

A total of 1141 samples from 75 countries were provided by the BIOMIN Mycotoxin Survey for measuring up to 800 analytes, including fungal and bacterial metabolites, pesticides, and veterinary drug residues using a LC-MS/MS multi-mycotoxin analysis method [24]. Samples were collected after instruction or by trained staff only from February 2014 until February 2019. For the present study, data from finished pig feed samples including 28 fungal metabolites were chosen for detailed analysis (see Table 1). The threshold *(t)* was set to be >1.0 μg/kg or the limit of detection (LOD), whichever was higher.

A minimum of 500 g of sample was submitted to the laboratory of the Institute of Bioanalytics and Agro-Metabolomics at the University of Natural Resources and Life Sciences Vienna (BOKU) in Tulln. After reception, samples were immediately milled, homogenized, and finally analyzed. Samples were extracted with a mixture of acetonitrile (ACN), water, and acetic acid (79:20:1, per volume) on a rotary shaker for 90 min. After centrifugation, the supernatant was transferred to a glass vial and diluted with a mixture of ACN, water, and acetic acid (20:79:1, per volume), and was injected into the LC-MS/MS system (electrospray ionisation and mass spectrometric detection employing a quadrupole mass filter). Quantification was done according to an external calibration using a multi-analyte stock solution.

The method was performed according to the guidelines from the Directorate General for Health and Consumer affairs of the European Commission, published in document No. 12495/2011 [70].

5.3.3. Statistics and Evaluation

The half-maximal inhibitory concentrations ($IC_{50}$) were calculated using GraphPad Prism (GraphPad Prism Version 7.03, San Diego, CA, USA). For calculation of the relative $IC_{50}$ value, data was log-transformed and fitted to a four-parameter logistic equation:

$$Y = Bottom + (Top - Bottom)/(1 + 10((LogIC50 - X)\ x\ Hillslope \tag{1}$$

The molar concentration of a substance that reduced viability to 50% between the top and the bottom plateau was calculated.

For the calculation of the absolute $IC_{50}$ value, data was log-transformed and following equation was used:

$$Y = Bottom + (Top - Bottom)/(1 + 10\left((LogIC50 - X)\ x\ HillSlope + \log\left(\frac{Top - Bottom}{Fifty - Bottom} - 1\right)\right) \tag{2}$$

Fifty = 50; Top = 100

The molar concentration of a substance that reduced viability to 50% of the maximum viability was calculated.

**Author Contributions:** B.N. conceived and designed the experiments; B.N. and V.R. performed the experiments; B.N., M.S., and E.M. analyzed the data; M.S. provided the analysis tool (LC-MS/MS method); B.N. wrote the paper; D.H., G.S., and E.M. reviewed the paper.

**Funding:** This research received funding from the Austrian Research Promotion Agency (Österreichische Forschungsförderungsgesellschaft FFG (grant numbers 853863 and 859603), as well as EFREtop (grant number 864743).

**Acknowledgments:** We would like to thank Philipp Fruhmann (University of Natural Resources and Life Sciences, Vienna) for the generous gift of the culmorin stock, which was produced according to Weber et al. [65].

**Conflicts of Interest:** B.N., V.R., G.S., and E.M. are employed by BIOMIN. However, this circumstance did not influence the design of the experimental studies or bias the presentation and interpretation of results. The other two authors, M.S. and D.H., declare no conflict of interest.

## References


1. Bérdy, J. Bioactive microbial metabolites. *J. Antibiot.* **2005**, *58*, C1. [CrossRef] [PubMed]
2. Commission Regulation (EC) No 1881/2006: Setting maximum levels for certain contaminantns in foodstuffs. *Off. J. Eur. Union* **2006**, *364*, 5–24.
3. EFSA. Scientific opinion on the risk for public and animal health related to the presence of sterigmatocystin in food and feed. *EFSA J.* **2016**, *11*, 3254.
4. EFSA. Scientific opinion on Ergot alkaloids in food and feed. *EFSA J.* **2012**, *10*, 158.
5. EFSA. Scientific opinion on the risks to human and animal health related to the presence of beauvericin and enniatins in food and feed. *EFSA J.* **2014**, *12*, 3802. [CrossRef]
6. Knutsen, H.K.; Alexander, J.; Barregård, L.; Bignami, M.; Brüschweiler, B.; Ceccatelli, S.; Cottrill, B.; Dinovi, M.; Grasl-Kraupp, B.; Hogstrand, C.; et al. Risks to human and animal health related to the presence of moniliformin in food and feed. *EFSA J.* **2018**, *16*, 5082.
7. Gruber-Dorninger, C.; Novak, B.; Nagl, V.; Berthiller, F. Emerging mycotoxins: Beyond traditionally determined food contaminants. *J. Agric. Food Chem.* **2017**, *65*, 7052–7070. [CrossRef] [PubMed]
8. Jestoi, M. Emerging fusarium-mycotoxins fusaproliferin, beauvericin, enniatins, and moniliformin—A review. *Crit. Rev. Food Sci. Nutr.* **2008**, *48*, 21–49. [CrossRef]
9. Fraeyman, S.; Croubels, S.; Devreese, M.; Antonissen, G. Emerging fusarium and alternaria mycotoxins: Occurrence, toxicity and toxicokinetics. *Toxins* **2017**, *9*, 228. [CrossRef]
10. Sulyok, M.; Krska, R.; Schuhmacher, R. A liquid chromatography/tandem mass spectrometric multi-mycotoxin method for the quantification of 87 analytes and its application to semi-quantitative screening of moldy food samples. *Anal. Bioanal. Chem.* **2007**, *389*, 1505–1523. [CrossRef]
11. Van der Fels-Klerx, H.J.; Klemsdal, S.; Hietaniemi, V.; Lindblad, M.; Ioannou-Kakouri, E.; van Asselt, E.D. Mycotoxin contamination of cereal grain commodities in relation to climate in North West Europe. *Food Addit. Contam. Part A* **2012**, *29*, 1581–1592. [CrossRef] [PubMed]
12. Van der Fels-Klerx, H.; Kandhai, M.; Brynestad, S.; Dreyer, M.; Börjesson, T.; Martins, H.; Uiterwijk, M.; Morrison, E.; Booij, C. Development of a European system for identification of emerging mycotoxins in wheat supply chains. *World Mycotoxin J.* **2009**, *2*, 119–127. [CrossRef]
13. Streit, E.; Schwab, C.; Sulyok, M.; Naehrer, K.; Krska, R.; Schatzmayr, G. Multi-mycotoxin screening reveals the occurrence of 139 different secondary metabolites in feed and feed ingredients. *Toxins* **2013**, *5*, 504–523. [CrossRef] [PubMed]
14. Hietaniemi, V.; Rämö, S.; Yli-Mattila, T.; Jestoi, M.; Peltonen, S.; Kartio, M.; Sieviläinen, E.; Koivisto, T.; Parikka, P. Updated survey of Fusarium species and toxins in Finnish cereal grains. *Food Addit. Contam. Part A* **2016**, *33*, 831–848. [CrossRef] [PubMed]
15. Lindblad, M.; Gidlund, A.; Sulyok, M.; Börjesson, T.; Krska, R.; Olsen, M.; Fredlund, E. Deoxynivalenol and other selected fusarium toxins in swedish wheat—Occurrence and correlation to specific fusarium species. *Int. J. Food Microbiol.* **2013**, *167*, 284–291. [CrossRef] [PubMed]
16. Juan, C.; Covarelli, L.; Beccari, G.; Colasante, V.; Mañes, J. Simultaneous analysis of twenty-six mycotoxins in durum wheat grain from Italy. *Food Control* **2016**, *62*, 322–329. [CrossRef]
17. De Souza, M.D.L.M.; Sulyok, M.; Freitas-Silva, O.; Costa, S.S.; Brabet, C.; Machinski, M., Jr.; Sekiyama, B.L.; Vargas, E.A.; Krska, R.; Schuhmacher, R. Cooccurrence of mycotoxins in maize and poultry feeds from Brazil by liquid chromatography/tandem mass spectrometry. *Sci. World J.* **2013**, *2013*, 427369. [CrossRef] [PubMed]
18. Kovalsky, P.; Kos, G.; Nährer, K.; Schwab, C.; Jenkins, T.; Schatzmayr, G.; Sulyok, M.; Krska, R. Co-occurrence of regulated, masked and emerging mycotoxins and secondary metabolites in finished feed and maize–An extensive survey. *Toxins* **2016**, *8*, 363. [CrossRef]
19. Goossens, J.; Pasmans, F.; Verbrugghe, E.; Vandenbroucke, V.; De Baere, S.; Meyer, E.; Haesebrouck, F.; De Backer, P.; Croubels, S. Porcine intestinal epithelial barrier disruption by the Fusarium mycotoxins deoxynivalenol and T-2 toxin promotes transepithelial passage of doxycycline and paromomycin. *BMC Vet. Res.* **2012**, *8*, 245. [CrossRef]
20. Ficheux, A.S.; Sibiril, Y.; Parent-Massin, D. Effects of beauvericin, enniatin b and moniliformin on human dendritic cells and macrophages: An invitro study. *Toxicon* **2013**, *71*, 1–10. [CrossRef]

21. Zouaoui, N.; Mallebrera, B.; Berrada, H.; Abid-Essefi, S.; Bacha, H.; Ruiz, M.J. Cytotoxic effects induced by patulin, sterigmatocystin and beauvericin on CHO-K1 cells. *Food Chem. Toxicol.* **2016**, *89*, 92–103. [CrossRef] [PubMed]
22. Bensassi, F.; Gallerne, C.; Sharaf El Dein, O.; Hajlaoui, M.R.; Bacha, H.; Lemaire, C. Cell death induced by the Alternaria mycotoxin Alternariol. *Toxicol. Vitr.* **2012**, *26*, 915–923. [CrossRef] [PubMed]
23. Jarolim, K.; Wolters, K.; Woelflingseder, L.; Pahlke, G.; Beisl, J.; Puntscher, H.; Braun, D.; Sulyok, M.; Warth, B.; Marko, D. The secondary Fusarium metabolite aurofusarin induces oxidative stress, cytotoxicity and genotoxicity in human colon cells. *Toxicol. Lett.* **2018**, *284*, 170–183. [CrossRef] [PubMed]
24. Malachová, A.; Sulyok, M.; Beltrán, E.; Berthiller, F.; Krska, R. Optimization and validation of a quantitative liquid chromatography-tandem mass spectrometric method covering 295 bacterial and fungal metabolites including all regulated mycotoxins in four model food matrices. *J. Chromatogr. A* **2014**, *1362*, 145–156. [CrossRef] [PubMed]
25. Vaclavikova, M.; Malachova, A.; Veprikova, Z.; Dzuman, Z.; Zachariasova, M.; Hajslova, J. "Emerging" mycotoxins in cereals processing chains: Changes of enniatins during beer and bread making. *Food Chem.* **2013**, *136*, 750–757. [CrossRef] [PubMed]
26. Vidal, A.; Ouhibi, S.; Ghali, R.; Hedhili, A.; De Saeger, S.; De Boevre, M. The mycotoxin patulin: An updated short review on occurrence, toxicity and analytical challenges. *Food Chem. Toxicol.* **2019**, *129*, 249–256. [CrossRef] [PubMed]
27. Kosalec, I.; Pepeljnjak, S. Chemistry and biological effects of gliotoxin. *Arh. Hig. Rada Toksikol.* **2004**, *55*, 313–320. [PubMed]
28. Kanora, A.; Maes, D. The role of mycotoxins in pig reproduction: A review. *Vet. Med.* **2009**, *54*, 565–576. [CrossRef]
29. Schierack, P.; Nordhoff, M.; Pollmann, M.; Weyrauch, K.D.; Amasheh, S.; Lodemann, U.; Jores, J.; Tachu, B.; Kleta, S.; Blikslager, A.; et al. Characterization of a porcine intestinal epithelial cell line for in vitro studies of microbial pathogenesis in swine. *Histochem. Cell Biol.* **2006**, *125*, 293–305. [CrossRef]
30. Nossol, C.; Barta-Böszörményi, A.; Kahlert, S.; Zuschratter, W.; Faber-Zuschratter, H.; Reinhardt, N.; Ponsuksili, S.; Wimmers, K.; Diesing, A.K.; Rothkötter, H.J. Comparing two intestinal porcine epithelial cell lines (IPECs): Morphological differentiation, function and metabolism. *PLoS ONE* **2015**, *10*, e0132323. [CrossRef]
31. Sebaugh, J.L. Guidelines for accurate EC50/IC50 estimation. *Pharm. Stat.* **2011**, *10*, 128–134. [CrossRef] [PubMed]
32. Pestka, J.J. Deoxynivalenol: Mechanisms of action, human exposure, and toxicological relevance. *Arch. Toxicol.* **2010**, *84*, 663–679. [CrossRef] [PubMed]
33. Paulick, M.; Winkler, J.; Kersten, S.; Schatzmayr, D.; Schwartz-Zimmermann, H.E.; Dänicke, S. Studies on the bioavailability of deoxynivalenol (DON) and DON sulfonate (DONS) 1, 2, and 3 in pigs fed with sodium sulfite-treated DON-contaminated maize. *Toxins* **2015**, *7*, 4622–4644. [CrossRef] [PubMed]
34. Han, J.W.; Ahn, S.H.; Park, S.H.; Wang, S.Y.; Bae, G.U.; Seo, D.W.; Kwon, H.K.; Hong, S.; Hoi, Y.; Lee, Y.W.; et al. Apicidin, a histone deacetylase inhibitor, inhibits proliferation of tumor cells via induction of p21(WAF1/Cip1) and gelsolin. *Cancer Res.* **2000**, *60*, 6068–6074. [PubMed]
35. Darkin-Rattray, S.J.; Gurnett, A.M.; Myers, R.W.; Dulski, P.M.; Crumley, T.M.; Allocco, J.J.; Cannova, C.; Meinke, P.T.; Colletti, S.L.; Bednarek, M.A.; et al. Apicidin: A novel antiprotozoal agent that inhibits parasite histone deacetylase. *Proc. Natl. Acad. Sci. USA* **1996**, *93*, 13143–13147. [CrossRef] [PubMed]
36. Park, J.S.; Lee, K.R.; Kim, J.C.; Lim, S.H.; Seo, J.A.; Lee, Y.W. A hemorrhagic factor (apicidin) produced by toxic Fusarium isolates from soybean seeds. *Appl. Environ. Microbiol.* **1999**, *65*, 126–130.
37. Pena, G.A.; Pereyra, C.M.; Armando, M.R.; Chiacchiera, S.M.; Magnoli, C.E.; Orlando, J.L.; Dalcero, A.M.; Rosa, C.A.R.; Cavaglieri, L.R. *Aspergillus fumigatus* toxicity and gliotoxin levels in feedstuff for domestic animals and pets in Argentina. *Lett. Appl. Microbiol.* **2010**, *50*, 77–81. [CrossRef] [PubMed]
38. Nieminen, S.M.; Mäki-Paakkanen, J.; Hirvonen, M.R.; Roponen, M.; Von Wright, A. Genotoxicity of gliotoxin, a secondary metabolite of *Aspergillus fumigatus*, in a battery of short-term test systems. *Mutat. Res.* **2002**, *520*, 161–170. [CrossRef]
39. Upperman, J.S.; Potoka, D.A.; Zhang, X.R.; Wong, K.; Zamora, R.; Ford, H.R. Mechanism of intestinal-derived fungal sepsis by gliotoxin, a fungal metabolite. *J. Pediatr. Surg.* **2003**, *38*, 966–970. [CrossRef]

40. Limón, M.C.; Rodríguez-Ortiz, R.; Avalos, J. Bikaverin production and applications. *Appl. Microbiol. Biotechnol.* **2010**, *87*, 21–29. [CrossRef]
41. Deshmukh, R.; Mathew, A.; Purohit, H.J. Characterization of antibacterial activity of bikaverin from Fusarium sp. HKF 15. *J. Biosci. Bioeng.* **2014**, *117*, 443–448. [CrossRef] [PubMed]
42. Fuska, J.; Proksa, B.; Fuskova, A. New potential cytotoxic and antitumor substances. I. In vitro effect of bikaverin and its derivatives on cells of certain tumors. *Neoplasma* **1975**, *22*, 335–338. [PubMed]
43. Font, G.; Prosperini, A.; Ruiz, M.J. Cytotoxicity, bioaccessibility and transport by Caco-2 cells of enniatins and beauvericin. *Toxicol. Lett.* **2011**, *205*, S159. [CrossRef]
44. Prosperini, A.; Juan-García, A.; Font, G.; Ruiz, M.J. Beauvericin-induced cytotoxicity via ROS production and mitochondrial damage in Caco-2 cells. *Toxicol. Lett.* **2013**, *222*, 204–211. [CrossRef] [PubMed]
45. Meca, G.; Font, G.; Ruiz, M.J. Comparative cytotoxicity study of enniatins A, A1, A2, B, B1, B4 and J3 on Caco-2 cells, Hep-G2 and HT-29. *Food Chem. Toxicol.* **2011**, *49*, 2464–2469. [CrossRef] [PubMed]
46. Fraeyman, S.; Meyer, E.; Devreese, M.; Antonissen, G.; Demeyere, K.; Haesebrouck, F.; Croubels, S. Comparative in vitro cytotoxicity of the emerging Fusarium mycotoxins beauvericin and enniatins to porcine intestinal epithelial cells. *Food Chem. Toxicol.* **2018**, *121*, 566–572. [CrossRef]
47. Springler, A.; Vrubel, G.J.; Mayer, E.; Schatzmayr, G.; Novak, B. Effect of Fusarium-derived metabolites on the barrier integrity of differentiated intestinal porcine epithelial cells (IPEC-J2). *Toxins* **2016**, *8*, 345. [CrossRef] [PubMed]
48. Broekaert, N.; Devreese, M.; Demeyere, K.; Berthiller, F.; Michlmayr, H.; Varga, E.; Adam, G.; Meyer, E.; Croubels, S. Comparative in vitro cytotoxicity of modified deoxynivalenol on porcine intestinal epithelial cells. *Food Chem. Toxicol.* **2016**, *95*, 103–109. [CrossRef]
49. Mahnine, N.; Meca, G.; Elabidi, A.; Fekhaoui, M.; Saoiabi, A.; Font, G.; Mañes, J.; Zinedine, A. Further data on the levels of emerging Fusarium mycotoxins enniatins (A, A1, B, B1), beauvericin and fusaproliferin in breakfast and infant cereals from Morocco. *Food Chem.* **2011**, *63*, 161–165. [CrossRef]
50. Devreese, M.; Broekaert, N.; De Mil, T.; Fraeyman, S.; De Backer, P.; Croubels, S. Pilot toxicokinetic study and absolute oral bioavailability of the Fusarium mycotoxin enniatin B1 in pigs. *Food Chem. Toxicol.* **2014**, *63*, 161–165. [CrossRef]
51. Meca, G.; Mañes, J.; Font, G.; Ruiz, M.J. Study of the potential toxicity of enniatins A, A 1, B, B 1 by evaluation of duodenal and colonic bioavailability applying an invitro method by Caco-2 cells. *Toxicon* **2012**, *59*, 1–11. [CrossRef]
52. Saleh, I.; Goktepe, I. The characteristics, occurrence, and toxicological effects of patulin. *Food Chem. Toxicol.* **2019**, *129*, 301–311. [CrossRef]
53. Puel, O.; Galtier, P.; Oswald, I.P. Biosynthesis and toxicological effects of patulin. *Toxins* **2010**, *2*, 613–631. [CrossRef]
54. Dvorska, J.E.; Surai, P.F.; Speake, B.K.; Sparks, N.H.C. Effect of the mycotoxin aurofusarin on the antioxidant composition and fatty acid profile of quail eggs. *Br. Poult. Sci.* **2001**, *42*, 643–649. [CrossRef]
55. Dvorska, J.E.; Surai, P.F.; Speake, B.K.; Sparks, N.H.C. Antioxidant systems of the developing quail embryo are compromised by mycotoxin aurofusarin. *Comp. Biochem. Physiol. C Toxicol. Pharmacol.* **2002**, *131*, 197–205. [CrossRef]
56. Tola, S.; Bureau, D.P.; Hooft, J.M.; Beamish, F.W.H.; Sulyok, M.; Krska, R.; Encarnação, P.; Petkam, R. Effects of wheat naturally contaminated with Fusarium mycotoxins on growth performance and selected health indices of red tilapia (*Oreochromis niloticus* × *O. mossambicus*). *Toxins* **2015**, *7*, 1929–1944. [CrossRef]
57. Uhlig, S.; Jestoi, M.; Kristin Knutsen, A.; Heier, B.T. Multiple regression analysis as a tool for the identification of relations between semi-quantitative LC-MS data and cytotoxicity of extracts of the fungus *Fusarium avenaceum* (syn. F. arthrosporioides). *Toxicon* **2006**, *48*, 567–579. [CrossRef]
58. Vejdovszky, K.; Warth, B.; Sulyok, M.; Marko, D. Non-synergistic cytotoxic effects of Fusarium and Alternaria toxin combinations in Caco-2 cells. *Toxicol. Lett.* **2016**, *241*, 1–8. [CrossRef]
59. Izhaki, I. Emodin—A secondary metabolite with multiple ecological functions in higher plants. *N. Phytol.* **2002**, *155*, 205–217. [CrossRef]
60. Springler, A.; Hessenberger, S.; Reisinger, N.; Kern, C.; Nagl, V.; Schatzmayr, G.; Mayer, E. Deoxynivalenol and its metabolite deepoxy-deoxynivalenol: Multi-parameter analysis for the evaluation of cytotoxicity and cellular effects. *Mycotoxin Res.* **2017**, *33*, 25–37. [CrossRef]

61. Fontaine, K.; Mounier, J.; Coton, E.; Hymery, N. Individual and combined effects of roquefortine C and mycophenolic acid on human monocytic and intestinal cells. *World Mycotoxin J.* **2015**, *9*, 51–62. [CrossRef]
62. Juan-Garcí, A.; Fernández-Blanco, C.; Font, G.; Ruiz, M.J. Toxic effects of alternariol by in vitro assays: A review. *Rev. Toxicol.* **2015**, *31*, 196–203.
63. Juan-García, A.; Juan, C.; König, S.; Ruiz, M.J. Cytotoxic effects and degradation products of three mycotoxins: Alternariol, 3-acetyl-deoxynivalenol and 15-acetyl-deoxynivalenol in liver hepatocellular carcinoma cells. *Toxicol. Lett.* **2015**, *235*, 8–16. [CrossRef]
64. Woelflingseder, L.; Warth, B.; Vierheilig, I.; Schwartz-Zimmermann, H.; Hametner, C.; Nagl, V.; Novak, B.; Šarkanj, B.; Berthiller, F.; Adam, G.; et al. The Fusarium metabolite culmorin suppresses the in vitro glucuronidation of deoxynivalenol. *Arch. Toxicol.* **2019**, *93*, 1729–1743. [CrossRef]
65. Weber, J.; Vaclavikova, M.; Wiesenberger, G.; Haider, M.; Hametner, C.; Fröhlich, J.; Berthiller, F.; Adam, G.; Mikula, H.; Fruhmann, P. Chemical synthesis of culmorin metabolites and their biologic role in culmorin and acetyl-culmorin treated wheat cells. *Org. Biomol. Chem.* **2018**, *16*, 2043–2048. [CrossRef]
66. Li, Y.C.; Ledoux, D.R.; Bermudez, A.J.; Fritsche, K.L.; Rottinghaus, G.E. Effects of moniliformin on performance and immune function of broiler chicks. *Poult. Sci.* **2000**, *79*, 26–32. [CrossRef]
67. Wattana-Amorn, P.; Charoenwongsa, W.; Williams, C.; Crump, M.P.; Apichaisataienchote, B. Antibacterial activity of cyclo(L-Pro-L-Tyr) and cyclo(D-Pro-L-Tyr) from Streptomyces sp. strain 22-4 against phytopathogenic bacteria. *Nat. Prod. Res.* **2016**, *30*, 1980–1983. [CrossRef]
68. Kosalec, I.; Ramić, S.; Jelić, D.; Antolović, R.; Pepeljnjak, S.; Kopjar, N. Assessment of tryptophol genotoxicity in four cell lines in vitro: A pilot study with alkaline comet assay. *Arh. Hig. Rada Toksikol.* **2011**, *62*, 41–49. [CrossRef]
69. Kosalec, I.; Šafranić, A.; Pepeljnjak, S.; Bačun-Družina, V.; Ramić, S.; Kopjar, N. Genotoxicity of tryptophol in a battery of short-term assays on human white blood cells in vitro. *Basic Clin. Pharmacol. Toxicol.* **2008**, *102*, 443–452. [CrossRef]
70. Pihlström, T. *Method Validation and Quality Control Procedures for Pesticide Residues Analysis in Food and Feed*; DG SANCO/12495/2011; European Commission Directorate-General for Health and Food Safety: Brussels, Belgium, 2011; pp. 1–41.

*toxins*

MDPI

*Article*

# BmTudor-sn Is a Binding Protein of Destruxin A in Silkworm Bm12 Cells

**Jingjing Wang, Weina Hu and Qiongbo Hu ***

Key Laboratory of Bio-Pesticide Innovation and Application of Guangdong Province, College of Agriculture, South China Agricultural University, Guangzhou 510642, China; wangjingjing@stu.scau.edu.cn (J.W.); hwn688094@163.com (W.H.)

* Correspondence: hqbscau@scau.edu.cn; Tel.: +86-20-8528-0308; Fax: +86-20-8528-0292

Received: 19 December 2018; Accepted: 23 January 2019; Published: 24 January 2019

**Abstract:** Destruxin A (DA), a hexa-cyclodepsipeptidic mycotoxin secreted by the entomopathogenic fungus *Metarhizium anisopliae*, was reported to have an insecticidal effect and anti-immunity activity. However, its molecular mechanism of action remains unclear. Previously, we isolated several potential DA-affinity (binding) proteins in the *Bombyx mori* Bm12 cell line. By docking score using MOE2015, we selected three proteins—BmTudor-sn, BmPiwi, and BmAGO2—for further validation. First, using Bio-Layer Interferometry in vitro, we found that BmTudor-sn had an affinity interaction with DA at 125, 250, and 500 μM, while BmPiwi and BmAGO2 had no interaction signal with DA. Second, we employed standard immunoblotting to verify that BmTudor-sn is susceptible to DA, but BmPiwi and BmAGO2 are not. Third, to verify these findings in vivo, we used a target engagement strategy based on shifts in protein thermal stability following ligand binding termed the cellular thermal shift assay and found no thermal stability shift in BmPiwi and BmAGO2, whereas a shift was found for BmTudor-sn. In addition, in BmTudor-sn knockdown Bm12 cells, we observed that cell viability increased under DA treatment. Furthermore, insect two-hybrid system results indicated that the key site involved in DA binding to BmTudor-sn was Leu704. In conclusion, in vivo and in vitro experimental evidence indicated that BmTudor-sn is a binding protein of DA in silkworm Bm12 cells at the 100 μM level, and the key site of this interaction is Leu704. Our results provide new perspectives to aid in elucidating the molecular mechanism of action of DA in insects and developing new biopesticide.

**Keywords:** Destruxin A; *Bombyx mori*; binding protein; BmTudor-sn; Bm12 cell

**Key Contribution:** BmTudor-sn is a Binding Protein of Destruxin A in Silkworm Bm12 cells by in vivo and in vitro experimental evidences, and the key site of this interaction is Leu704.

## 1. Introduction

Destruxins are cyclodepsipeptidic mycotoxins, and there are 39 analogues [1]. Destruxin A (DA, Figure 1A), the common analogue secreted by the entomopathogenic fungus *Metarhizium anisopliae*, has a strong insecticidal effect and anti-immunity activity, which includes breaking the balance between calcium and hydrogen ions and subsequently affecting the function of phagocytosis and encapsulation in hemocyte [2,3]. Because of the immunosuppression activity of DA in insects, the majority of studies have focused on the mechanism of action of the effect of DA on the immune-related pathway or stress reaction (response), such as changes to the transcriptome [4] and proteome [5] or immune regulation by microRNA [6] in *Plutella xylostella*. There have been various studies on the effects of DA, including its impact on transcriptome [7], proteome, transcription factor, and antibacterial peptide expression [8] in *Bombyx mori* and its influence on the Toll or Imd pathway in *Bemisia tabaci* [9]. However, for drug research or development, it is important to look for direct targets, most of which are proteins, in appropriate tissues or cells. In order to clarify the molecular mechanism more directly, previously, we screened and isolated DA-binding proteins in ovary-derived Bm12 cells using a label-free small molecule drug target identification method called drug affinity responsive target stability (DARTS) [10]. The DARTS results indicated that DA greatly induced heat shock proteins (HSPs) in cultured cells, and we successfully demonstrated that DA binds to an HSP in vitro by molecular interaction validation [11]. However, evidence from only one approach is not sufficient, especially for studies only performed in vitro.

Here, we selected three proteins, BmTudor-sn, BmPiwi, and BmAGO2, from the DARTS analysis based on their molecular docking score and determined whether these proteins are DA binding proteins through a series of in vivo and in vitro experiments. In brief, BmPiwi and BmAGO2 belong to the Argonaute family [12], which plays a vital role in germ cell development and represent a core component of the RNA interference (RNAi) pathway and function in transcriptional regulation [13]. Meanwhile, BmTudor-sn, a multifunctional protein containing four staphylococcal nuclease domains and a Tudor domain, participates in cellular pathways involved in gene regulation, cell growth, and development and interacts with Argonaute proteins [14], and it is known as stress granule protein in *Bombyx mori* [15]. These three proteins are all critical components in the RNAi pathway [16]. Notably, few studies have associated DA with germ line-derived proteins that are involved in several important physiological processes. In addition, this study may provide novel insights to exploit new targets and pathways for the development of pesticides.

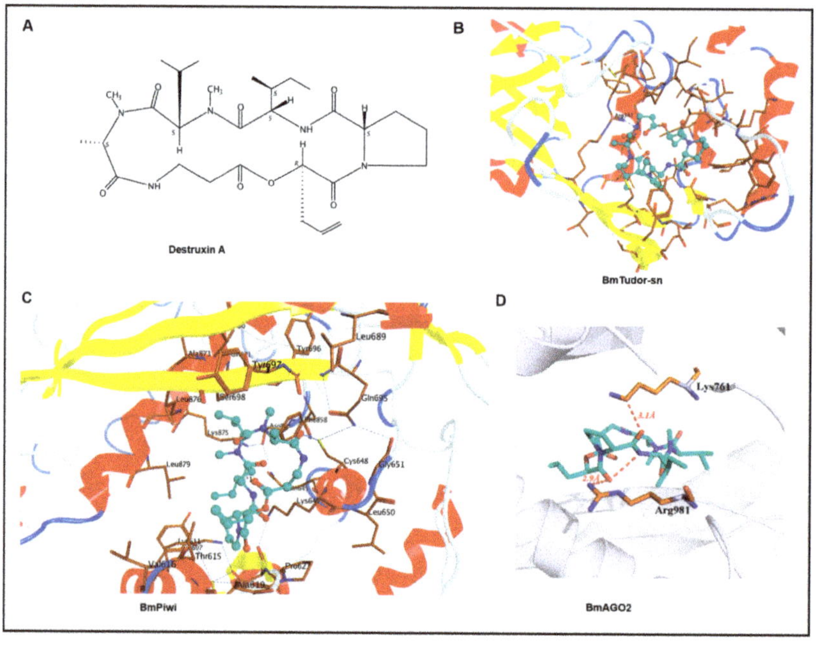


**Figure 1.** Binding pose of Destruxin A (DA) with BmTudor-sn, BmPiwi, and BmAGO2. DA is colored in cyan, and the surrounding residues in the binding pockets are colored in orange. The backbone of the receptor is depicted as spectrum ribbon. (**A**) The structure of DA. (**B**) The binding poses of DA with BmTudor-sn. (**C**) The binding mode of DA with BmPiwi. (**D**) The binding patterns of DA with BmAGO2.

## 2. Results

### 2.1. Molecular Docking

Faced with hundreds of isolated proteins from the DARTS analysis, molecular docking was a convenient and efficient method to screen for proteins that are of research value. Ultimately, BmTudor-sn, BmPiwi, and BmAGO2 protein were selected from hundreds of candidates because of their relatively high binding scores and because they play crucial roles in many physiological processes in *Bombyx mori*.

Through molecular docking, we obtained the binding modes of DA with the BmTudor-sn, BmPiwi, and BmAGO2 proteins. The estimated binding free energies indicated by GBVI/WSA dG scoring are listed in Table 1. A lower binding free energy suggests a higher binding affinity. The ligands and DA had docking scores that ranged from −9.1947 to −11.002 kcal/mol, suggesting a good binding affinity with these proteins. The binding modes of DA with BmTudor-sn, BmPiwi, and BmAGO2 are depicted in Figure 1. DA fits the pocket well in terms of the shape in the binding sites. For the BmTudor-sn docking pattern, the Arg343 side chain of the SN3 domain could have a hydrogen bond interaction with the carbonyl group of DA, which contains a number of carbonyl groups that might form hydrogen bonds with nearby basic amino acids. For the BmPiwi binding mode, the carbonyl in DA, which is regarded as a hydrogen bond donor, forms one hydrogen bond with the side chain of Cys648 in BmPiwi, which forms other hydrogen bonds with Gln695 and Gly651. At the bottom of the binding pocket, hydrogen bonds are formed between Cys614 and several residues around it. For the binding mode of DA with BmAGO2, one oxygen atom of the carbonyl near the pyrrolidine of DA, which is regarded as a hydrogen bond donor, forms one hydrogen bond with the side chain of Arg981 in BmAGO2 and forms another intramolecular hydrogen bond with a nitrogen atom. The other oxygen atom of the carbonyl near the pyrrolidine of DA, which is regarded as a hydrogen bond donor, forms one hydrogen bond with the side chain of Lys761 in BmAGO2.

**Table 1.** The docking score of DA against BmTudor-sn, BmPiwi, and BmAGO2.

| Proteins | Docking Score (kcal/mol) |
|---|---|
| BmTudor-sn | −11.002 |
| BmPiwi | −10.8577 |
| BmAGO2 | −9.1947 |

### 2.2. Assessing the Interaction of DA with BmTudor-sn, BmPiwi, and BmAGO2 by Bio-Layer Interferometry (BLI) In Vitro

The determination of the affinity constant between heterologously expressed recombinant proteins with a small molecule through in vitro biophysical approaches is a generally accepted and frequently used method for target validation. In this study, we selected bio-layer interferometry [17] because it is label free, has high sensitivity, and can be performed in real-time to assess the binding affinity. Recombinant proteins were expressed and purified from eukaryotic expression in lepidoptera *Spodoptera frugiperda* 9 (Sf9) cells because of their similar tertiary structure with native proteins. The BLI analysis results indicated that DA interacts with BmTudor-sn at concentrations of 125 μm, 250 μm, and 500 μm but not BmPiwi or BmAGO2 (Figure 2A,B). And the affinity constant KD is $5.87 \times 10^{-4}$M. These results possibly contradict the above docking results, which indicated that DA formed hydrogen bonds with the three proteins.

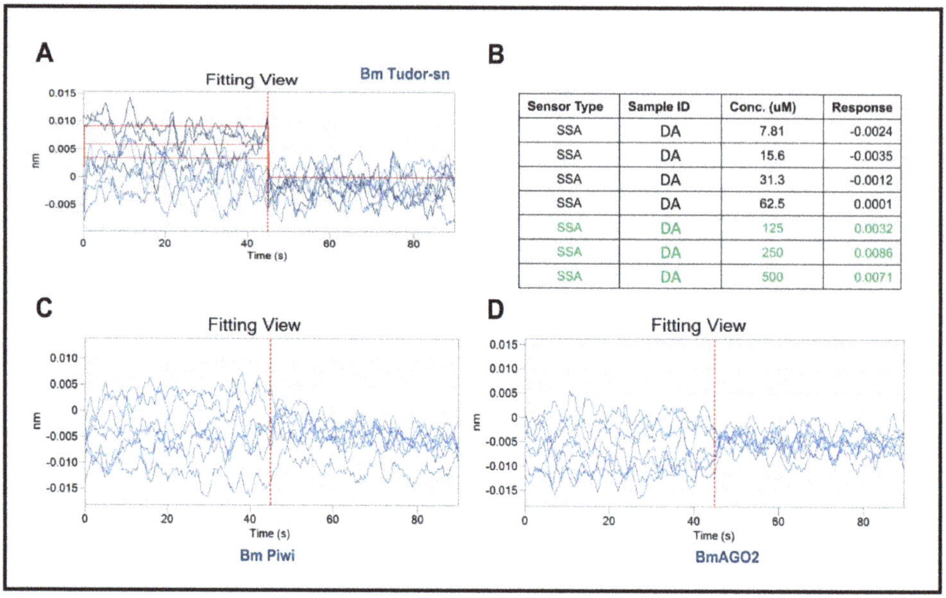


**Figure 2.** Results of recombinant proteins interacting with DA using BLI. (**A**) Data analysis with software showing there are interactions between BmTudor-sn and DA. (**B**) Molecular interaction kinetic data of BmTudor-sn with DA. (**C**,**D**) Processed data indicated no interaction of BmPiwi or BmAGO2 with DA.

### *2.3. Assessing the Interaction of DA with BmTudor-sn through Protein Stability and RNAi In Vivo*

DARTS is based on the principle that protein folding stability is more resistant to protease and heat treatments under conformational modifications caused by small molecules or other ligands. Notably, false-positive DARTS results will be obtained with the high expression of proteins caused by drug treatment and the stress response thus, it was necessary to confirm that BmTudor-sn was not completely hydrolyzed by proteolysis. The immunoblotting results (Figure 3A) clearly indicated that BmTudor-sn, but not BmPiwi and BmAGO2, was stable with DA treatment in a dosage-dependent manner under proteolysis, which suggested that BmTudor-sn is a DA binding protein. Additional evidence was obtained using a method that directly monitored target engagement based on the shift in protein thermal stability induced by a small molecule, which is termed the cellular thermal shift assay (CETSA) [18]. As depicted in Figure 3B, the thermal stability of BmTudor-sn increased following DA binding modification, as indicated by the binding protein solubility in the supernatant being positively correlated with the temperature gradient. These protein stability shift assay results provided sufficient evidence to demonstrate that BmTudor-sn is a binding protein of DA in Bm12 cells. Then, cytotoxicity and viability assays were performed following DA treatment with BmTudor-sn knockdown, and the results revealed that viability increased by approximately 20% (Figure 3C).

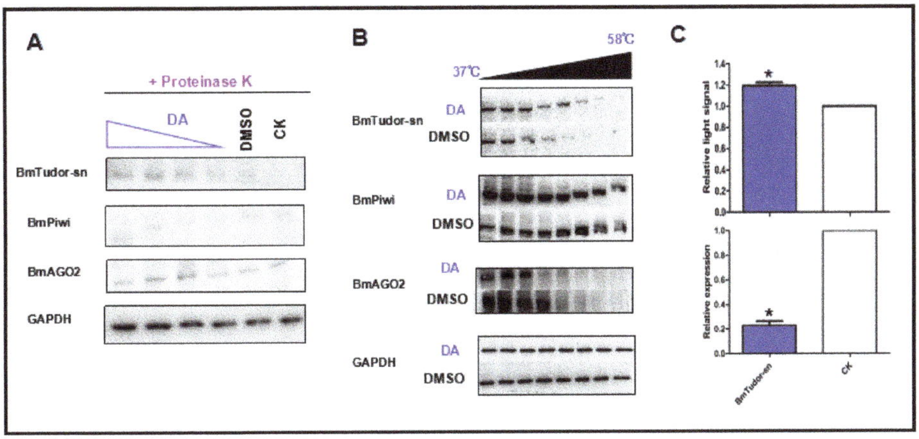


**Figure 3.** Protein stability shift assay by immunoblotting and CETSA results indicated that DA specifically binds to BmTudor-sn but not BmPiwi or BmAGO2. (**A**) Immunoblotting results demonstrating that BmTudor-sn stability was influenced by interacting with DA in a dosage-dependent manner. (**B**) CETSA showing that BmTudor-sn thermal stability was subject to thermal gradient treatment after adding DA. (**C**) BmTudor-sn knock down cells showed higher viability under DA treatment. Significant differences between columns are indicated by an * ($p < 0.05$) according to $t$ test.

### *2.4. Screening Key Amino Acid Sites of Interaction between DA and BmTudor-sn Using an Insect Two-Hybrid (I2H) System*

The above experiments assessed and verified the interaction of DA with BmTudor-sn. However, the exact interaction sites were not clear. Here, we evaluated the binding site in vivo using the insect two-hybrid (I2H) protein-protein interaction method [19] (Figure 4). This method was used to assess key sites where DA disrupted the interaction of BmTudor-sn with BmAGO1 in the Spodoptera frugiperda 9 (Sf9) cell line. Six mutants were prepared according to optimal docking sites, and 0.02 and 0.2 μg/mL DA treatments were selected based on our previous results. The results clearly indicated that for the 0.02 and 0.2 μg/mL treatments, the signals for 2 mutants, Ser707Ala and leu704Ala, and 3 mutants, Ser701Ala, Leu704Ala, and Tyr708Ala, respectively, were each different from the wild type signal, which suggested that the binding mode is dependent on the DA dosage. Apparently, DA interacts with BmTudor-sn at both concentrations at Leu704. At the protein domain level, the differences in the mutants were both in the Tudor domain (Ser707, Leu704, Ser701, Tyr708) rather than the SN3 (Lys492) and SN4 (Lys582) domains. In addition, DA impeded the protein pair interaction at Ser707 and Tyr708 and promoted it at Leu704 and Ser701 based on the increase or decrease in the signal, respectively.

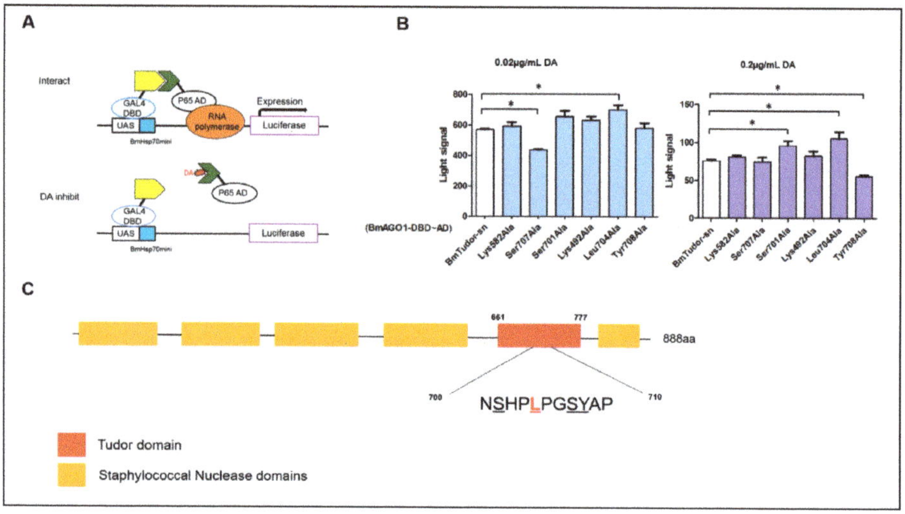


**Figure 4.** Key amino acid sites of interaction between DA and BmTudor-sn. (**A**) Schematic of the principle of the insect two-hybrid (I2H) system [19]. (**B**) Differences in the mutants with the 0.02 and 0.2 μg/mL DA treatments. Significant differences between columns are indicated by an * ($p < 0.05$) according to DMRT. (**C**) Sketch of the domain structure of BmTudor-sn and the key amino acid sites of the Tudor domain. The text continues here.

## 3. Discussion

In drug research and development, it is important to clearly determine the mechanism of action of small molecules in cells, the most common target of which are binding proteins [20]. Previously, we attempted to elucidate the mechanism for DA using different approaches, such as analyzing phenotype differences and changes in the transcriptome[7] and proteome [21]. Unfortunately, because DA has no active group, it is not possible to bond affinity chromatography tags for use in chemical proteomics. With DARTS, we have the ability to bond DA with potential proteins. However, DARTS can return false-positive results when highly expressed proteins are not digested completely by protease [22]. Indeed, BmTudor-sn, BmPiwi, and BmAGO2 proteins were upregulated by DA 2-3-fold at the transcriptional level. Immunoblotting is typically used for verification [23], and the dosage-dependent blot protein is the binding protein. Based on this, we confirmed that BmTudor-sn is a binding protein of DA but not BmPiwi or BmAGO2.

DARTS analysis revealed dozens of potential binding proteins, and it was necessary to determine which were the most probable. Molecular docking is a reasonable, efficient, and convenient strategy to narrow down candidates among all proteins compared to other methods such as heterologous expression and kinetic analysis, which require verification one by one. However, it seems paradoxical in this study that proteins with the top docking scores were not the binding protein [24]. Actually, docking is a completely theoretical speculation, and other experiments are required to draw a conclusion. Here, BLI kinetic analysis in vitro and CETSA in vivo were performed to address these drawbacks, demonstrating that DA binds to BmTudor-sn rather than BmPiwi or BmAGO2. BLI is a recently developed, frequently used bio-molecular interaction analysis method based on optical interference signals and is a fast, real-time method that uses a small amount of sample. Meanwhile, CETSA is a small molecule target engagement strategy based on protein thermal stability shifts caused by ligand binding, and it has been successfully used to identify several target proteins in drug studies in recent years [25]. Moreover, in the BLI analysis, we found that DA bound to BmTudor-sn at the 100 μM level, and this result agreed with the DARTS experiment in which BmTudor-sn only appeared in the 200 μg/mL treatment with a specific proteinase and not at the lower dosage and with other proteinases. Furthermore, the CETSA results demonstrated that BmTudor-sn showed thermal stability with the 200 μg/mL treatment and not at the lower dose. I2H was first used to study protein-protein interactions20, and with it, we screened the key amino acid sites of the protein-ligand complex using different mutants because of its convenience and sensitivity and because a purified protein was not required. I2H was also practical for comparing the drug inhibition rates of protein pairs.

DA has been previously reported to play a role in immune related pathways and in inducing the immunosuppression phenotype in insects [26]. The majority of studies have focused on these roles, while few have addressed the mechanism of action in cells. Therefore, previously, we assessed the ion concentration inside and outside the cell [2] and found that DA strongly induced the expression of heat shock proteins (HSPs) in cells and bound to one of them in vitro [11], and here, we showed that BmTudor-sn is a DA binding protein. Tudor-sn, a multifunctional protein, was reported to regulate downstream expression and slice RNAi under normal conditions and participate in the formation of stress granules and processing bodies under stress [15]. This may also explains why BmTudor-sn only appeared in the high concentration treatment in DARTS. Another question is whether DA binds to Tudor-sn in humans. DA is one of fungal toxins generated by the commercial biopesticide *M. anisopliae*, which also produces Destruxin B (DB), and DB was reported to have clear anti-cancer activity [27]. Interestingly, we previously showed that DB is more sensitive to V-ATPase than DA in silkworm hemocytes, and this ion channel is known to be the most probable target of DA. However, DA likely does not bind to Tudor-sn in humans because Tudor-sn has different functions in different species.

In conclusion, in vivo and in vitro experimental evidence indicated that BmTudor-sn is a binding protein of DA in silkworm Bm12 cells at the 100 μM level, and the key amino acid site of this interaction is Leu704.

## 4. Materials and Methods

### 4.1. Cell Lines and Culture

The silkworm Bm12 cell line was donated by Professor Cao Yang (College of Animal Science at South China Agricultural University) and cultured in TNM-FH culture medium (Hyclone, Pittsburgh, MA, USA) and 10% fetal bovine serum (Gibco, Waltham, MA, USA). The *Spodoptera frugiperda* 9 (Sf9) cell line was cultured in SFX culture medium (Hyclone) with 5% fetal bovine serum. Cells were cultured at 27 °C and maintained at over a period of 2–4 days. Cells in the logarithmic phase were used for the experiment.

### 4.2. Destruxin A and Treatment

Destruxin A (DA) was isolated and purified from the *Metarhizium anisopliae* var. anisopliae strain MaQ10 in our laboratory [28]. A DA stock solution of 10,000 μg/mL was made up from 1 mg of DA and 100 μL of dimethyl sulfoxide (DMSO, Sigma-Aldrich, Darmstadt, Germany). To begin treatment, the DA stock solution was added to a cell well at a final concentration of 200 μg/mL DA. The control group was only supplemented with 0.1% DMSO.

### 4.3. Homology Modeling and Molecular Docking

Homology modeling was conducted in MOE v2015.1001. The structure was determined by homology modeling of the target sequence. Template crystal structures were identified using NCBI BLAST and downloaded from the RCSB Protein Data Bank. The Protonate module of MOE v2015.1001 was used to calculate the protonation state at pH = 7. Ten independent intermediate models were built. These different homology models were obtained from the mutational selection of different loop candidates and side chain rotamers. Then, the intermediate model that scored the highest according to the GB/VI scoring function was chosen as the final model and subjected to further energy minimization using the AMBER12: EHT force field.

MOE Dock was used for molecular docking simulations. The 2D structure of the ligand was drawn in ChemBioDraw 2014 and converted to 3D in MOE v2015.1001 through energy minimization with the MMFF94x force field. The protein structures were constructed by homology modeling. The Site Finder module in MOE was used to predict the potential binding pockets. Then, the protonation state of the protein and the orientation of the hydrogens were optimized using LigX at a pH of 7 and temperature of 300 K. Prior to docking, the force field of AMBER12: EHT and the implicit solvation model of Reaction Field (R-field) were selected. The docking workflow followed the "induced fit" protocol, in which the side chains of the receptor pocket were allowed to move according to ligand conformations, with a constraint on their positions. The weight used for tethering side chain atoms to their original positions was 10. For each ligand, all docked poses were ranked by London dG scoring first, and a force field refinement was then carried out on the top 30 poses followed by a rescoring of GBVI/WSA dG.

### 4.4. Bio-Layer Interferometry (BLI)

All proteins were prepared by eukaryotic expression in the Sf9 cell line. These were tagged with His-tag and purified by nickel affinity chromatography. BLI analysis was performed on a ForteBio OctetQK System (K2, Pall Fortebio Corp, Menlo Park, CA, USA). Generally, the protein samples were coupled with a biosensor for immobilization. Serial not gradient dilutions of DA (500, 250, 125, 62.5, 31.25, 15.63, and 7.813 μM) were used for treatment. PBST buffer (0.05% Tween20, 5% DMSO) was used for the reference and dilution buffers. The working procedure was baseline for 60 s, association for 60 s, and dissociation for 60 s. Finally, the raw data were processed with Data Analysis Software (9.0, Pall Fortebio Corp, Menlo Park, CA, USA).

### 4.5. Immunoblot and Cellular Thermal Shift Assay (CETSA)

The Bm12 cell line was used to conduct the CETSA and immunoblot experiments. Cells were treated with DA. For immunoblotting, cell extracts from different DA treatments, collected after incubation with RIPA lysis buffer, were digested with proteinase K and then heated in water at 90 °C for 5 min. Samples were analyzed using SDS-PAGE and transferred to PVDF membranes. The membranes were then incubated in skim milk powder, followed by incubation with primary and HRP antibodies. ECL was added to the chemiluminescence reaction. For CETSA, Bm12 cells, treated with 200 μg/mL DA, were divided into 8 aliquots, heated at 37–58 °C, and lysed by a freeze-thaw cycle. The supernatants of the lysed cells were used for the western blot analysis as described above.

### 4.6. RNAi and Viability and Toxicity Assessment

SiRNAs were prepared by synthesis in vitro. The sequence of *BmTudor-sn* siRNA is 5′-CCAAAGGACCGCCAACAAUTT-3′ and 5′-AUUGUUGGCGGUCCUUUGGTT-3′. SiRNA and FuGENE transfection reagent were each diluted in serum-free medium and then mixed. The mixture was added to Bm12 cells after the DA treatment. Viability and toxicity assessment were performed following the manufacturer's instructions.

### 4.7. Insect Two Hybrid (I2H) System

BmTudor-sn and mutants were cloned into the I2H vector pIE-AD, and BmAGO1 was cloned into the I2H vector pIE-DBD using the Gateway system. These vectors and the luciferase vector were co-transfected into the Sf9 cell line and treated with DA at 0.02 and 0.2 μg/mL. The luciferase activities in the cell extracts were determined using a Luciferase Reporter Assay System (Promega, Beijing, China) and Synergy™ H1 (BioTek, Winooski, VT, USA).

**Author Contributions:** J.W. designed and completed the experiments and wrote the paper. W.H. completed the isolation and characterization of proteins. Q.H. conceived and designed the experiments and revised the paper.

**Funding:** This research is supported by National Natural Science Foundation of China (31772184 and 31272057) and Guangdong Province Science and Technology Project (2016B020234005).

**Conflicts of Interest:** The authors declare no conflict of interest.

## References

1. Pedras, M.S.C.; Zaharia, L.I.; Ward, D.E. The destruxins: Synthesis, biosynthesis, biotransformation, and biological activity. *Phytochemistry* **2002**, *59*, 579–596. [CrossRef]
2. Chen, X.R.; Hu, Q.B.; Yu, X.Q.; Ren, S.X. Effects of destruxins on free calcium and hydrogen ions in insect hemocytes. *Insect Sci.* **2014**, *21*, 31–38. [CrossRef] [PubMed]
3. Fan, J.Q.; Chen, X.R.; Hu, Q.B. Effects of Destruxin A on Hemocytes Morphology of Bombyx mori. *J. Integr. Agric.* **2013**, *12*, 1042–1048. [CrossRef]
4. Shakeel, M.; Xu, X.; Xu, J.; Zhu, X.; Li, S.; Zhou, X.; Yu, J.; Xu, X.; Hu, Q.; Yu, X.; Jin, F. Identification of immunity-related genes in Plutella xylostella in response to fungal peptide destruxin A: RNA-Seq and DGE analysis. *Sci. Rep.* **2017**, *7*, 10966. [CrossRef] [PubMed]
5. Han, P.; Jin, F.; Dong, X.; Fan, J.; Qiu, B.; Ren, S. Transcript and protein profiling analysis of the Destruxin A-induced response in larvae of Plutella xylostella. *PLoS ONE* **2013**, *8*, e60771. [CrossRef] [PubMed]
6. Shakeel, M.; Xu, X.; Xu, J.; Li, S.; Yu, J.; Zhou, X.; Xu, X.; Hu, Q.; Yu, X.; Jin, F. Genome-Wide Identification of Destruxin A-Responsive Immunity-Related MicroRNAs in Diamondback Moth, Plutella xylostella. *Front. Immunol.* **2018**, *9*, 185. [CrossRef] [PubMed]
7. Gong, L.; Chen, X.; Liu, C.; Jin, F.; Hu, Q. Gene expression profile of Bombyx mori hemocyte under the stress of destruxin A. *PLoS ONE* **2014**, *9*, e96170. [CrossRef] [PubMed]
8. Hu, W.; He, G.; Wang, J.; Hu, Q. The Effects of Destruxin A on Relish and Rel Gene Regulation to the Suspected Immune-Related Genes of Silkworm. *Molecules* **2016**, *22*, 41. [CrossRef] [PubMed]
9. Zhang, C.; Yan, S.Q.; Shen, B.B.; Ali, S.; Wang, X.M.; Jin, F.L.; Cuthbertson, A.G.S.; Qiu, B.L. RNAi knock-down of the Bemisia tabaci Toll gene (BtToll) increases mortality after challenge with destruxin A. *Mol. Immunol.* **2017**, *88*, 164–173. [CrossRef]
10. Lomenick, B.; Hao, R.; Jonai, N.; Chin, R.M.; Aghajan, M.; Warburton, S.; Wang, J.; Wu, R.P.; Gomez, F.; Loo, J.A.; et al. Target identification using drug affinity responsive target stability (DARTS). *Proc. Natl. Acad. Sci. USA* **2009**, *106*, 21984–21989. [CrossRef]
11. Zhang, H.; Hu, W.; Xiao, M.; Ou, S.; Hu, Q. Destruxin A induces and binds HSPs in Bombyx mori Bm12 cells. *J. Agric. Food Chem.* **2017**, *65*, 9849–9853. [CrossRef] [PubMed]
12. Wang, G.H.; Jiang, L.; Zhu, L.; Cheng, T.C.; Niu, W.H.; Yan, Y.F.; Xia, Q.Y. Characterization of Argonaute family members in the silkworm, Bombyx mori. *Insect Sci.* **2013**, *20*, 78–91.
13. Höck, J.; Meister, G. The Argonaute protein family. *Genome Biol.* **2008**, *9*, 210.
14. Gutierrezbeltran, E.; Denisenko, T.V.; Zhivotovsky, B.; Bozhkov, P.V. Tudor staphylococcal nuclease: Biochemistry and functions. *Cell Death Differ.* **2016**, *23*, 1739–1748. [CrossRef] [PubMed]
15. Zhu, L.; Tatsuke, T.; Mon, H.; Li, Z.; Xu, J.; Lee, J.M.; Kusakabe, T. Characterization of Tudor-sn-containing granules in the silkworm, Bombyx mori. *Insect Biochem. Mol. Biol.* **2013**, *43*, 664–674. [CrossRef] [PubMed]
16. Zhu, L.; Tatsuke, T.; Li, Z.; Mon, H.; Xu, J.; Lee, J.M.; Kusakabe, T. Zoology, Molecular cloning of BmTUDOR-SN and analysis of its role in the RNAi pathway in the silkworm, Bombyx mori (Lepidoptera: Bombycidae). *Appl. Entomol. Zool.* **2012**, *47*, 207–215. [CrossRef]
17. Abdiche, Y.; Dan, M.; Pinkerton, A.; Pons, J. Determining kinetics and affinities of protein interactions using a parallel real-time label-free biosensor, the Octet. *Anal. Biochem.* **2008**, *377*, 209–217. [CrossRef]
18. Martinez Molina, D.; Jafari, R.; Ignatushchenko, M.; Seki, T.; Larsson, E.A.; Dan, C.; Sreekumar, L.; Cao, Y.; Nordlund, P. Monitoring drug target engagement in cells and tissues using the cellular thermal shift assay. *Science* **2013**, *341*, 84–87. [CrossRef]
19. Mon, H.; Sugahara, R.; Hong, S.M.; Lee, J.M.; Kamachi, Y.; Kawaguchi, Y.; Kusakabe, T. Analysis of protein interactions with two-hybrid system in cultured insect cells. *Anal. Biochem.* **2009**, *392*, 180–182. [CrossRef]
20. Ziegler, S.; Pries, V.; Hedberg, C.; Waldmann, H. Target identification for small bioactive molecules: Finding the needle in the haystack. *Angew. Chem.* **2013**, *52*, 2744–2792. [CrossRef]

21. Fan, J.; Han, P.; Chen, X.; Hu, Q. Comparative proteomic analysis of Bombyx mori hemocytes treated with Destruxin A. *Arch. Insect Biochem. Physiol.* **2014**, *86*, 33–45. [PubMed]
22. Lomenick, B.; Olsen, R.W.; Huang, J. Identification of direct protein targets of small molecules. *ACS Chem. Biol.* **2011**, *6*, 34. [CrossRef] [PubMed]
23. Chin, R.M.; Fu, X.; Pai, M.Y.; Vergnes, L.; Hwang, H.; Deng, G.; Diep, S.; Lomenick, B.; Meli, V.S.; Monsalve, G.C.; et al. The metabolite alpha-ketoglutarate extends lifespan by inhibiting the ATP synthase and TOR. *Nature* **2014**, *510*, 397–401. [CrossRef] [PubMed]
24. Chen, Y.C. Beware of docking! *Trends Pharmacol. Sci.* **2015**, *36*, 78–95. [CrossRef] [PubMed]
25. Jafari, R.; Almqvist, H.; Axelsson, H.; Ignatushchenko, M.; Lundbäck, T.; Nordlund, P.; Martinez Molina, D. The cellular thermal shift assay for evaluating drug target interactions in cells. *Nat. Protoc.* **2014**, *9*, 2100–2122. [CrossRef] [PubMed]
26. Pal, S.; Leger, R.J.S.; Wu, L.P. Fungal Peptide Destruxin A Plays a Specific Role in Suppressing the Innate Immune Response in Drosophila melanogaster. *J. Biol. Chem.* **2007**, *282*, 8969–8977. [CrossRef] [PubMed]
27. Wu, C.C.; Chen, T.H.; Liu, B.L.; Wu, L.C.; Chen, Y.C.; Tzeng, Y.M.; Hsu, S.L. Destruxin B Isolated from Entomopathogenic Fungus Metarhizium anisopliae Induces Apoptosis via a Bcl-2 Family-Dependent Mitochondrial Pathway in Human Nonsmall Cell Lung Cancer Cells. *Evid. Based Complement. Alternat. Med.* **2013**, *2013*, 548929.
28. Hu, Q.B.; Ren, S.X.; Wu, J.H.; Chang, J.M.; Musa, P.D. Investigation of destruxin A and B from 80 Metarhizium strains in China, and the optimization of cultural conditions for the strain MaQ10. *Toxicon* **2006**, *48*, 491–498. [CrossRef]

MDPI
St. Alban-Anlage 66
4052 Basel
Switzerland
Tel. +41 61 683 77 34
Fax +41 61 302 89 18
www.mdpi.com

*Toxins* Editorial Office
E-mail: toxins@mdpi.com
www.mdpi.com/journal/toxins

www.ingramcontent.com/pod-product-compliance
Lightning Source LLC
LaVergne TN
LVHW070401100526
838202LV00014B/1365
* 9 7 8 3 0 3 9 3 6 9 2 6 3 *